Y0-BDW-801

Contents

Handbook of Early Language Impairment in Children: Nature

Thomas L. Layton, Ph.D., CCC-SLP
Professor, Communication Sciences and Disorders
North Carolina Central University, Durham

Elizabeth R. Crais, Ph.D., CCC-SLP
Associate Professor
University of North Carolina at Chapel Hill

Linda R. Watson, Ed.D., CCC-SLP
Clinical Associate Professor
University of North Carolina at Chapel Hill

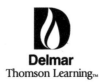

Delmar
Thomson Learning™

Africa • Australia • Canada • Denmark • Japan • Mexico
New Zealand • Philippines • Puerto Rico • Singapore
Spain • United Kingdom • United States

MW

NOTICE TO THE READER

Publisher does not warrant or guarantee any of the products described herein or perform any independent analysis in connection with any of the product information contained herein. Publisher does not assume, and expressly disclaims, any obligation to obtain and include information other than that provided to it by the manufacturer.

The reader is expressly warned to consider and adopt all safety precautions that might be indicated by the activities described herein and to avoid all potential hazards. By following the instructions contained herein, the reader willingly assumes all risks in connection with such instructions.

The publisher makes no representations or warranties of any kind, including but not limited to the warranties of fitness for particular purpose or merchantability, nor are any such representations implied with respect to the material set forth herein, and the publisher takes no responsibility with respect to such material. The publisher shall not be liable for any special, consequential or exemplary damages resulting, in whole or in part, from the reader's use of, or reliance upon, this material.

Delmar Staff
Business Unit Director: William Brottmiller
Executive Editor: Cathy L. Esperti
Development Editor: Deb Flis
Executive Marketing Manager: Dawn Gerrain
Project Editor: Stacey Prus
Production Coordinator: John Mickelbank
Art/Design Coordinator: Mary Colleen Liburdi

ISBN: 0 8273 7523 9

11/21/02

List of Illustrations

List of Tables

Preface

This book grew out of our collaborative efforts to conduct a graduate seminar in language disorders that was based on etiological categories. As is probably true of most programs in speech and hearing sciences, our curriculum is rich with possibilities to learn about a variety of disabilities in young children; however, few courses present in-depth views of these individual disabilities. Although we agree with the widely held view that each child should be viewed as an individual, we also recognize the importance of understanding specific disorders and the unique characteristics and issues that may be associated with each. Thus, we began to develop the current book to be used by graduate students in our language seminar, with a broader view to helping practicing professionals keep current in a number of etiological areas.

We soon discovered that the amount of information available clearly exceeded a single volume. Therefore, we decided to divide the material into two books: one that covered the basic nature and description of children with language impairments (the current text), and a second volume, *Handbook of Early Language Impairment in Children: Assessment and Intervention* (Watson, Crais, & Layton, 2000), which provides the most current thinking on how to assess and treat these children.

The focus of the two books is on the younger child (i.e., the infant, toddler, and preschool-age child), although some information is also presented on school-age children. The narrow focus is deliberate because of the need for material in this area. Because of the continuity of development into the school years, however, some information is presented on school-age children as well. To exclude these older children would lessen the understanding of the nature of each area. For example, attention deficit/hyperactivity disorder is typically not diagnosed until a child is in school, although some symptoms are present during the preschool years (see Chapter 3, "Attention Deficit/Hyperactivity Disorder in Young Children). In addition, we believe it is important for professionals working with young children who have language impairments to be informed about the longer developmental course and prognosis for these children. Such understanding can have important implications for determining priorities for intervention during the early years of development, counseling families of young children, and planning transitions of children to different systems of intervention services as they grow older.

AUDIENCE

The initial audience intended for *Handbook of Early Language Impairment in Children: Nature* and *Handbook of Early Language Impairment in Children: Assessment and Intervention* is graduate students in speech-language pathology; however, students and professionals in other disciplines involved in early intervention will also find the books relevant and important. We believe the two books can fill an important void in the libraries of professionals who serve children with disabilities. Both books are valuable reference guides. In highlighting issues related to working with young children in "family-friendly" ways, the current two volumes can provide guidance in these areas. Where possible, the information provided is based on the existing research literature, particularly for those areas with long histories of research in early intervention. However, because of the rapidly changing nature of the field, clinical judgment and anecdotal information are also provided for the reader's consideration.

ORGANIZATION

CHAPTER 1 lays out the major issues regarding the diagnosis and characteristics of language impairment in young children. Rescorla and Lee provide a description of the two most common subtypes of specific language impairment: the pure expressive type and the mixed receptive-expressive type. They also discuss the possible overlapping diagnoses of children labeled late talkers and those identified as specifically language impaired. The chapter provides up-to-date information on the language, cognitive, neuromotor, and social-behavioral characteristics of these children. Finally, there is an overview of theories of the etiologies of specific language impairment.

CHAPTER 2 covers communication deficits in children with psychiatric disorders. Baltaxe's vast experience in working with children with such problems adds much to her ability to provide comprehensive information. The chapter updates the professional's understanding of the critical overlap between children with psychiatric disorders and those with communication deficits. This chapter also ties well into Chapter 3, on attention deficit/hyperactivity disorder (AD/HD), and Chapter 4, on pervasive developmental disorders.

In CHAPTER 3, Giddan and Milling pull together a large amount of research in a coherent and concise manner. With the emergence of recent federal guidelines for serving children with attention-deficit/hyperactivity disorders, many professionals are seeking a clearer understanding of these deficits in young children. This chapter explains the differences between children with AD/HD who are predominantly inattentive, those who are hyperactive-impulsive, and those whose diagnosis is not otherwise specified (i.e., when inattention or hyperactivity-impulsivity are not present). The five current theories for explaining the development and persistence of AD/HD are also presented. The authors' approach for assessment and treatment concludes the chapter.

CHAPTER 4, by Watson and Ozonoff, provides an overview of the research on children with pervasive developmental disorders and its relation to communication disorders. The current subtypes of pervasive developmental disorders are described, including autistic disorder, childhood disintegrative disorder, Rett's disorder, Asperger's disorder, and pervasive developmental disorder—not otherwise specified. Reflecting a body of literature on intervention specific to this population, this chapter includes information on early intervention strategies for children with these disorders.

In CHAPTER 5, Spiridigliozzi, Lachiewicz, Mirrett, and McConkie-Rosell present research on the motor, cognitive, and communication skills of children with fragile X syndrome, with the last sections detailing the authors' own experiences with these children and their families. In contrast to previous work, which focused primarily on boys, this chapter provides a succinct account for both boys and girls with fragile X syndrome.

CHAPTER 6 covers the early and advanced stages of play, cognitive, and communication development in children with Down syndrome. Layton addresses the issues of family involvement in the identification process and the development of early literacy concepts. The last sections include a discussion of imaginary companions among children with Down syndrome and how the dialogues with these companions may be a valuable source for diagnosing communication skills in this population.

CHAPTER 7, by Blosser and Depompei, details the causes, types, and terms associated with traumatic brain injury (TBI) in children. Numerous tables and figures are provided to show clear examples of TBI. Especially important in this chapter is the authors' outline of the assessment and intervention issues across three phases. They explain what is happening at each phase and what to do, as well as provide a case study of a child in each of the phases.

CHAPTER 8 updates the reader on the latest understanding of children with Landau-Kleffner syndrome. Despite the assumption that this is a rare condition, it has been identified more frequently than any other type of acquired childhood aphasia. Harrison provides an account of the past four decades of research in this area, the current thinking on treatment, and the value of a multidisciplinary assessment approach with these children.

CHAPTER 9, on the effects of prenatal substance use, presents an office scenario in which professionals are consulting with the mother of a boy who was prenatally exposed to alcohol. The tenor of that meeting sets the stage for the chapter, which targets the deleterious effects of prenatal exposure to two substances, alcohol and cocaine. In the initial section of the chapter, Sparks covers the terminology, referral strategies, assessment, and intervention for children with alcohol-related disorders. The second half of the chapter mirrors the same content areas for prenatal cocaine exposure.

CHAPTER 10 provides an extensive review of the causes of the human immunodeficiency virus (HIV), its transmission, and its effect on the cognitive, motor, and communication skills of children affected by it. Scott and Layton also review the currently available literature that details linguistic function within the pediatric population with HIV. The value of a multidisciplinary assessment approach and the role of the speech-language pathologist on that team also are explained.

CHAPTER 11 concludes the book with an overview of the diagnosis and treatment needs of children who are deaf or hearing impaired. Kretschmer and Kretschmer argue that early identification and appropriate intervention should provide for a near-typical development of communication skills in these children later in life. Also provided is an overview of the available communication modes (e.g., spoken or signed English, American Sign Language, or some other combination) from which each family must choose.

CASE STUDIES

The use of case studies throughout the chapters should help the reader tie the various discussions of development, etiological characteristics, assessment, and intervention to real-life experiences. Due to the nature of the text, the case studies are focused primarily on highlighting these aspects as they relate to the children's communication skills. Although we strongly advocate the use of an interdisciplinary approach with all children, because of space limitations we could not provide for each child all the relevant information for each discipline that might be involved in each case study. Readers should bear in mind that there is a wide range of developmental patterns, family contexts, and potentially appropriate approaches to assessment and intervention among the populations of young children with language impairments. The case studies presented in this volume are examples illustrating development in particular children, specific family issues, or a possible approach to assessment or intervention applied to a given child. The case studies provided here represent the authors' views of favored or typical practices in their particular area but are, in no way, meant to imply that they are the best or only methods avail-

able. The authors represented in this text are professionals with clear exper-
tise in research and/or clinical practice in their respective areas; consequently,
they provide direct links between research and practice.

Obviously, this brief introduction can only provide some of the information contained in the chapters, but hopefully it gives the reader a sense of the
content and the direction for current and future research and clinical activities in this area. We believe the volumes provide a great deal of important information on the cognitive, motor, and communication deficits in young
children with language impairments. We sincerely hope that we have provided
readers with information that can be directly applied to their interactions with
young children with communication deficits and their families.

Contributors

Christiane A. M. Baltaxe, Ph.D., Professor, Department of Psychiatry, University of California, Los Angeles

Jean L. Blosser, Ed.D., CCC-SLP, Interim Associate Provost, University of Akron, Akron, Ohio

Elizabeth R. Crais, Ph.D., CCC-SLP, Associate Professor, Division of Speech and Hearing Sciences, University of North Carolina, Chapel Hill

Roberta DePompei, Ph.D., CCC-SLP, Professor, School of Communicative Disorders, University of Akron, Akron, Ohio

Jane J. Giddan, M.A., CCC-SLP, Medical College of Ohio, Toledo, Ohio

Melody Harrison, Ph.D., CCC-SLP, Associate Professor, Division of Speech and Hearing Sciences, University of North Carolina, Chapel Hill

Laura W. Kretschmer, Ed.D., CCC-A, Professor, Department of Communication Sciences and Disorders, University of Cincinnati, Cincinnati, Ohio

Richard R. Kretschmer, Jr., Ed.D., Professor, Division of Special Education, University of Cincinnati, Cincinnati, Ohio

Ave M. Lachiewicz, M.D., Assistant Clinical Professor, Department of Pediatrics, Duke University Medical Center, Durham

Thomas L. Layton, Ph.D., CCC-SLP, Professor, Communication Sciences and Disorders, North Carolina Central University, Durham, North Carolina

Eliza Carlson Lee, M.A., doctoral candidate, Department of Psychology, Bryn Mawr College, Bryn Mawr, Pennsylvania

Allyn McConkie-Rosell, Ph.D., Certified Genetic Counselor; Clinical Associate, Division of Medical Genetics, Department of Pediatrics, Duke University Medical Center, Durham, North Carolina

Leonard Milling, Ph.D., Medical College of Ohio, Toledo

Penny Mirrett, Ph.D., CCC-SLP, Project Director, Frank Porter Graham Child Development Center, University of North Carolina, Chapel Hill

Sally Ozonoff, Ph.D., Associate Professor, Department of Psychology, University of Utah, Salt Lake City

Leslie A. Rescorla, Ph.D., Professor, Department of Psychology, Bryn Mawr College, Bryn Mawr, Pennsylvania

Shirley N. Sparks, M.S., CCC-SLP, Associate Professor Emeritus, Department of Speech Pathology and Audiology, Western Michigan University, Kalamazoo; also currently affiliated with the Department of Early Childhood Special Education, Santa Clara University, Santa Clara, California

Gail A. Spiridigliozzi, Ph.D., Assistant Clinical Professor of Psychiatry and Behavioral Sciences and Pediatrics, Duke University Medical Center, Durham, North Carolina

Genine Sander Scott, M.A., CCC-SLP, Speech-Language Pathologist, Chapel Hill, North Carolina

Linda R. Watson, Ed.D., CCC-SLP, Clinical Associate Professor, Division of Speech and Hearing Sciences, University of North Carolina, Chapel Hill

Reviewers

Mary Beth Armstrong, Ph.D., CCC-SLP, Assistant Professsor and Clinical Supervisor, University of Montevallo, Birmingham, Alabama

Frances P. Billeaud, M.A, CCC-SLP, ASHA Fellow, Director of Clinical Activities, Department of Communicative Disorders, University of Southwestern Louisiana, Lafayette

Mavis Donahue, Ed.D., Professor and Chair, Special Education, University of Illinois at Chicago

Judith F. Duchan, Ph.D., Professor, Communications Disorders Program, State University College at Buffalo, Buffalo, New York

Rhea Paul, Ph.D., Professor, Department of Communication Disorders, Southern Connecticut State University, and Fellow, Yale Child Study Center, New Haven

Clare Melanie Schuele, Ph.D., Visiting Assistant Professor, Case Western Reserve University, Cleveland

Rosalind R. Scudder, Ph.D., Professor, Department of Communicative Disorders and Sciences, Wichita State University, Wichita, Kansas

Language Impairment in Young Children

Leslie A. Rescorla, Ph.D.
Professor
Bryn Mawr College
Bryn Mawr, Pennsylvania
and
Eliza Carlson Lee, M.A.
Doctoral Candidate
Bryn Mawr College
Bryn Mawr, Pennsylvania

Key Terms

attention deficit/hyperactivity
  disorder (AD/HD)
familial aggregation
late talkers
linguistic deficit accounts
major domains of language

neurological soft signs
normal distribution account
perceptual deficit accounts
specific language impairment (SLI)
subtypes

Overview

One of the most common reasons why children under the age of 5 are referred for evaluation and/or intervention is that they are manifesting delay in expressive language. For many children, this expressive language delay is secondary to another condition (Tallal, 1988; Whitehurst & Fischel, 1994). Some young children who are slow to talk may have a hearing loss, a seizure condition, or a brain lesion. Others may be mentally retarded, with delayed language development being just one of many symptoms of below-average developmental progress. A small number of children with language delay have pervasive developmental disorder, with delayed language accompanied by deficits in social relatedness and oddities in play and behavior. Finally, some children show delays in language as well as other areas of development as a result of environmental deprivation, extreme neglect, or abuse.

When language delay is found in the absence of any other condition presumed to be primary (i.e., when all of the primary conditions can be excluded), the diagnostic term of choice in current practice is **specific language impairment (SLI)**. Although the term SLI is relatively new, in the field of communication disorders the notion of diagnosis by exclusion is quite old (Kamhi, 1998). For example, the influential Proceedings of the Institute on Childhood Aphasia held in 1960 (Johnston, 1988) defined this condition as an "impairment of language function (expressive and receptive)" that was not "associated primarily with" mental deficiency, hearing impairment, central nervous system (CNS) damage to the peripheral speech mechanism, emotional disturbance, or social-emotional factors. Other terms that have been used for this condition are "developmental aphasia" (Benton, 1964), "developmental language disorder" (Tallal, 1988), and "specific language delay" (Whitehurst & Fischel, 1994).

SLI is not a unitary disorder. Rather, it consists of at least two, and possibly three, major **subtypes**, depending on whether the delay is in language comprehension (receptive), language production (expressive), or both. The two universally accepted subtypes are a pure expressive type and a mixed receptive-expressive type. According to the nosology used in the *Diagnostic and Statistical Manual of Mental Disorders, Fourth Edition (DSM-IV)* (American Psychiatric Association [APA] 1994), the expressive type has an estimated prevalence of about 3 percent to 5 percent, and the mixed receptive-expressive type, of about 3 percent. More controversial is the existence of the pure receptive type, a subtype that is not included in the *DSM-IV.*

Although the *DSM-IV* does not cite empirical studies as references for its estimates, a number of large-scale epidemiological studies have provided various prevalence estimates. However, findings from these studies are quite discrepant, due to variations in subject age, assessment tools, and diagnostic criteria. Three of the early prevalence studies involved 3-year-olds. For example, Stevenson and Richman (1976) reported that about 3 percent of their sample of 705 British children had delayed expressive language; however, fewer than 1 percent would meet the exclusionary criteria for SLI. Fundudis, Kolvin, and Garside (1980) estimated the rate of speech and language impairment in their sample of British 3-year-olds to be 4 percent, but it is not clear from their report how many of these youngsters would meet the criteria for SLI. The Dunedin epidemiological study of 3-year-olds in New Zealand (Silva, 1980) indicated language delay prevalence rates of 3 percent for the pure receptive type, 2.5 percent for the pure expressive, and 3 percent for the mixed receptive-expressive, but what proportion of these youngsters met the exclusionary criteria for SLI is not reported.

Two more recent studies have examined the prevalence of SLI in 5-year-old children. Beitchman's epidemiological study (Beitchman, Nair, Clegg, Ferguson, & Patel, 1986) of Canadian kindergarten children reported a prevalence rate of receptive and/or expressive language impairment of 12.6 percent; however, this group included an unknown number of children who would not be diagnosed as SLI because of low IQs or other primary conditions. The best estimate of SLI at age 5 comes from the recent epidemiological study reported by Tomblin and his colleagues (Tomblin et al., 1997). From an initial sample of more than 7,000 kindergarten children, a two-stage screening and diagnostic process yielded a prevalence rate of 7.4 percent for SLI. All these children had performance Intelligence Quotients (IQs) above 85; were monolingual English speakers without any history of autism, neurological impairment, or sensory problems; and tested –1.25 standard deviations (SDs) or more below age norms on at least two of five language composite measures.

In the last few years, an important distinction has been made in the communication disorders literature between children with SLI and **late talkers**. Late talkers are young children (e.g., under age 4) who are delayed in their expressive language skills despite normal nonverbal cognitive ability, adequate hearing, and typical (e.g., nonautistic) personality development. Some studies of late talkers have involved children with expressive language delay only (Fischel, Whitehurst, Caulfield, & DeBaryshe, 1989; Rescorla, Roberts, & Dahlsgaard, 1997; Rescorla & Schwartz, 1990), whereas other cohorts have included some late talkers with delayed receptive language as well (Paul, 1993; Thal & Tobias, 1992; Thal, Tobias, & Morrison, 1991). Researchers have recently begun to differentiate late talkers from children with SLI because, despite the fact that exactly the same diagnostic criteria apply to both groups, research suggests that relatively few late talkers continue to manifest significant language delays after age 4 or 5 (Paul, 1996; Whitehurst & Fischel, 1994), even though as a group, late talkers may continue to be inferior in language skills to children with normal language histories (Rescorla, 1993).

Because this distinction between children with SLI and late talkers is a relatively recent one, no clear convention has yet been established in the field as to the age at which a child with delayed language should be given the diagnosis of SLI as opposed to being called a late talker. However, because many late talkers seem to outgrow their language delay by age 4 and some research indicates that many children diagnosed with SLI at age 4 continue to manifest language impairments into the school years, we will, for the purposes of this chapter, refer to children identified with language delay before age 4 as late talkers and denote children diagnosed with language delays at age 4 or later as having SLI.

DIAGNOSTIC ISSUES

Because delayed language development first becomes evident in the preschool years, this chapter will focus primarily on the process by which late talkers become diagnosed. However, many of the same considerations apply to the diagnosis of SLI in children age 4 or older. In order to diagnose a child as a late talker and to categorize him or her as to subtype, a variety of assessment tools must be employed. Although some of these tools consist of standardized tests, other tools may include parent report instruments, rating scales, or clinical observation. For the diagnosis of children age 4 and older as SLI, a similar process is involved, but the tests used and the criteria employed may differ somewhat.

Clearly, the first task in diagnosing a child as a late talker is to ascertain that he or she has significantly delayed language development. An initial picture of a toddler's expressive language can be obtained by use of a variety of parent report, screening instruments, such as Rescorla's Language Development Survey (LDS) (Rescorla, 1989), or the MacArthur Communicative Development Inventory (CDI): Words and Sentences (Fenson et al., 1993). For example, on the LDS, a child of about 24 months with a reported vocabulary of fewer than 50 words or no word combinations would fall at about the 15th percentile for his or her age, and hence would be considered to have a possible delay in expressive language. Similarly, one could identify a cutoff point on the CDI at the 10th to 15th percentile as a "red flag" for referring the child for a speech and language evaluation.

Using a tool such as the LDS or the CDI: Words and Sentences to make an initial identification of a possible language delay would target children with a pure expressive delay as well as those with a mixed expressive-receptive delay. Obviously, a child who has only a receptive language delay would not be identified by the use of such expressive language screening tools. Such a youngster might come to professional attention because of parental concern that he or she was not understanding language, despite apparently normal expressive language. Were the child under the age of 16 months, his or her language comprehension could be assessed using the MacArthur Communicative Development Inventory: Words and Gestures (Fenson et al., 1993), which does include a receptive language section; however, few developmental specialists advocate the identification of language delay at such a young age. Because children in the period from 12 to 24 months vary widely in their rate of expressive language development, concern about a child being a late talker is generally not indicated until at least 24 months, provided he or she appears to be developing typically in all other respects (comprehension, gestures, play, phonology, imitation, social interaction).

Once a possible expressive language delay has been identified (through screening and/or parent report), a formal assessment of the child's expressive and receptive language needs to be conducted. Typically it must be determined whether the child scores below some established cutoff (e.g., 1.5 standard deviations below the mean on a standardized test or a 20 percent delay on nonstandardized measures). This process will be discussed in detail. However, first it is important to mention the procedures necessary to rule out the various primary conditions that may result in a significant language delay, whether in a late talker under the age of 4 or a child with SLI at age 4 or older. The following procedures help in the process of excluding various primary conditions that might cause delayed language development.

1. Audiometric testing must establish that hearing is within normal thresholds (e.g., better than or equal to 15 db); oral-motor examination must determine that there are no structural abnormalities impeding speech development; and various neurological tests, such as an electroencephalogram (EEG), magnetic resonance imaging (MRI), or computerized axial tomography (CAT) may be used to demonstrate the lack of significant CNS pathology, such as a congenital or acquired lesions, cerebral palsy, seizures, or a tumor.

2. An IQ test must be used to establish that the child has normal nonverbal intelligence and is therefore not mentally retarded. Intelligence tests for children under 4 that allow nonverbal ability to be assessed independent of language skills include the Stanford-Binet Intelligence Scale: Fourth Edition (Thorndike, Hagen, & Sattler, 1986); The Bayley II Scales of Infant Development–II (Bayley, 1993); the Kaufman Assessment Battery for Children (K-ABC) (Kaufman & Kaufman, 1983) and the Leiter International Performance Scale–R (Roid & Miller, 1997). For children age 4 and older, some of these same tests continue to be useful; the Wechsler Preschool and Primary Scale of Intelligence–Revised (WPPSI-R), (Wechsler, 1989); the McCarthy Scales of Children's Abilities (McCarthy, 1972); and the Columbia Mental Maturity Scale (Burgmeister, Blum, & Lorge, 1972) can also be employed after age 4.

3. Clinical observation and/or a rating scale such as the Childhood Autism Rating Scale (CARS), (Schopler, Reichler, & Renner, 1988), can be used to determine that the child does not have pervasive developmental disorder.

4. Family information must be obtained to rule out environmental deprivation, physical/emotional neglect, or child abuse as contributing factors to the observed language delay.

Once it is established that a child has a language delay and that hearing loss, neurological impairment, mental retardation, autism, and environmental deprivation, and/or abuse can be excluded as contributory factors, an in-depth characterization of the child's communication and/or language must be made. For young children with little productive language, assessment must include an examination of various aspects of communication such as functions and means of communication, use of eye gaze, gestures, affective signaling, social interaction, and vocalizations. In addition, domains related to communication, such as functional and symbolic play, fine and gross motor, and self-help skills, must be examined. For profiling a child's skills across multiple domains related to communication, tools such as the Communication and Symbolic Behavior Scales (Wetherby & Prizant, 1993) or the Infant-Toddler Language Scale (Rossetti, 1990) can be useful. Other tools, such as the Assessment, Evaluation, and Programming System for Children (Bricker, 1993) or the Battelle Developmental Inventory (Newborg, Stock, Wnek, Guidubaldi, & Svinicki, 1984), can provide information about related domains.

For children who have moved beyond the early stages of communication and have acquired a broader productive language repertoire, it is imperative to collect the relevant language test data in order to classify the language delay as to subtype and to establish a significant discrepancy between expected and actual language skills. This classification is important for children who are late talkers under the age of 4 and for children age 4 or older with SLI. To accomplish this purpose, language tests must be used that allow the computation of separate scores for receptive and expressive language. In addition, it is highly desirable to use tests that allow for separate scores in the various domains of language (e.g., phonology, vocabulary, grammar, pragmatics), particularly when working with a child older than age 4 whose language skills are somewhat further developed than those typically seen in late-talking toddlers.

Many commonly used language tests for children under the age of 4, such as the Preschool Language Scale–3 (Zimmerman, Steiner, & Pond, 1991), the Reynell Developmental Language Scales (Reynell & Gruber, 1985), or the Sequenced Inventory of Communicative Development (SICD)–Revised (Hedrick, Prather, & Tobin, 1984), yield only aggregate scores for receptive and expressive language. On such a test, a child with relatively good vocabulary can score in the average range despite a very significant delay in syntactic development (e.g., a 4-year-old speaking in 2- to 4-word phrases) or in morphological skills (e.g., a 3½-year old who uses few verb inflections). Therefore, if one is using a broad language test such as the Reynell or the SICD to diagnose a child under the age of 4 as a late talker, it is desirable to use some additional tests that tap only one specific domain of language, such as the Expressive One-Word Picture Vocabulary Test–R (Gardner, 1990) or the Peabody Picture Vocabulary Test–III (Dunn & Dunn, 1997) for vocabulary, and the Patterned Elicitation Syntax Test (PEST) (Young & Perachio, 1983) for syntax. Alternatively, one can use an omnibus language test such as the Clinical Evaluation of Language Fundamentals–Preschool (CELF Preschool) (Wiig, Secord, & Semel, 1992), which is standardized for children aged 3 to 6, generates both receptive and expressive composites; has standard scores for subtests in areas such as vocabulary, verbal memory, and morphology; and provides a set of guidelines for the interpretation of test results (e.g., when it is appropriate to interpret subtests versus when the composite scores suffice).

For children age 4 or older, a larger variety of language tests are available that have subtests allowing for more in-depth analysis of language skills by domain. The most recently renormed test of this type is the Test of Language Development–Primary–Third Edition (TOLD-3:P) (Newcomer & Hammill, 1997). In the major epidemiological study of SLI in 5-year-olds being conducted by Tomblin and colleagues (Tomblin et al., 1997; Tomblin, Records, & Zhang, 1996), five subtests of the TOLD-2:P (Newcomer & Hammill, 1991) plus two narrative measures were used to establish a 2 × 3 cell matrix yielding five composites, two by modality (comprehension and expression) and three by language domain (vocabulary, grammar, and narrative).

A major issue in the SLI field is how to determine a child's "expected" language skills for purposes of calculating a discrepancy between expected and actual skills (i.e., should expected language level be based on the child's chronological age or nonverbal cognitive ability). Another issue in the field is whether it is acceptable to use age-level scores to determine a significant language discrepancy (which has been common practice in the past and is permitted in the documentation of developmental delay for purposes of early intervention in many states), or whether norm-referenced standard scores should be used exclusively for this purpose. Third, it is also not clear whether the same degree of discrepancy should serve as the diagnostic standard at different ages (i.e., to diagnose a 30-month-old as a late talker versus a 5-year-old as having SLI).

As Aram, Morris, and Hall (1993) stated, procedures for establishing discrepancy vary tremendously in all three of these respects, whether it is the standard used to establish expected language skill (chronological age, grade level, mental age, or nonverbal IQ), the type of score to be used (age level vs. standard score), or the cutpoint employed to determine a discrepancy between predicted and actual language skill (e.g., 6 months vs. one year, one SD vs. 2 SDs). Aram and her colleagues (Aram et al., 1993) provide striking evidence of how this variation in criteria affects diagnostic consensus. Specifically, only 59 percent of the 252 children diagnosed as having SLI by clinicians in five major sites met the minimal research diagnostic criterion of 1 SD discrepancy between nonverbal IQ and composite language score.

In the past five years, several diagnostic standards addressing these issues have been proposed. In their review of the late talker literature, Whitehurst and Fischel (1994) suggest that the diagnosis of specific receptive-expressive language delay should not be made unless the child scores at least –1.5 SDs below average in both receptive and expressive skills, one of these scores is at least –2 SDs below average, and nonverbal IQ is within 1 SD of average. They suggest that the criteria for specific expressive delay should be nonverbal IQ and receptive language within 1 SD of average and an expressive delay of at least 2 SDs. This standard is stricter than the one used for establishing eligibility for early intervention in most states, for which a criterion of –1.5 SDs is generally used to establish the presence of a language delay in need of remediation (Bagnato & Neisworth, 1994). In Tomblin's recent epidemiological study, a score of –1.25 SDs below age expectations on two or more of five language composites was used as the criterion for SLI; Tomblin et al. (1996) identify this as the EpiSLI diagnostic standard. In one of the most recent commentaries on this issue, Kamhi (1998) argues for a differentiation of general developmental language disorders (DLD) from SLI; the former he would diagnose by an IQ within 2 SDs of average and any composite language score 1 SD below the mean, whereas the latter condition, which he estimates to comprise only 20 percent of DLD, would be identified by some, more specific criteria, such as normal receptive language but delayed expressive language, or evident morphosyntactic delays.

In sum, based on findings from these and other studies, recommended practice at this time seems to be to use standard scores rather than age levels to compare a child's language skills to those of chronological agemates, to use an IQ cutoff of 1 SD to establish normal nonverbal ability (e.g., a nonverbal IQ of at least 85), and to employ a discrepancy standard of –1.25 or –1.50 SDs below age expectations to establish language delay. Clearly, scores within 1 SD of average in either receptive or expressive language should be interpreted as falling in the normal range.

CHARACTERISTICS OF CHILDREN WITH LANGUAGE DELAYS

There is now a considerable body of research dealing with the characteristics of children with language delays in the domains of (1) language deficits, (2) cognitive abilities, (3) neuromotor/perceptual skills, and (4) social-behavioral development. It is important in considering this literature to try to distinguish between studies dealing with late talkers and research involving children aged 4 or older who have been diagnosed with SLI.

Language Deficits

Research on the language deficits manifested by late talkers and children with SLI generally focuses on four **major domains of language**: phonology; semantic/lexical skills; syntax and morphology; and pragmatics. The most common question that has been explored in this research is whether children with SLI manifest delayed versus deviant development.

Phonology.   Several studies of late talkers have demonstrated that young children who are slow to talk tend to have reduced volubility and more limited phonetic repertoires than typically developing toddlers. In particular, late talkers use fewer consonants than age-matched peers with normal language development (Mirak & Rescorla, 1998; Paul & Jennings, 1992; Rescorla & Ratner, 1996; Stoel-Gammon, 1989; Whitehurst, Smith, Fischel, Arnold, & Lonigan, 1991). However, late talkers appear to acquire a mastery of consonants in approximately the same sequence as typically developing children. In addition, late talkers appear to manifest the same kind of phonological processes that contribute to articulation errors in younger, typically developing children; namely, cluster reduction, final consonant deletion, and substitutions. Studies with two different groups of late talkers (Mirak & Rescorla, 1998; Paul & Jennings, 1992; Rescorla & Ratner, 1996) have demonstrated that these children are especially different from age-matched, typically developing peers in their ability to use consonants at the ends of words.

Follow-up studies of late talkers indicate that, as a group, they continue to be delayed phonologically until at least age 4. For example, in Rescorla's sample, by age 3 the late talkers were no longer less voluble than typically developing agemates at 3, but they had mastered fewer consonants, showed more phonological processes, and were less intelligible than children in the comparison group (Roberts, Rescorla, Giroux, & Stevens, 1998). Paul (1993) reported that 60 percent of her sample of late talkers were below the 10th percentile on an articulation test at age 3, and 34 percent were still below the 10th percentile on a measure of articulation at age 4. However, by second grade, mean score on Shriberg and Kwiatowski's (1982) measure of percent consonants correct was above 94%, indicating good speech intelligibility for the former late talkers.

Not all children age 4 and older who have been diagnosed with SLI have impaired phonology, and many children with perfectly normal language manifest articulatory problems. However, children with SLI do have elevated rates of phonological disorder relative to typically developing agemates (Bishop & Edmundson, 1987; Paul & Shriberg, 1982). For example, in the Beitchman study (Beitchman et al., 1986), 28 percent of 5-year-olds with speech-language impairments had speech problems only, 44 percent had language problems only, and 29 percent had both, indicating that about 40 percent of the children with language impairments also had speech problems. Tallal (1988) has suggested that children with SLI may differ from typically developing youngsters in that they manifest a more protracted period during which competing phonological representations for the same sound coexist in free variation.

Semantic/Lexical Skills.   Late talkers are generally first identified because they lag behind age expectations in vocabulary acquisition. For example, the late talkers in Rescorla's longitudinal sample (Rescorla et al., 1997) had a mean of 20 words on Rescorla's (1989) LDS at the intake age of 24 to 31 months, in contrast to a mean reported vocabulary of 226 words in the comparison group of toddlers. This is strikingly similar to the intake mean LDS scores of 29 versus 204 words for late talkers versus typically developing toddlers found in Paul's longitudinal study (Paul, Murray, Clancy, & Andrews, 1997). Very small vocabularies were also reported in Whitehurst's sample of late talkers identified at around age 2 (Fischel et al., 1989).

Longitudinal research suggests that vocabulary delays manifested by late talkers tend to resolve by ages 3 to 4 (Ellis Weismer, Murray-Branch, & Miller, 1994; Fischel et al., 1989; Paul, 1993; Rescorla et al., 1997; Thal et al., 1991). For example, in the sample of late talkers followed by Whitehurst and his colleagues (Whitehurst, Fischel, Arnold, & Lonigan, 1992), 88 percent of the group scored in the average range on the Expressive One-Word Picture Vocabulary Test (EOWPVT) (Gardner, 1979) at ages 3–6. In Rescorla's (Rescorla et al., 1997) longitudinal study, mean score on the EOWPVT was in the average range at age 3, with only 21 percent of the late talkers scoring more than 1 SD below age expectations by age 3 follow-up. However, late talkers still scored significantly below comparison peers, with whom they had been matched at intake on socioeconomic status (SES) and nonverbal ability, at ages 3 and 4 on the EOWPVT.

A laboratory training study of 3-year-old late talkers revealed that when compared with language-matched peers, they showed few significant differences in either the lexical types displayed (Leonard, Camarata, Rowan, & Chapman, 1982) or the rate and process by which novel lexical items were acquired (Leonard et al., 1982).

Results of vocabulary laboratory studies in children with SLI are somewhat equivocal, but they suggest greater impairments in the production than the comprehension of lexical items. In a study with 4- to 5-year-olds with SLI, Dollaghan (1987) found no differences in comprehension relative to age-matched peers after a single presentation of a novel word ("koob"), (i.e., a "fast-mapping" procedure); however, only one of the 11 subjects with SLI could produce the word correctly, whereas 7 of the comparison children could do so. On the other hand, using a "quick incidental learning" (QUIL) procedure, Rice, Buhr, and Oetting (1992) found 5-year-olds with SLI to perform worse than typically developing agemates, but similar to language-matched younger children, in learning novel words. In a recent study by Ellis Weismer and Hesketh (1996) involving 7-year-olds with SLI and typically developing agemates, much larger group differences were found for the production versus the comprehension of novel words (e.g., children with SLI comprehended 70 percent of the targets and produced 20 percent of them, whereas their agemates comprehended 83 percent and produced 43 percent). Gathercole and Baddeley (1990) found 8-year-old children with language disorders to be significantly worse at the verbatim repetition of nonwords relative to performance by 6-year-old vocabulary-matched, typically developing children, particularly when the stimuli were three or four syllables long; additional experiments suggested that the deficit was not in speech perception or in articulation, but rather in phonological memory.

A recent study by Kiernan and Gray (1998) examined the learning of novel vocabulary items by 4-year-olds with SLI and age-matched controls using a play-based, supported-learning context. As a group, the children with SLI learned to produce significantly fewer of the terms (which were obscure labels for pirate or knight paraphernalia). Further analyses indicated, however, that only 27 percent of the children with language impairments had poorer word learning skills, with the other 73 percent performing comparably to the typically developing children. It should also be noted that the children with impaired production comprehended most of the terms they failed to produce.

Syntax and Morphology. The first sign of syntactic delay in late talkers is that the child is slow to develop word combinations (Fischel et al., 1989; Rescorla et al., 1997; Rescorla & Schwartz, 1990). That is, while typically developing children manifest word combinations by age 2, many late talkers do not begin combining words until age 3.

Follow-up studies of late talkers indicate that they tend to lag behind in measures of syntax and morphology until ages 4 or 5. For example, Paul (1993) found that 60 percent of her sample of late talkers scored below the 10th percentile in Developmental Sentence Score (Lee, 1974) at age 3, and 47 percent scored at this level at age 4. In Rescorla's sample of late talkers followed up to age 3 (Rescorla et al., 1997), 53 percent scored more than 1.50 SDs below age expectations in mean length of ulterance (MLU), and 58 percent scored at this level on the Index of Productive Syntax (IPSyn), (Scarborough, 1990). At age 4, the corresponding figures were 32 percent and 62 percent, respectively (Rescorla & Dahlsgaard, 1995). Rescorla's (1993) sample of late talkers did not score in the average range on tests of syntactic competence until age 5.

Most of the work on syntax and morphology in children with language impairments has been done with children age 4 and older who have been diagnosed with SLI. The general conclusion from research conducted in the 1970s and 1980s was that children with SLI acquired syntax in roughly the same fashion as typically developing children, albeit at a slower rate (Tallal, 1988). That is, they appeared to use normal phrase structure rules, as well as standard rules for embedding clauses (Tallal, 1988). Tallal's study of a large group of children with SLI suggested a high degree of similarity in the rate and sequence of syntax acquisition when comparisons were made to language-matched peers (Curtiss, Katz, & Tallal, 1992), although Tallal (1988) suggested that children with SLI may produce ungrammatical utterances at higher rates.

It is well documented that children with SLI have particular difficulty with the acquisition of grammatical morphology (Bortolini, Caselli, & Leonard, 1997; Clahsen, 1989, 1991; Cleave & Rice, 1997; Crago & Gopnik, 1994; Johnston & Kamhi, 1984; Leonard, Bortolini, Caselli, McGregor, & Sabbadini, 1992; Leonard, Sabbadini, Volterra, & Leonard, 1988; Rice & Oetting, 1993; Rice & Wexler, 1996; Rice, Wexler, & Cleave, 1995). A great deal of research indicates that children with SLI have more problems with morphological inflections than younger, typically developing children matched on MLU level. Morphemes that appear to be particularly problematic for English-speaking children with SLI are third person singular -s, past -ed, copula forms (is, are), auxiliaries (is, do, does), possessive -'s, and articles (a, the), (Roberts & Leonard, 1997). Crosslinguistic studies of children with SLI learning Italian, Hebrew, and German suggest that the omission of grammatical morphemes is a more circumscribed problem in those morphologically complex languages, being confined to fewer forms than are found in English (Dromi, Leonard, & Shteiman, 1993; Leonard et al., 1992).

Pragmatics.   The main focus of studies looking at pragmatics in late talkers has been conversational interaction between the child and the caregiver. For example, data reported by Paul and Shiffer (1991) indicated that late talkers engaged in fewer joint attention interchanges with their mothers than did age-matched peers. More recently, Rescorla and Merrin (1998) reported that late-talking toddlers produced fewer initiations and responses than their age-matched peers in a mother-child play session, but did not differ from typically developing peers in the proportion of initiations versus responses, nor in the proportion of interactions that involved joint attention.

Studies of pragmatics in children age 4 and older diagnosed with SLI indicate roughly normal pragmatic development when compared to their developmental language age (Tallal, 1988). Research findings on pragmatics frequently show that children with SLI are less communicatively interactive than age-matched peers (Watson, 1977), but that they are quite comparable to younger, language-matched youngsters. For example, Fey and Leonard (1984) found that children with SLI did not show deficits in conversational participation when compared with linguistically matched controls. Similarly, reviews by Fey and Leonard (1984) and Lahey (1988) suggest that children with SLI differ in pragmatic skills in numerous ways from age-matched controls but show few pragmatics differences when compared with language-matched younger children.

Cognitive Abilities

By definition, late talkers and children with SLI have normal intelligence, as measured by nonverbal portions of standardized intelligence tests. However, research has shown that despite normal performance on nonverbal IQ tests, some children with language impairments have deficits and/or delays in several nonverbal cognitive areas, including gesture/symbolic play, conceptual reasoning, and rate of information processing and responding (Johnston, 1994).

Gesture/Symbolic Play.   In a study of language and gesture in 18- to 32-month-old late talkers in which children were asked to reproduce single gestures that had been modeled with toys and objects, Thal and Bates (1988) found that late talkers produced significantly fewer recognitory gestures (e.g., "drinking" from a toy cup) than age-matched controls, but the same number as language-matched controls. A follow-up study of these late talkers 1 year later showed that gesture production correlated significantly with language comprehension and that performance on gesture tasks predicted which children remained language delayed at follow-up and which children "caught up" (Thal et al., 1991).

Rescorla and Goossens (1992) studied play schemes in late talkers. They reported that, when compared with typically developing agemates, late talkers showed as much engagement with toys and similar levels of functional play, but they engaged in less higher level play than their agemates (e.g., play directed to a doll, sequences of play schemes, symbolic substitution); they also demonstrated less variety in their play scheme repertoire.

A study by Terrell, Schwartz, Prelock, and Messick (1984) examined play behaviors on the Symbolic Play Test (Lowe & Costello, 1976) in late talkers with a mean age of about 3 years. Their results showed that the late talkers, all of whom were in the single-word stage, exhibited significantly more mature and complex play skills than the language-matched controls, who were single-word speakers with a mean age of 19 months. However, the late talkers' level of play fell significantly below what would be expected given their chronological age. In a subsequent study, Terrell & Schwartz (1988) found that 3- to 4-year-old late talkers speaking at about a 2-year-old age level engaged in more concrete, and less symbolic (e.g., object substitution), play than agemates, but they did not differ from language-matched controls in object substitutions. However, a more recent study of symbolic play in 3- to 5-year-olds with expressive language delay by Kushnir and Blake (1996) reported no significant differences, when compared to typically developing agemates, in number or variety of play schemes, in sequence length, or in object substitutions.

A recent review of play behavior in children with language impairment by Casby (1997) argues that research does not support the notion that children with language impairments have a general deficit in symbolic competence. He concludes that many studies find no differences in play behavior when late talkers are matched with typically developing children on language level. Furthermore, he suggests that even when significant differences in play are found relative to age-matched controls, these differences tend to be frequency differences, not qualitative ones (i.e., the children with language impairments do display symbolic and representational play behavior, but less often than typically developing children). Most importantly, Casby (1997) argues that it is very difficult to avoid the confounding of language skill and play level in research of this kind. Specifically, late talkers and children with SLI who have receptive language deficits may fail to comprehend task instructions in play procedures, whereas youngsters with expressive language deficits may have difficulty narrating and explaining their play behavior in a way that allows observers to appreciate its complexity.

Categorization/Rule Learning.   Another possible cognitive deficit that has been explored in children with language impairments is the ability to classify, categorize, or induce rules (Ellis Weismer, 1991; Kamhi, 1981; Kamhi, Catts, Koenig, & Lewis, 1984; Kamhi, Nelson, Lee, & Gholson, 1985; Nelson, Kamhi, & Apel, 1987). For example, Kamhi (1981) used six Piagetian tasks with three groups of children: 5-year-old children with specific language impairment, mental age–matched controls, and language-matched controls. The tasks included sorting geometric shapes, arranging small toys according to a model, and determining the relative quantity of two sets of checkers. In each task, the children with SLI performed below the mental age–matched comparison group, but above the language-matched younger children.

Somewhat contrary findings have been reported, however, by Connell and Stone (1994). Their study involved 5- to 6-year-olds with SLI and age-matched, typically developing children. The children were taught a nonlinguistic conceptual rule in a computer-based concept identification task (e.g., they had to induce that the target was hidden behind either the small, square, dotted, or lower figure). The authors reported no group differences in the ability to induce a rule in this task, whereas children with SLI had been less skilled at inducing pseudo-morpheme rules in a parallel task conducted by the same authors (Connell & Stone, 1992). Although the authors concluded that their data suggest that the difficulty of children with SLI have in rule induction may be specific to language tasks, they caution that more complex tasks with more rules to be learned might have shown a significant group difference, implying that children with SLI may only begin to look inferior to agemates when task complexity is great, multiple tasks are given, or cognitive flexibility across tasks is required.

A recent study by Kiernan and colleagues (Kiernan, Snow, Swisher, & Vance, 1997) examining the issue of conceptual deficit in children with language impairments compared 4- to 6-year-old children with SLI and age-matched controls and found results quite consistent with those of Connell and Stone (1994). In this study, a rule induction–rule shift procedure modeled on the Wisconsin Card Sorting Test (Berg, 1948) was used. The results indicated that children with SLI did not differ from controls in trials to criterion on the induction of the first rule, on the within-dimensional shift (e.g., from red to blue), or on the extradimensional shift (e.g., from red to small). The authors conclude that their study provided no supporting evidence for the hypothesis that children with SLI have nonverbal rule-induction deficits, and they suggest that the difficulties of children with SLI in learning morphosyntactic patterns is "language-specific."

Rate of Processing/Responding.   A third cognitive area in which children with language impairments have been shown to have deficits is in the rate of processing and responding. A large body of work by Tallal and her colleagues (Johnston, Stark, Mellits, & Tallal, 1981; Tallal, 1988; Tallal, Dukette, & Curtiss, 1989; Tallal, Stark, Kallman, & Mellits, 1981; Tallal, Stark, & Mellits, 1985) indicates significant differences between typically developing children and children with SLI in the ability to discriminate between two tones and to determine sequential order when two tones are presented in rapid sequence. Furthermore, the degree of temporal perceptual deficits correlated highly with the degree of receptive language impairment, $r = 89$, $p < .001$ (Tallal et al., 1985). From such studies, Tallal (1988) concluded that children with SLI are specifically impaired in their ability to process rapidly presented information.

The novel vocabulary study by Ellis Weismer and Hesketh (1996) reviewed earlier provides corroborating evidence for the hypothesis that children with SLI have problems in rapid temporal processing. In that study, a faster than normal presentation rate had a much larger negative impact for the children with SLI than for their typically developing agemates; interestingly, however, this effect was only found for production probes, and not for comprehension. In addition, more children with SLI than typically developing children benefited from slower than normal presentation rates, an effect found in both comprehension and production probes.

Deficits in producing speeded responses, as well as in processing rapidly presented incoming information, have been noted in children with SLI. For example, Kail and Leonard (1986) reported that children with SLI named pictures and recognized words more slowly than agemates. Nonverbal cognitive tasks have also been used to show that children with SLI may have problems with the rapid execution of mental tasks. For example, scanning short-term memory and mentally rotating shapes have been found to take longer for children with SLI than typically developing youngsters (Johnston & Ellis Weismer, 1983; Sininger, Klatzky, & Kirchner, 1989).

In an ingenious reanalysis of 22 pairs of means from several previous studies, Kail (1994) demonstrated that school-age children with SLI needed about 30 percent more time to perform a variety of cognitive tasks than their typically developing peers. Virtually the same time coefficient was found in all these comparisons, regardless of whether the task was picture naming, recognition memory for pictures, picture discrimination, or digit recognition memory.

In summary, the sampling of studies reviewed here shows that children with SLI often show deficits in nonverbal cognitive abilities relative to their age-matched peers. This is particularly true when tasks are lengthy and complex or when speeded performance is essential. However, much research also shows no difference in nonverbal cognitive abilities between children with SLI and their agemates, suggesting that sample characteristics or task parameters are crucial in determining whether the performance of children with SLI will be similar to, or deficient from, that of age-matched, typically developing peers. Perhaps the most robust finding in this area of research is that children with SLI appear to engage in information processing somewhat more slowly than typically developing children.

Neuromotor Skills

Although, by definition, late talkers and children with SLI have no obvious or significant CNS disorder, it is also the case that language impairment is often considered to be one of several **neurological soft signs**. This suggests that delays in language development could result from a primary motoric problem at the neurological level (Tallal, 1988).

One possibility that has been explored in late talkers is that some neurological condition may make it more difficult to control the speech organs (Whitehurst & Fischel, 1994). Thus, Whitehurst and colleagues (Whitehurst et al., 1992) asked parents of late talkers and of typically developing controls about their children's history of chewing problems, choking, and drooling.

Drooling and choking were reported significantly more often for the late talkers, supporting the hypothesis that oral-motor problems are associated with slow language development in some children (Whitehurst & Fischel, 1994).

Gross motor development has also been studied in late talkers. Paul (1991) found that her late talkers did not differ from typically developing children on the motor subscale of the Vineland Adaptive Behavior Scales (Sparrow, Balla, & Cicchetti, 1984). In their review of the late talker literature, Whitehurst and Fischel (1994) reported that late talkers generally do not seem to have gross motor difficulties.

Research with children age 4 or older manifesting SLI suggests the presence of a variety of mild motor difficulties. For example, as part of a longitudinal study on language and motor development, Bishop and Edmundson (1987) examined the fine motor skills of 4-year-olds with SLI using a task in which the children moved pegs from one row to another using each hand. The children with language delays were slower than the typically developing language controls. A follow-up at age 5½ of the children with language delays showed that improvement in language abilities correlated highly with improvement on the peg task, suggesting a developmental lag in both language and neuromotor skills that resolves by about age 5. At 8½ years of age, the children with continuing language impairment were still slower than the typically developing controls on the peg task.

In a study of behavioral characteristics of 81 children with SLI aged 4 years old, Tallal and colleagues (Tallal et al., 1989) found that the items *twitches, accident prone,* and *clumsy* on the Child Behavior Checklist (CBCL), (Achenbach, 1991), discriminated between the children with language impairments and the typically developing children. Additional evidence of an underlying neurological delay or deficit associated with language impairment is revealed in the epidemiological study of kindergarten children by Beitchman and his colleagues (Beitchman, Hood, Rochon, Peterson, Mantini, et al., 1989). They reported that children who had poor language abilities also had the lowest scores on measures of visual-motor integration.

The studies reviewed here show that some children with SLI are deficient in motor and/or visual-motor skills. The neuromotor deficits reported in children with language impairments provide support for the hypothesis that SLI is related to a more general neurodevelopmental problem, at least in some children (Tallal, 1988).

Social-behavioral development

Given the importance of language in the development of social skills and behavioral regulation, a child with limited language ability would likely experience difficulties in these areas. In fact, a growing body of research has provided evidence of an association between language impairment and psychosocial problems.

Social Functioning. The social functioning of late talkers and children with SLI has been somewhat neglected in research until recent years (Fujiki & Brinton, 1994). In a study of toddlers with delayed expressive language development, Paul (1991) assessed the children's socialization skills using the Vineland Adaptive Behavior Scales (Sparrow et al., 1984) and found that 62 percent of the late talkers scored more than 6 months below age level, whereas none of the typically developing group scored this low. An item analysis showed that the late talkers performed more poorly than the control group on the nonverbal, as well as the verbal, items (Paul, 1991).

Deficits in the social skills of children age 4 or older with SLI have also been reported. Despite having relatively normal pragmatics skills given their language level, children with SLI are at a social disadvantage in group settings with age-matched peers. In a study of peer interactions, preschool children with language impairments and typically developing children were observed in free and structured play situations (Siegel, Cunningham, & van der Spuy, 1985). The children with language delays initiated less than typically developing children, and the typically developing children frequently attempted to establish dominance and control over the children with SLI. A study by Rice, Sell, and Hadley (1991) reported that 4-year-old children with SLI were less likely to initiate interactions with peers and had shorter responses to the initiations of their peers and teachers than children with normal language skills. Finally, Fujiki and Brinton (1994) pointed out that children with SLI sometimes use language in ways that directly result in social problems. These socially penalizing linguistic behaviors often consist of pragmatic misuses of language that result in negative reactions from peers and adults (Fujiki & Brinton, 1994; Rice, Hadley, & Alexander, 1993).

These findings lend support to Rice's conclusion concerning the "social consequences account of language impairment" (Rice et al., 1991). In this account, children with SLI are limited in their abilities to interact with peers. They tend to restrict their social interactions, which in turn limits their opportunities to learn important communication skills from their peers. Children with language impairments, therefore, are vulnerable to a "negative spiral of social/communication failure beginning in the preschool years" (Rice et al., 1991, p. 1305).

An even more ominous finding reported by Rice and her colleagues is that children with SLI are rated by kindergarten teachers as less bright, less likable, less socially mature, and less likely to succeed in kindergarten than typically developing agemates (Rice et al., 1993). Kindergarten children with SLI are also less likely to be promoted to regular first grade (Rice et al., 1993). In some cases, retention may be recommended because the child has significant learning problems, but in other cases limited verbal ability may cause teachers to underestimate the intellectual ability and social maturity of a child with SLI who is actually ready for first grade.

Behavioral Adjustment. Studies have also shown that children with language impairments are more likely to have behavioral and attentional problems than children with normal language development. In Paul's (1991) study of 2-year-olds, mothers of late talkers reported significantly more problem behaviors than did mothers of typically developing agemates, with late talkers perceived as overly active and more difficult to manage than typically developing peers. Several epidemiological studies have demonstrated elevated rates of behavior problems in 3-year-old children with language delays (Richman, Stevenson, & Graham, 1982; Silva, McGee, & Williams, 1983); however, as was noted previously, only some of the children with language impairments in these samples met the exclusionary criteria for SLI.

In the large study of kindergarten children with language impairment conducted by Beitchman and his colleagues (Beitchman et al., 1986; Beitchman, Hood, & Inglis, 1990), it was reported that 59 percent of the children with the lowest language abilities were diagnosed with **attention deficit/hyperactivity disorder (AD/HD)**. In the group of children with receptive language impairments, all of the children who had a psychiatric disorder were diagnosed with AD/HD (Beitchman, Hood, Rochon, & Peterson, 1989; Beitchman, Hood, Rochon, Peterson, Mantini, et al., 1989). Similarly, in the study by Tallal and her colleagues (Tallal, Dukette, et al., 1989), which identified children as SLI at age 4, the items on the Child Behavior Checklist (Achenbach, 1991) that differentiated the children with SLI from their typically developing peers included *acts too young, can't concentrate, twitches, confused,* and *accident prone,* all of which might be seen as characteristics of AD/HD. Finally, Cantwell and colleagues (Baker & Cantwell, 1982; Cantwell & Baker, 1987), who studied psychiatric disorders in school-age children with speech and language disorders, found that AD/HD was the most frequently occurring disorder in children with receptive SLI or combined receptive/expressive SLI.

THEORIES OF ETIOLOGY

Many theories have been proposed to explain why some children become late talkers or manifest SLI. Over the years, familial factors have been the subject of much study. In addition, recent theorizing about the etiology of SLI has been dominated by three major accounts, which we refer to as **perceptual deficit accounts, linguistic deficit accounts,** and the **normal distribution account**. Each of these approaches to explaining the etiology of SLI will be summarized.

Familial Factors

Familial factors include both parent-child interaction characteristics and genetic disposition.

Parent-Child Interaction Characteristics.   One of the first lines of research on the etiology of SLI focused on the language-learning environments of children with language impairments. This work examined the verbal interactions between mothers and their children with language impairments, focusing on maternal responsiveness, dyadic synchrony, and conversational structure (Chapman, 1981; Conti-Ramsden & Friel-Patti, 1983; Cunningham, Siegel, van der Spuy, Clark, & Bow, 1985; Lasky & Klopp, 1982; Mosely, 1990; Rescorla & Fechnay, 1996; Snow, 1984; Wubert, Inglis, Kriegsmann, & Mills, 1975). A few studies suggested that children with language impairments experience a negative conversational environment. For example, Wubert and colleagues (Wubert et al., 1975) reported that mothers of 2- to 5-year-old children with language impairments were more critical, controlling, and punitive and less interactive than mothers of typically developing children. However, most research indicates no major differences in the communicative environment of children with language impairments (Cunningham et al., 1985; Lasky & Klopp, 1982; Rescorla & Fechnay, 1996), whether the children in question are late talkers or older children with SLI. In addition, the evidence that the characteristics of parent-child interaction affect normal language development is weak, and investigators do not agree on the type of communicative environment that is optimal, even for typically developing children (Leonard, 1987). Therefore, this line of research has made limited contributions to the search for the etiology of SLI.

Genetics.   In recent years, there has been increased interest in the search for a possible genetic role in the etiology of SLI. One of the first suggestions of a biological basis for SLI comes from the extreme gender imbalance of the disorder. Data consistently indicate higher rates of SLI among male children (Bishop & Edmundson, 1987; Paul, 1991; Rescorla et al., 1997; Silva, 1980; Stevenson & Richman, 1976; Whitehurst & Fischel, 1994); however, many of these studies are quite old, and none surveyed children over the age of 4. It should be noted that the two most recent prevalence studies, both of which used kindergarten children, showed no strong male preponderance. Beitchman and colleagues (1986) found that language disorders were slightly more common among girls than boys, and Tomblin (Tomblin et al., 1997) found that 41 percent of the 216 children diagnosed as SLI were female.

A twin study by Bishop (1992) provides stronger evidence of a genetic basis for SLI. Specifically, in a sample of 61 twin pairs in which at least one twin had a current or past SLI, a higher concordance rate was reported in the monozygotic (MZ) twins than the dizygotic (DZ) twins (67 percent versus 32 percent, respectively). A more recent study by Bishop and her colleagues (Bishop, North, & Donlan, 1995) reported a concordance of 46 percent for 27 DZ twin pairs and 70 percent for 63 MZ twin pairs for a variety of language impairments. Most recently, Tomblin and Buckwalter (1998), using a large battery of different language tests, found concordance rates of 96 percent and 69 percent for MZ and DZ twins, respectively, suggesting a strong genetic component to language impairment.

Other support for genetic factors in the etiology of SLI comes from studies of the **familial aggregation** of language disorders, including SLI. Familial aggregation has received relatively little study in samples of late talkers. Paul (1991) reported that a family history of language or learning problems was much more likely in her late talkers than in her typically developing age-matched controls. On the other hand, Whitehurst and colleagues (Whitehurst et al., 1991) found no difference in family history of speech, language, and school problems when late talkers were compared with typically developing children. It should be recalled that the children in Whitehurst's sample all had normal receptive language, whereas about one-quarter of Paul's (1991) group had receptive as well as expressive delays.

In studies of children age 4 and older who have been diagnosed with SLI, significant familial aggregations of language impairment have been consistently reported. For example, Lahey and Edwards (1995) examined 53 children with SLI aged 4 to 9 years. It was found that 60 percent of the families had at least one other family member with a history of language or learning impairment, with 26 percent of mothers, 22 percent of fathers, and 29 percent of siblings having such history. Somewhat surprisingly, the group representing the pure expressive subgroup (26 percent of the sample) had significantly higher familial aggregations than the mixed receptive-expressive group.

Bishop and Edmundson (1986) collected family history data for 56 children with language impairments and an SES-matched control group of children with typical language development. The parents of the children with language impairments reported that 46 percent had relatives with a history of speech, language, or reading disorders, a rate much higher than the 15 percent reported in the typically developing group.

Work by Tallal, Ross, and Curtiss (1989) indicated that 77 percent of families with a child who had SLI reported at least one first-degree relative with a history of language, speech, or hearing problems or with low school achievement, relative to a rate of 46 percent in families of typically developing agemates. Tomblin (1989) found that over half of his sample reported a family history of language problems, with the brothers of children with language impairment being more likely to be affected than the sisters.

A recent study by Spitz, Tallal, Flax, and Benasich (1997) examined familial aggregation prospectively. Ten toddlers who had at least one sibling (or one parent) diagnosed with language impairment and a comparison group of 10 agemates with no such family history were compared in their language and nonverbal abilities. Toddlers with positive family history for language problems had somewhat lower receptive and expressive language scores and lower cognitive ability scores than agemates with no such family history. Half the toddlers with positive family history had language scores at least 1.5 SDs below age level, whereas no children in the other group performed this poorly.

Three Major Theoretical Accounts of SLI

Three major accounts have dominated theorizing regarding the etiology of SLI: perceptual deficit accounts, linguistic deficit accounts, and the normal distribution account.

Perceptual Deficit Accounts. Perceptual deficit accounts are based on evidence that some children with SLI perform below their age level on auditory processing tasks. As described earlier, the work of Tallal and her colleagues (Tallal, 1988; Tallal et al., 1981; Tallal & Piercy, 1973) has shown that children with SLI have difficulty discriminating and sequencing rapid acoustic events. The language difficulties experienced by children with SLI are attributed to this auditory-processing deficit. According to this account, children with SLI are impaired in their ability to learn language because of a deficiency in their processing of the incoming speech stream.

Another version of a perceptual deficit account is the surface account proposed by Leonard (1989, 1994). Leonard's account is also concerned with the processing demands of the language acquisition process; however, this view focuses on explaining the morphological deficits of children with SLI. According to Leonard (1989, 1994), children with SLI experience extreme difficulty in producing certain grammatical morphemes, such as the affix -*s*. These morphemes pose problems for the child with SLI because they are non-stressed, unsalient morphemes and are difficult to perceive. Leonard's account assumes that this presents a challenge to the limited processing capacity of the child with SLI. As a result, Leonard predicts that children with SLI will have more difficulty with unstressed morphological markers, such as plurals and verb agreement markings, than their language-matched peers (Leonard, 1994; Leonard, Eyer, Bedore, & Grela, 1997; Rice, 1994).

Linguistic Deficit Accounts. Linguistic deficit accounts of SLI postulate an inherited deficit in one or more of the underlying linguistic mechanisms that support normal language acquisition (e.g., in "universal grammar"). Each of the various linguistic deficit models that has been proposed (Clahsen, 1989, 1991; Gopnik, 1990; Gopnik & Crago, 1991; Rice, 1994; Rice et al., 1995; Rice & Oetting, 1993; Rice & Wexler, 1996) hypothesizes that SLI is attributable to missing or aberrant elements of universal grammar in the child's linguistic endowment that will interfere with the acquisition of morphological features such as those for number, tense, gender, animacy, or aspect. For instance, Ullman and Gopnik (1994) argued that children with SLI may have a specific genetic predisposition that results in "feature blindness," namely, an inability to form automatic, implicit grammatic rules for number, person, and tense marking.

A major linguistic account formulated in recent years by Rice and her colleagues is that children with SLI have an extended period in which they manifest the "optional infinitive" (Rice et al., 1995; Rice & Wexler, 1996). That is, they inconsistently apply tense and person markers on verbs such as -ed, -s, be, and do; however, when they do supply them, they do so correctly.

It is important to underscore the fact that linguistic deficit accounts and perceptual deficit accounts explain the difficulty of children with SLI with morphemes such as third-person regular -s in fundamentally different ways. In perceptual deficit accounts, the underlying language mechanism is assumed to be intact and the problem lies in a limited processing capacity, whereas in linguistic deficit models, the problem is more fundamental because the source of the impairment is in the underlying biological mechanism that is responsible for grammatical competence.

Normal Distribution Account.   Both the perceptual deficit and linguistic deficit accounts suggest that SLI is due to a specific deficit. However, the great heterogeneity among youngsters with SLI suggests that no single deficit will account entirely for this disorder. For example, how can the perceptual deficit account explain the existence of pure expressive type SLI, where the child has normal receptive language skill and therefore apparently perceives low-stress morphophonemic items without difficulty yet fails to produce them consistently? In addition, neither the perceptual deficit nor the linguistic deficit accounts can fully explain why the accuracy of performance of children with SLI on various grammatical morphemes is often as high as 80 percent. If these accounts were correct, one would assume the target feature to be absent from the children most, or all, of the time.

More important, it is unclear how either the perceptual deficit or linguistic deficit models can account for the language history shown by many children with SLI. Although research now indicates that only a small fraction of late talkers go on to be diagnosable with SLI by age 5, this fraction does show a continuous pattern of language impairment. This pattern starts off with slow vocabulary development before age 2; is characterized by small vocabularies, limited phonological repertoires, and delayed word combinations between ages 24 and 30 months; and then is marked by delayed and protracted development in both syntax and morphology between ages 2 and 5. Neither a perceptual deficit account nor a linguistic deficit account explains why many children with SLI first show language problems at ages 24 to 30 months, which is before much grammatical development has occurred in most normal children.

Considerations such as these suggest that a multidimensional account of SLI is needed. Perhaps the clearest existing account along these lines is one put forth by Leonard (1987, 1991), based on Gardner's (1983) theory of multiple intelligences, which we refer to here as the "normal distribution" account. This account suggests that children with SLI are not necessarily impaired but are simply less skilled in their language abilities than others, just as some individuals are less skilled than others in music, spatial, or athletic ability. Children with specific language impairment may simply represent the low end of the normal distribution of language ability. This limited language ability results in both slower development and poorer asymptotic performance.

Elaborating on the normal distribution account, one might argue that language ability can be conceptualized as an aggregate ability based on many subskills, each of which also varies in its distribution across individuals (e.g., auditory perception and discrimination, phonological memory, associative ability, word retrieval skill, inferencing ability). Presumably, these various subskills are subserved by diverse brain mechanisms. Therefore, the suboptimal functioning of these constituent skills supporting language is ultimately rooted in the neurological functioning of children with SLI.

This kind of normal distribution account seems well equipped to handle the diversity found in children with SLI. Because language is a complex skill supported by many different abilities, a child might perform at the low end of the average range in language for various reasons; similarly, this suboptimal language functioning might be demonstrated on some tasks and not on others. In addition, this account is perhaps best able to explain the probabilistic nature of language performance by children with SLI. Because their language system is less efficient, they do not perform as consistently as typically developing children on a variety of language tasks. Therefore, they make more errors, omit more obligatory morphemes, fail to retrieve lexical items when under pressure, need additional time for verbal formulation, and require more learning trials to acquire new lexical entries.

OUTCOME

Most late-talking toddlers seem to outgrow their language problems, with only 10 to 15 percent displaying significant deficits in expressive language by second grade (Paul, Hernandez, Taylor, & Johnson, 1996). However, late talkers seem to be quite variable in the rapidity with which their language problems resolve. For example, in Paul's longitudinal study, the percentage of late talkers falling below the 10th percentile on Developmental Sentence Score (Lee, 1974) was 60 percent at age 3, 47 percent at age 4, 37 percent in kindergarten, 27 percent in first grade, and 14 percent in second grade (Paul, 1993; Paul et al., 1996).

A similar pattern was found in Rescorla's sample of late talkers, in which 53 percent scored more than 1.50 SDs below age expectations in MLU at age 3, and 32 percent scored this poorly by age 4 (Rescorla & Dahlsgaard, 1995; Rescorla et al., 1997). Rescorla's group of late talkers did not score in the average range on tests of syntactic competence until age 5 (Rescorla, 1993). They continued to obtain lower scores on almost all language measures through age 8 as compared to children with whom they had been matched as toddlers in SES and nonverbal ability, despite the fact that their scores were generally in the average range (Rescorla, 1993).

A few studies have also reported academic outcomes of late talkers. For example, Paul and colleagues (Paul et al., 1997) summarized school achievement scores of two subgroups of late talkers, those whose Developmental Sentence Score (Lee, 1974) was above the 10th percentile (84 percent), and the remaining 16 percent who still had poor expressive language skills. The subgroups did not differ from each other—nor did they differ from comparison children with no history of language problems—in reading decoding, reading comprehension, or spelling, with mean scores of the late talkers in the average range. Converging results were reported by Whitehurst and Fischel (1994), who found that the 22 late talkers whom they followed up at age 7 did not differ in standardized tests of reading from age-based normative patterns. In Rescorla's sample of late talkers, there were also no differences in reading performance through age 7, but by age 8 the late talkers had significantly lower reading scores than the comparison group children, despite the fact that they scored in the average range (Rescorla & Dahlsgaard, 1995).

Preschool children with SLI manifest variable outcomes in terms of their later language skills. For example, 44 percent of 4-year-olds with SLI attained a "good outcome" by age 5½ in Bishop and Edmundson's (1987) sample (as opposed to 11 percent with a "good outcome" in children with language impairments with concomitant below-average nonverbal skills). Thus, although some preschool children with SLI continue to manifest significant language problems, many function in the average range by age 5 (Bishop & Adams, 1990; Bishop & Edmundson, 1986; Whitehurst & Fischel, 1994). However, they quite commonly remain less skilled in language functioning than in other areas of development (Whitehurst & Fischel, 1994).

A number of prospective studies have looked at academic outcomes of preschool children with SLI. Whereas children with pure articulation disorder generally have a good reading outcome (Bishop & Adams, 1990; Catts, Hu, Larrivee, & Swank, 1994), children whose preschool language is marked by semantic and syntactic delay are at high risk for showing reading problems in the primary grades (Bishop & Adams, 1990; Catts et al., 1994; Menyuk et al., 1991; Tallal, 1988). Language outcome by age 5 appears to be one of the best predictors of later academic outcomes, with children who have caught up in language by age 5 showing normal reading outcomes (Bishop & Adams, 1990). In a study by Catts and his colleagues (Catts et al., 1994), 50 percent of kindergartners with semantic-syntactic SLI had reading problems at the end of first or second grade. Children with SLI often manifest a deficit in phonological awareness, namely, a problem in detecting and operating on the phonemes in words. This phonological awareness deficit is often the best predictor of later reading difficulty (Catts et al., 1994; Magnusson & Naucler, 1990; Menyuk et al., 1991). Children with a history of SLI often continue to require special services in school well into adolescence, and they show below-average skills in many areas even as adults, with deficits being especially apparent in language, reading, spelling, and writing (Aram, Ekelman, & Nation, 1984; Hall & Tomblin, 1978; Tomblin, Freese, & Records, 1992).

SLI also has negative implications for social and behavioral outcomes, as was summarized in a review by Fujiki and Brinton (1994). For example, many children with SLI have significant deficits in social skills and consequently are often viewed negatively by peers, parents, and teachers. Furthermore, children with SLI manifest higher rates of psychiatric disorders as they get older, particularly conduct disorders and AD/HD (Baker & Cantwell, 1982).

CASE STUDIES: JOSH, TOMMY, LARRY

The wide variability in outcome of late talkers, even when only expressive language is delayed, can be illustrated by case studies of three boys drawn from Rescorla's (1993) longitudinal sample of children identified between 24 and 31 months of age. The three boys were very comparable at intake, but their expressive language delay improved at very different rates. Furthermore, improvement varied widely across the different domains of language, highlighting the importance of detailed and specific language assessment. By age 6, two of the three boys had essentially average language skills. They were all normal readers at age 8, although one had deficits in written language.

Josh, a second child, was identified as a late talker at 25 months. His mother (a psychologist), his father (an economist), and his older brother all had normal language histories. Josh had a history of chronic otitis media and received ear tubes at 20 months of age. At intake, Josh had a reported vocabulary of ten words on the LDS (Rescorla, 1989); he scored at the 15-month level on expressive language on the Reynell Developmental Language Scales (Reynell, 1977), but at the 26-month age level in receptive language. Josh received no speech-language therapy. At age 3, he had an MLU of only 2.91, and his IPSyn (Scarborough, 1990) score was 1.5 SDs below age expectations. However, by age 4, Josh's MLU had increased to 4.25 and his MLU was within one-half SD of normal. His score on the Patterned Elicitation Syntax Test (PEST) (Young & Perachio, 1983) at age 4 was at the 5th percentile, but it had risen to the 56th percentile by age 5. He scored above average (116) on the Stanford-Binet Intelligence Scale: Fourth Edition (Thorndike et al., 1986) verbal factor, but below age expectations in nonverbal skills (86). Josh's TOLD-P:2 (Newcomer & Hamill, 1991) scores at age 6 ranged from a 6 (9th percentile) on Oral Vocabulary to a 13 (84th percentile) on Grammatic Completion and Grammatic Understanding. At age 7, he scored a 4 (2nd percentile) on the CELF-R (Semel, Wiig, & Secord, 1987) Formulated Sentences subtest and a 6 (9th percentile) on Word and Sentence Structure. By age 8, his CELF-R scores ranged from a 7 (16th percentile) to a 14 (91st percentile), with the poorest performance on Formulated Sentences and Sentence Assembly. Josh's reading on the Woodcock-Johnson Psychoeducational Battery Tests of Achievement (Woodcock & Johnson, 1989) ranged from a 98 (45th percentile) on Word Attack to a 123 (94th percentile) on Passage Comprehension.

Tommy, also a second child, was 24 months at intake, with an LDS (Rescorla, 1989) reported vocabulary of five words. His mother (a nurse) and his older sister had no history of language problems, but his father (a draftsman) has a severe sensorineural hearing loss and consequent weak language skills and poor articulation. Tommy's maternal uncle had a history of language delay. Tommy scored at the 15-month age level in expressive language, but at the 23 month level in receptive language on the Reynell Developmental Language Scales (Reynell, 1977). His expressive language delay was still marked at age 3, despite therapy initiated at 30 months. At age 3, his MLU was 1.22 and his IPSyn (Scarborough, 1990) was more than 4 SDs below average. At age 4, Tommy was still quite language-delayed, with an MLU of 3.17 and an IPSyn score 4 SDs below average. He scored at the 5th percentile on the PEST (Young & Perachio, 1983) at both age 4 and 5, but his Stanford-Binet Intelligence Scale: Fourth Edition (Thorndike et al., 1986) verbal and nonverbal scores were average at age 5. By age 6, Tommy's scores on the TOLD-P:2 (Newcomer & Hamill, 1991) ranged from 7 (16th percentile) to 15 (95th percentile). On the CELF-R (Semel et al., 1987), administered at age 7, Tommy scored a 14 (91st percentile) and a 15 (95th percentile) on Sentence and Word Structure but only a 5 (5th percentile) on Formulated Sentences. By age 8, his CELF-R scores ranged from a 4 (2nd percentile) on Formulated Sentences to a 10 (50th percentile) on Word Associations, with six of his seven scores below 10. However, Tommy was an outstanding reader at age 8, with his Woodcock-Johnson Psychoeducational Battery Tests of Achievement (Woodcock & Johnson, 1989) scores ranging from 113 (81st percentile) on Word Attack to 135 (99th percentile) on Passage Comprehension.

Larry, a third child, was 30 months old at the time of intake. His mother and father, both physicians, reported no history of language delay in the family. When first diagnosed as a late talker, Larry had a reported vocabulary on the LDS (Rescorla, 1989) of about 30 words and was producing a few word combinations. His expressive language was at the 18-month level according to the Reynell Developmental Language Scales (Reynell, 1977), but his receptive language score on the Reynell scale was at the 33-month age level. Larry's expressive language was still very delayed at age 3, with his MLU more than 3 SDs below age level and his IPSyn (Scarborough, 1990) score more than 5 SDs below age expectations. He still used very few word combinations and was performing at the 23-month level on the Reynell. At age 4, Larry was still almost 3 SDs below age level in MLU and 8 SDs below age expectations on the IPSyn, and his intelligibility was poor. On the Patterned Elicitation Syntax Test (PEST), (Young & Perachio, 1983), given at age 5, Larry scored at the 5th percentile. Despite his severe expressive language delay, also at age 5, Larry had a Verbal Reasoning score of 105 and an Abstract/Visual Reasoning score of 95 on the Stanford-Binet Intelligence Scale: Fourth Edition (Thorndike et al., 1986). Larry's TOLD-P:2 (Newcomer & Hamill, 1988) scores at age 6 ranged from 0 on Sentence Imitation to 12 (75th percentile) on Picture Vocabulary, with scores of 8 (25th percentile) on Oral Vocabulary and Grammatic Understanding and 9 (37th percentile) on Grammatic Completion. By age 7, just before he entered first grade, Larry was still omitting auxiliary, third-person, and future-tense forms in his spontaneous speech. At age

8, Larry's CELF-R (Semel, Wiig, & Secord, 1987) scores ranged from 3 (1st percentile) in Formulated Sentences to 9 (37th percentile) on Linguistic Concepts, with six of his seven subtest scores at 8 (25th percentile) or below. However, he scored in the average range or above on the Letter-Word Identification, Word Attack, and Passage Comprehension subtests of the Woodcock-Johnson Psychoeducational Battery Tests of Achievement (Woodcock & Johnson, 1989), (with scores of 99 to 116, which ranged from the 47th to 86th percentiles). Larry had many years of private speech therapy, attended special preschool and kindergarten programs for children with language impairments, and by second grade was gradually spending more and more time in mainstream classes. Larry continued to receive speech and language services into middle school, as well as special education support for written language. It was clear by the time Larry was about 6 years old that he had the most severe and enduring language disorder of all the late talkers in the sample.

SUMMARY

Specific language impairment (SLI) is diagnosed when a child demonstrates a substantial delay in language in the presence of normal nonverbal ability and no other significant condition is presumed to be primary (e.g., hearing loss, neurological disorder, mental retardation, or pervasive developmental disorder). When a child under the age of 4 presents with this condition, it has become customary to label the youngster as a late talker, in recognition of the data emerging over the last decade showing that most of these children do not seem to have significant language problems by age 5. The term *SLI* is thus recommended for use only for a child aged 4 or older. The two most commonly accepted types of SLI are a pure expressive type (estimated prevalence of 3 percent to 5 percent) and a mixed receptive-expressive type (estimated prevalence of 3 percent).

Late talkers are characterized by slow vocabulary acquisition between ages 1 and 3, limited phonetic repertoires and reduced vocalization before age 3, poor articulation until about age 4, and syntactical and morphological delays until ages 4 or 5. Late talkers appear to be delayed rather than deviant in their language development, and they typically do not differ from typically developing agemates in many aspects of social interaction and communicative intent, at least in the case of children whose receptive language skills are normal. In the primary grades, late talkers appear to function in the average range on most language and academic tests, although in some studies they have been found to score less well than agemates from similar backgrounds and with normal language histories on a variety of linguistic, prereading, and reading measures.

Preschool children with SLI have a variable outcome, with those who continue to manifest language problems after age 5 typically manifesting significant learning problems as well as social and behavioral difficulties throughout their school careers. School-age children with diagnoses of learning disabilities and/or attention deficit/hyperactivity disorder quite commonly have a history of SLI, and for many such children, language deficits continue to be present in higher-level skills.

It is not yet well understood whether late talkers and preschool children with SLI are manifesting the same basic condition at different levels of severity, or if these two groups are quite distinct. Studies of both groups suggest that the later the age of identification or the more persistent the delay, the more severe the underlying condition can be presumed to be and, therefore, the less optimistic the outcome to be expected.

Although the etiology of SLI is unknown, familial prevalence data and twin studies suggest a genetic predisposition. Whether the fundamental cause of SLI is a specific grammatical deficit, a temporal-processing problem, or nonspecific and varied weaknesses in many skills subserving language is unclear at this time. There is also little consensus as to whether the same etiological explanation will apply to both late-talking toddlers and preschool children with SLI. Systematically differentiating between these two conditions and determining how they are related is an important goal for future research. Specifically, it now seems clear that only a small minority of late-talking toddlers turn out at age 5 to have SLI; however, we still know relatively little about how to identify this at-risk subgroup. Furthermore, we do not know at this time the percentage of 5-year-olds with SLI who were late talkers at ages 2 to 4, nor is it clear how those children might differ in their language and academic skills, their family history, and their prognosis from 5-year-olds with SLI who developed typically in language until age 4 or 5.

References

Achenbach, T. M. (1991). *Manual for The Child Behavior Checklist/4-18 and 1991 Profile.* Burlington: University of Vermont, Department of Psychiatry.

American Psychiatric Association (1994). *Diagnostic and statistical manual of mental disorders* (4th ed.). Washington, D.C.: Author.

Aram, D. M., Ekelman, B., & Nation, J. (1984). Preschoolers with language disorders: 10 years later. *Journal of Speech and Hearing Research, 27,* 232–244.

Aram, D. M., Morris, R., & Hall, N. E. (1993). Clinical and research congruence in identifying children with specific language impairment. *Journal of Speech and Hearing Research, 36,* 580–591.

Bagnato, S. J., & Neisworth, J. T. (1994). A national study of the social and treatment "invalidity" of intelligence testing for early intervention. *School Psychology Quarterly, 9,* 81–102.

Baker, L., & Cantwell, D. (1982). Psychiatric disorders in children with different types of communication disorders. *Journal of Communication Disorders, 15,* 113–126.

Bayley, N. (1993). *The Bayley II Scales of Infant Development–II.* San Antonio: Psychological Corporation.

Beitchman, J. H., Hood, J., & Inglis, A. (1990). Psychiatric risk in children with speech and language disorders. *Journal of Abnormal Child Psychiatry, 18*(3), 283–296.

Beitchman, J. H., Hood, J., Rochon, J., & Peterson, M. (1989). Empirical classification of speech and language impairment in children: II. Behavioral characteristics. *Journal of the American Academy of Child and Adolescent Psychiatry, 28*(1), 118–123.

Beitchman, J. H., Hood, J., Rochon, J., Peterson, M., Mantini, T., & Majumdar, S. (1989). Empirical classification of speech/language impairment in children: I: Identification of speech/language categories. *Journal of the American Academy of Child and Adolescent Psychiatry, 28,* 112–117.

Beitchman, J. H., Nair, R., Clegg, M., Ferguson, B., & Patel, P. (1986). Prevalence of psychiatric disorders in children with speech and language disorders. *Journal of the American Academy of Child Psychiatry, 25,* 538–535.

Benton, A. L. (1964). Developmental aphasia and brain damage. *Cortex, 1,* 40–52.

Berg, E. A. (1948) A simple objective technique for measuring flexibility in thinking. *Journal of General Psychology, 39,* 15–22.

Bishop, D. V. M. (1992). The biological basis of specific language impairment. In P. Fletcher & D. Hall (Eds.), *Speech and language disorders in children* (pp. 2–17). London: Whurr.

Bishop, D. V. M., & Adams, C. (1990). A prospective study of the relationship between specific language impairment, phonological disorders, and reading retardation. *Journal of Child Psychology and Psychiatry, 31,* 1027–1050.

Bishop, D. V. M., & Edmundson, A. (1986). Is otitis media a major cause of specific developmental language disorders? *British Journal of Disorders of Communication, 21,* 321–388.

Bishop, D. V. M, & Edmundson, A. (1987). Specific language impairment as a maturational lag: Evidence from longitudinal data on language and motor development. *Developmental Medicine and Child Neurology, 29,* 442–459.

Bishop, D. V. M., North, T., & Donlan, C. (1995). Genetic basis of specific language impairment: Evidence from a twin study. *Developmental Medicine and Child Neurology, 37,* 56–71.

Bortolini, U., Caselli, M. C., & Leonard, L. B. (1997). Grammatical deficits in Italian-speaking children with specific language impairment. *Journal of Speech, Language, and Hearing Research, 40,* 809–820.

Bricker, D. (1993). *Assessment, Evaluation, and Programming System for Children: AEPS measurement for children birth to three years* (Vol. 1). Baltimore: Brookes.

Burgmeister, B., Blum, L., & Lorge, I. (1972). *Columbia Mental Maturity Scale* (3rd ed.). New York: Psychological Corporation.

Cantwell, D., & Baker, L. (1987). *Developmental speech and language disorders.* New York: Guilford.

Casby, M. W. (1997). Symbolic play of children with language impairment. *Journal of Speech, Language, and Hearing Research, 40,* 468–479.

Catts, H. C., Hu, C., Larrivee, L., & Swank, L. (1994). Early identification of reading disabilities in children with speech-language impairment. In R. V. Watkins & M. L. Rice (Eds.), *Specific language impairments in children: Current directions in research and intervention* (pp. 145–160). Baltimore: Brookes.

Chapman, R. S. (1981). Mother-child interaction in the second year of life. In R. L. Schiefelbusch and D. D. Bricker (Eds.), *Early language: Acquisition and intervention* (pp. 201–250). Baltimore: University Park Press.

Clahsen, H. (1989). The grammatical characterization of developmental dysphasia. *Linguistics, 27,* 897–920.

Clahsen, H. (1991). *Child language and developmental dysphasia: Linguistic studies of the acquisition of German.* Philadelphia: Benjamins.

Cleave, P. L., & Rice, M. L. (1997). An examination of the morpheme BE in children with specific language impairment: The role of contractibility and grammatical form class. *Journal of Speech and Hearing Research, 40,* 480–492.

Connell, P. J., & Stone, C. A. (1992). Morpheme learning of children with specific language impairment under controlled conditions. *Journal of Speech and Learning Research, 25,* 844–852.

Connell, P. J., & Stone, C. A. (1994). The conceptual basis for morpheme learning problems in children with specific language impairment. *Journal of Speech and Hearing Research, 37,* 389–398.

Conti-Ramsden, G., & Friel-Patti, S. (1983). Mothers' discourse adjustments to language-impaired and non–language-impaired children. *Journal of Speech and Hearing Disorders, 48,* 360–367.

Crago, M., & Gopnik, M. (1994). From families to phenotypes: Theoretical and clinical implications of research into the genetic basis of specific language impairment. In R. V. Watkins & M. L. Rice (Eds.), *Specific language impairments in children: Current directions in research and intervention* (pp. 35–51). Baltimore: Brookes.

Cunningham, C. E., Siegel, L. S., van der Spuy, H. I. J., Clark, M. L., & Bow, S. J. (1985). The behavioral and linguistic interactions of specifically language-delayed and normal boys with their mothers. *Child Development, 56,* 1389–1403.

Curtiss, S., Katz, W., & Tallal, P. (1992). Delay versus deviance in the language acquisition of language-impaired children. *Journal of Speech and Hearing Research, 35,* 373–383.

Dollaghan, C. (1987). Fast mapping in normal and language-impaired children. *Journal of Speech and Hearing Disorders 52,* 218–222.

Dromi, E., Leonard, L., & Shteiman, M. (1993). The grammatical morphology of Hebrew-speaking children with specific language impairment: Some competing hypotheses. *Journal of Speech and Hearing Research, 36,* 760–771.

Dunn, L. M., & Dunn, L. M. (1997). *Peabody Picture Vocabulary Test–Third Edition.* Circle Pines, Minn.: American Guidance Service.

Ellis Weismer, S. (1991). Hypothesis-testing abilities of language-impaired children. *Journal of Speech and Hearing Research, 34,* 1329–1338.

Ellis Weismer, S., & Hesketh, L. J. (1996). Lexical learning by children with specific language impairment: Effects of linguistic input presented at varying speaking rates. *Journal of Speech and Hearing Research, 39,* 177–190.

Ellis Weismer, S., Murray-Branch, J., & Miller, J. (1994). A prospective longitudinal study of language development in late talkers. *Journal of Speech and Hearing Research, 37,* 852–867.

Fenson, L., Dale, P. S., Reznick, J. S., Thal, D., Bates, E., Hartung, J., Pethick, S., & Reilly, J. S. (1993). *Guide and technical manual for the MacArthur Communicative Development Inventories.* San Diego: Singular Press.

Fey, M., & Leonard, L. (1984). Partner age as a variable in the conversational performance of specifically-language impaired and normal children. *Journal of Speech and Hearing Research, 27,* 413–423.

Fischel, J., Whitehurst, G., Caulfield, M., & DeBarysche, B. (1989). Language growth in children with expressive language delay. *Pediatrics, 82,* 218–227.

Fujiki, M., & Brinton, B. (1994). Social competence and language impairment in children. In R. V. Watkins & M. L. Rice (Eds.), *Specific language impairments in children: Current directions in research and intervention* (pp. 123–143). Baltimore: Brookes.

Fundudis, T., Kolvin, I., & Garside, R. F. (1980). A follow-up of speech retarded children. In L. A. Hersov, M. Berger, & A. R. Nichols (Eds.), *Language and language disorders in children* (pp. 97–113). New York: Pergamon.

Gardner, H. (1983). *Frames of mind.* New York: Basic Books.

Gardner, M. F. (1979). *Expressive One–Word Picture Vocabulary Test.* Novato, Calif.: Academic Therapy.

Gardner, M. F. (1990). Expressive One-Word Picture Vocabulary Test–Revised. Novato, Calif.: Academic Therapy.

Gathercole, S., & Baddeley, A. D. (1990). Phonological memory deficits in language disordered children: Is there a causal connection? *Journal of Memory and Language, 29,* 336–360.

Gopnik, M. (1990). Feature blindness: A case study. *Language Acquisition, 1,* 139–164.

Gopnik, M., & Crago, M. B. (1991). Familial aggregation of developmental language disorder. *Cognition, 39,* 1–50.

Hall, K., & Tomblin, J. B. (1978). A follow-up study of children with articulation and language disorders. *Journal of Speech and Hearing Disorders, 43,* 227–241.

Hedrick, D. L., Prather, E. M., & Tobin, A. R. (1984). *Sequenced Inventory of Communicative Development–Revised.* Seattle: University of Washington Press.

Johnston, J. (1988). Specific language disorders in the child. In N. Lass, J. Northern, L. McReynolds, & D. E. Yoder (Eds.), *Handbook of speech-language pathology and audiology* (pp. 685–715). Philadelphia: B.C. Decker.

Johnston, J. R. (1994). Cognitive abilities in children with language impairment. In R. V. Watkins and M. L. Rice (Eds.), *Specific language impairments in children* (pp. 107–121). Baltimore: Brookes.

Johnston, J. R., & Ellis Weismer, S. (1983). Mental rotation abilities in language-disordered children. *Journal of Speech and Hearing Research, 26,* 397–403.

Johnston, J. R., & Kamhi, A. G. (1984). Syntactic and semantic aspects of the utterances of language-impaired children: The same can be less. *Merrill-Palmer Quarterly, 30,* 65–85.

Johnston, R. B., Stark, R. E., Mellits, E. D., & Tallal, P. (1981). Neurological status of language-impaired and normal children. *Annals of Neurology, 10,* 159–163.

Kail, R. (1994). A method for studying the generalized slowing hypothesis in children with specific language impairment. *Journal of Speech and Hearing Research, 37,* 418–421.

Kail, R., & Leonard, L. B. (1986). *Word-finding abilities in children with specific language impairment. Monographs of the American Speech-Language-Hearing Association,* No. 25. Rockville, Md.: American Speech-Language-Hearing Association.

Kamhi, A. (1981). Nonlinguistic symbolic and conceptual abilities of language-impaired and normally developing children. *Journal of Speech and Hearing Research, 24,* 446–453.

Kamhi, A. (1998). Trying to make sense of developmental language disorders. *Language, Speech, and Hearing Services in Schools, 29,* 35–44.

Kamhi, A. G., Catts, H. W., Koenig, L. A., & Lewis, B. A. (1984). Hypothesis-testing and nonlinguistic symbolic abilities in language-impaired children. *Journal of Speech and Hearing Disorders, 49,* 169–176.

Kamhi, A. G., Nelson, L. K., Lee, R. F., & Gholson, B. (1985). The ability of language-disordered children to use and modify hypotheses in discrimination learning. *Applied Psycholinguistics, 6,* 435–452.

Kaufman, A. S., & Kaufman, N. L. (1983). *The Kaufman Assessment Battery for Children (K–ABC).* Circle Pines, Minn.: American Guidance Service.

Kiernan, B., & Gray, S. (1998). Word learning in a supported-learning context by preschool children with specific language impairment. *Journal of Speech, Language, and Hearing Research, 41,* 161–171.

Kiernan, B., Snow, D., Swisher, L., & Vance, R. (1997). Another look at nonverbal rule induction in children with SLI: Testing a flexible reconceptualization hypothesis. *Journal of Speech, Language, and Hearing Research, 40,* 75–82.

Kushnir, C. C., & Blake, J. (1996). The nature of the cognitive deficit in specific language impairment. *First Language, 16,* 21–40.

Lahey, M. (1988). *Language disorders and language development.* New York: Macmillan.

Lahey, M., & Edwards, J. (1995). Specific language impairment: Preliminary investigation of factors associated with familial history and with patterns of language performance. *Journal of Speech and Hearing Research, 38,* 643–657.

Lasky, E., & Klopp, K. (1982). Parent-child interactions in normal and language-disordered children. *Journal of Speech and Hearing Disorders, 47,* 7–18.

Lee, L. (1974). *Developmental Sentence Analysis.* Evanston, Ill.: Northwestern University Press.

Leonard, L., Bortolini, U., Caselli, M. C., McGregor, K. K., & Sabbadini, L. (1992). Morphological deficits in children with specific language impairment: The status of features in the underlying grammar. *Language Acquisition, 2,* 151–179.

Leonard, L., Camarata, S., Rowan, L. E., & Chapman, K. (1982). The communicative functions of lexical usage by language impaired children. *Applied Psycholinguistics, 3,* 109–125.

Leonard, L., Sabbadini, L., Volterra, V., & Leonard, J. S. (1988). Some influences on the grammar of English- and Italian-speaking children with specific language impairment. *Applied Psycholinguistics, 9,* 39–57.

Leonard, L., Schwartz, R. G., Chapman, K., Rowan, L. E., Prelock, P. A., Terrell, B., Weiss, A. L., & Messick, C. (1982). Early lexical acquisition in children with specific language impairment. *Journal of Speech and Hearing Research, 23,* 554–564.

Leonard, L. B. (1987). Is specific language impairment a useful construct? In S. Rosenberg (Ed.), *Advances in applied psycholinguistics: Volume 1. Disorders of first-language development* (pp. 1–39). New York: Cambridge University Press.

Leonard, L. B. (1989). Language learnability and specific language impairment in children. *Applied Psycholinguistics, 10,* 179–202.

Leonard, L. B. (1991). Specific language impairment as a clinical category. *Language, Speech, and Hearing Services in Schools, 22,* 66–68.

Leonard, L. B. (1994). Some problems facing accounts of morphological deficits in children with specific language impairments. In R. V. Watkins & M. L. Rice (Eds.), *Specific language impairments in children: Current directions in research and intervention* (pp. 91–105). Baltimore: Brookes.

Leonard, L. B., Eyer, J. A., Bedore, L. M., & Grela, B. G. (1997). Three accounts of grammatical morpheme difficulties of English-speaking children with specific language impairment. *Journal of Speech and Hearing Research, 40,* 741–753.

Lowe, M., & Costello, A. J. (1976). *The Symbolic Play Test.* Windsor, U.K.: NFER-Nelson Publishing.

Magnusson, E., & Naucler, K. (1990). Reading and spelling in language-disordered children—linguistic and metalinguistic prerequisites: Report on a longitudinal study. *Clinical Linguistics and Phonetics, 4,* 49–61.

McCarthy, D. (1972). *The McCarthy Scales of Children's Abilities.* New York: Psychological Corporation.

Menyuk, P., Chesnick, M., Liebergott, J., Korngold, B., D'Agostino, R., & Belanger, A. (1991). Predicting reading problems in at-risk children. *Journal of Speech and Hearing Research, 34,* 893–903.

Mirak, J., & Rescorla, L. (1998). Phonetic skills and vocabulary in toddlers with specific expressive language impairment (SLI-E): Concurrent and predictive relationships. *Applied Psycholinguistics.*

Mosely, M. J. (1990). Mother-child interaction with preschool language-delayed children: Structuring conversations. *Journal of Communication Disorders, 23,* 187–203.

Nelson, L., Kamhi, A., & Apel, K. (1987). Cognitive strengths and weaknesses in language impaired children: One more look. *Journal of Speech and Hearing Disorders, 52,* 36–43.

Newborg, J., Stock, J., Wnek, L., Guidubaldi, J., & Svinicki, J. (1984). *The Batelle Developmental Inventory.* Allen, Tex.: DLM/Teaching Resources.

Newcomer, P. L., & Hammill, D. (1991). *Test of Language Development–Primary: 2.* Austin, Tex.: Pro-Ed.

Newcomer, P. L. & Hammill, D. (1997). *Test of Language Development–Primary: 3.* Austin, Tex.: Pro-Ed.

Paul, R. (1991). Profiles of toddlers with slow expressive language development. *Topics in Language Disorders, 11*(4), 1–13.

Paul, R. (1993). Patterns of development in late talkers: Preschool years. *Journal of Communication Disorders, 15,* 7–14.

Paul, R. (1996). Clinical implications of the natural history of slow expressive language development. *American Journal of Speech-Language Pathology, 5,* 5–21.

Paul, R., Hernandez, R., Taylor, L., & Johnson, K. (1996). Narrative development in late talkers: Early school age. *Journal of Speech and Hearing Research, 39,* 1295–1303.

Paul, R., & Jennings, P. (1992). Phonological behaviors in toddlers with slow expressive language development. *Journal of Speech and Hearing Research, 35,* 99–107.

Paul, R., Murray, C., Clancy, K., & Andrews, D. (1997). Reading and metaphonological outcomes in late talkers. *Journal of Speech, Language, and Hearing Research, 40,* 1037–1047.

Paul, R., & Shiffer, M. E. (1991). Communicative initiations in normal and late-talking toddlers. *Applied Psycholinguistics, 12,* 419–431.

Paul, R., & Shriberg, L. (1982). Associations between phonology and syntax in speech-delayed children. *Journal of Speech and Hearing Research, 25,* 536–547.

Rescorla, L. (1989). The Language Development Survey: A screening tool for delayed language in toddlers. *Journal of Speech and Hearing Disorders, 54,* 587–599.

Rescorla, L. (1993, March). *Outcome of toddlers with specific expressive language delay (SELD) at ages 3, 4, 5, 6, 7, and 8.* Paper presented at the biennial meeting of the Society for Research in Child Development, New Orleans.

Rescorla, L., & Dahlsgaard, K. (1995). *Language and reading outcomes at ages 5–8 for toddlers with specific language impairment.* Poster presented at the biennial meeting for the Society for Research in Child Development, Indianapolis.

Rescorla, L., & Fechnay, T. (1996). Mother-child synchrony and communicative reciprocity in late-talking toddlers. *Journal of Speech and Hearing Research, 39,* 200–208.

Rescorla, L., & Goossens, M. (1992). Symbolic play development in toddlers with expressive specific language impairment (SLI-E). *Journal of Speech and Hearing Research, 35,* 1290–1302.

Rescorla, L., & Merrin, L. (1998). Communicative intent in late talking toddlers. *Applied Psycholinguistics, 19* (3), 393–414.

Rescorla, L., & Ratner, N. B. (1996). Phonetic profiles of toddlers with specific expressive language impairment (SLI-E). *Journal of Speech and Hearing Research, 39,* 153–165.

Rescorla, L., Roberts, J., & Dahlsgaard, K. (1997). Late talkers at 2: Outcome at age 3. *Journal of Speech and Hearing Research, 40,* 556–566.

Rescorla, L., & Schwartz, E. (1990). Outcome of toddlers with expressive language delay. *Applied Psycholinguistics, 11,* 393–407.

Reynell, J. K. (1977). Reynell Developmental Language Scales, revised edition. Windsor, U.K.: NFER–Nelson.

Reynell, J. K., & Gruber, C. (1985). *The Reynell Developmental Language Scales.* Los Angeles: Western Publishing Company.

Rice, M. L. (1994). Grammatical categories of children with specific language impairment. In R. V. Watkins & M. L. Rice (Eds.), *Specific language impairments in children: Current directions in research and intervention* (pp. 69–89). Baltimore: Brookes.

Rice, M. L., Buhr, J. C., & Oetting, J. B. (1992). Speech-language-impaired children's quick incidental learning of words: The effect of a pause. *Journal of Speech and Hearing Research, 35*(5), 1040–1048.

Rice, M. L., Hadley, P. A., & Alexander, A. L. (1993). Social biases toward children with speech and language impairments: A correlative causal model of language limitations. *Applied Psycholinguistics, 14,* 445–471.

Rice, M. L. & Oetting, J. B. (1993). Morphological deficits of children with SLI: Evaluation of number marking and agreement. *Journal of Speech and Hearing Research, 36,* 1249–1257.

Rice, M. L., Sell, M. A., & Hadley, P. A. (1991). Social interactions of speech- and language-impaired children. *Journal of Speech and Hearing Research, 34,* 1299–1307.

Rice, M. L., & Wexler, K. (1996). Toward tense as a clinical marker of specific language impairment in English-speaking children. *Journal of Speech and Hearing Research, 39,* 1239–1257.

Rice, M. L., Wexler, K., & Cleave, P. (1995). Specific language impairment as a period of extended optional infinitive. *Journal of Speech and Hearing Research, 38,* 850–863.

Richman, N., Stevenson, J., & Graham, P. (1982). *Preschool to school: A behavioral study.* New York: Academic.

Roberts, J., Rescorla, L., Giroux, J., & Stevens, L. (1998). Phonological skills of children with specific expressive language impairment (SLI-E): Outcome at age 3. *Journal of Speech, Language, and Hearing Research, 41*(2), 374–384.

Roberts, S. S., & Leonard, L. B. (1997). Grammatical deficits in German and English: A crosslinguistic study of children with specific language impairment. *First Language, 17,* 131–150.

Roid, G. H. & Miller, L. J. (1997). *Leiter International Performance Scale–Revised.* Wood Dale, Ill.: Stoelting Co.

Rossetti, L. (1990). *Infant-Toddler Language Scale.* East Moline, Ill.: Linguisystems.

Scarborough, H. S. (1990). Index of Productive Syntax. *Applied Psycholinguistics, 11,* 1–12.

Schopler, E., Reichler, R. J., & Renner, B. R. (1988). *The Childhood Autism Rating Scale.* Los Angeles: Western Publishing Company.

Semel, E. M., Wiig, E. H., & Secord, W. (1987). *Clinical Evaluation of Language Fundamentals–Revised.* San Antonio: Psychological Corporation.

Shriberg, L. & Kwiatkowski, J. (1982). Phonological disorders III: A procedure for assessing severity of involvement. *Journal of Speech and Hearing Disorders, 47,* 256–270.

Shriberg, L. D. & Kwiatkowski, J. (1994). Developmental phonological disorders I: A clinical profile. *Journal of Speech and Hearing Research, 37,* 1100–1126.

Siegel, L. S., Cunningham, C. E., & van der Spuy, H. I. J. (1985). Interactions of language-delayed and normal preschool boys with their peers. *Journal of Child Psychology and Psychiatry, 26*(1), 77–83.

Silva, P. A. (1980). The prevalence, stability, and significance of developmental language delay in preschool children. *Developmental Medicine and Child Neurology, 22,* 768–777.

Silva, P. A., McGee, R., & Williams, S. M. (1983). Developmental language delay from three to seven and its significance for low intelligence and reading difficulties at seven. *Developmental Medicine and Child Neurology, 25,* 783–793.

Sininger, Y. S., Klatzky, R. L., & Kirchner, D. M. (1989). Memory-scanning speed in language-disordered children. *Journal of Speech and Hearing Research, 32,* 289–297.

Snow, C. E. (1984). Parent-child interaction and the development of communicative ability. In R. L. Schiefelbusch & J. Picker (Eds.), *The acquisition of communicative competence* (pp. 69–107). Baltimore: University Park Press.

Sparrow, S., Balla, D., & Cicchetti, D. (1984). *Vineland Adaptive Behavior Scales.* Minneapolis: American Guidance Service.

Spitz, R. V., Tallal, P., Flax, J., & Benasich, A. A. (1997). Look who's talking: A prospective study of familial transmission of language impairments. *Journal of Speech, Language, and Hearing Research, 40,* 990–1001.

Stevenson, J., & Richman, N. (1976). The prevalence of language delay in a population of three-year-old children and its association with general retardation. *Developmental Medicine and Child Neurology, 18,* 431–441.

Stoel-Gammon, C. (1989). Prespeech and early speech development in two late talkers. *First Language, 9,* 207–224.

Tallal, P. (1988). Developmental language disorders. In J. F. Kavanaugh & T. J. Truss, Jr. (Eds.), *Learning disabilities: Proceedings of the national conference* (pp. 181–272). Parkton, Md.: York Press,

Tallal, P., Dukette, K., & Curtiss, S. (1989). Behavioral/emotional profiles of preschool language-impaired children. *Development and Psychopathology, 1,* 51–67.

Tallal, P., & Piercy, M. (1973). Defects of non-verbal auditory perception in children with developmental aphasia. *Nature, 241,* 468–469.

Tallal, P., Ross, R., & Curtiss, S. (1989). Familial aggregation in specific language impairment. *Journal of Speech and Hearing Disorders, 54,* 167–173.

Tallal, P., Stark, R., Kallman, C., & Mellits, D. (1981). A re-examination of some non-verbal perceptual abilities of language-impaired and normal children as a function of age and sensory modality. *Journal of Speech and Hearing Research, 24,* 351–357.

Tallal, P., Stark, R., & Mellits, D. (1985). Identification of language-impaired children on the basis of rapid perception and production skills. *Brain and Language, 25,* 314–322.

Terrell, B., & Schwartz, R. (1988). Object transformations in the play of language-impaired children. *Journal of Speech and Hearing Disorders, 53,* 459–466.

Terrell, B. Y., Schwartz, R. G., Prelock, P. A., and Messick, C. J. (1984). Symbolic play in normal and disordered children. *Journal of Speech and Hearing Research, 27,* 424–429.

Thal, D., & Bates, E. (1988). Language and gesture in late talkers. *Journal of Speech and Hearing Research, 31,* 115–123.

Thal, D. & Tobias, S. (1992). Communicative gestures in children with delayed onset of oral expressive vocabulary. *Journal of Speech and Hearing Research, 35,* 1281–1289.

Thal, D., Tobias, S., & Morrison, D. (1991). Language and gesture in late talkers: A 1 year follow-up. *Journal of Speech and Hearing Research, 34,* 604–612.

Thorndike, R. L., Hagen, E. P., & Sattler, J. M. (1986). *Stanford-Binet Intelligence Scale–Fourth Edition.* Chicago: Riverside Publishing.

Tomblin, J. B. (1989). Familial concentration of developmental language impairment. *Journal of Speech and Hearing Research 54*(2), 287–295.

Tomblin, J. B., & Buckwalter, P. R. (1998). Heritability of poor language achievement among twins. *Journal of Speech and Hearing Research, 41,* 188–199.

Tomblin, J. B., Freese, P. R., & Records, N. L. (1992). Diagnosing specific language impairment in adults for the purpose of pedigree analysis. *Journal of Speech and Hearing Research 35,* 832–843.

Tomblin, J. B., Records, N. L., Buckwalter, P., Zhang, X., Smith, E., & O'Brien, M. (1997). Prevalence of specific language impairment in kindergarten children. *Journal of Speech, Language, and Hearing Research, 40,* 1245–60.

Tomblin, J. B., Records, N. L., & Zhang, X. (1996). A system for the diagnosis of specific language impairment in kindergarten children. *Journal of Speech and Hearing Research, 39,* 1284–1294.

Ullman, M., & Gopnik, M. (1994). Past tense production: Regular, irregular, and nonsense verbs. *McGill Working Papers in Linguistics, 10,* 81–118.

Watson, L. (1977). Conversational participation by language deficient and normal children. In J. Andrews & M. Burns (Eds.), *Selected papers in language and phonology* (Vol. 2, pp. 104–109). Evanston, Ill.: Institute for Continuing Education.

Wechsler, D. (1989). *The Wechsler Preschool and Primary Scale of Intelligence–Revised (WPPSI-R).* San Antonio: Psychological Corporation.

Wetherby, A., & Prizant, B. (1993). *Communication and Symbolic Behavior Scales.* Chicago: Riverside.

Whitehurst, G. J. & Fischel, J. E. (1994). Early developmental language delay: What, if anything, should the clinician do about it? *Journal of Child Psychology and Psychiatry, 35*(4), 613–648.

Whitehurst, G. J., Fischel, J. E., Arnold, D. S., & Lonigan, C. J. (1992). Evaluating outcomes with children with expressive language delay. In S. F. Warren & J. Reichle (Eds.), *Causes and effects in communication and language intervention* (Vol. 1, pp. 277–313). Baltimore: Brookes.

Whitehurst, G., Smith, M., Fischel. J., Arnold, D., & Lonigan, C. (1991). The continuity of babble and speech in children with specific expressive language delay. *Journal of Speech and Hearing Research, 34,* 1121–1129.

Wiig, E. H., Secord, W., & Semel, E. M. (1992). *The Clinical Evaluation of Language Fundamentals–Preschool.* San Antonio: Psychological Corporation.

Woodcock, R., & Johnson, M. B. (1989). *Woodcock-Johnson Psychoeducational Battery–Revised.* Chicago, Ill.: Riverside Publishing Company.

Wubert, M., Inglis, S., Kriegsmann, E., & Mills, B. (1975). Language delay and associated mother-child interaction. *Developmental Psychology, 11,* 61–70.

Young, E. C., & Perachio, J. J. (1983). *The Patterned Elicitation Syntax Test (PEST).* Tucson, Ariz.: Communication Skill Builders.

Zimmerman, I. L., Steiner, V., & Pond, R. E. (1991). *The Preschool Language Scale–3.* San Antonio: Psychological Corporation.

Emotional, Behavioral, and Other Psychiatric Disorders of Childhood Associated with Communication Disorders

Christiane A. M. Baltaxe, Ph.D.
Professor
University of California, Los Angeles

Key Terms

associated features
behavioral disorder
comorbidity
differential diagnosis
emotional disorder
essential features

interdisciplinary
mental disorder
multiaxial coding
psychiatric disorder
psychosocial stressors
transdisciplinary

Overview

Over the past decade communication specialists as well as mental health professionals have become increasingly sensitized to an unusually close association between communication disorders and psychiatric disorders. Earlier studies, case reports, and observations had suggested a curiously close relationship between communication disorders and psychiatric disorders (Affolder, Brubaker, & Bischofberger, 1974; Fundudis, Kolvin, & Garside, 1979; Solomon, 1961; Stevenson & Richman, 1976, 1978). More recently, several large-scale, well-controlled studies have shown that about half the children initially referred for speech and language services also have, or will develop, a diagnosable emotional, behavioral, or other psychiatric disorder (Baker & Cantwell, 1985, 1987a, 1987b; Beitchman, Hood, & Inglis, 1990; Beitchman, Hood, Rochon, & Peterson, 1989a, 1989b; Beitchman, Nair, Clegg, Ferguson, & Patel, 1986a, 1986b; Beitchman, Peterson, & Clegg, 1988; Cantwell & Baker, 1980, 1985, 1987a, 1987b, 1991b, 1992).

When emotional, behavioral, or other psychiatric problems are the primary reason for referral, very high rates of communication disorders are found to co-occur with these disorders (Baltaxe, in press; Baltaxe & Simmons, 1988a, 1991; Cohen, Davine, Horodesky, Lipsett, & Isaacson, 1993; Gualtieri, Koriath, Von Bourgondien, & Saleeby, 1983; Trautman, Giddan, & Jurs, 1990). Most studies have shown communication impairments in two-thirds or more of the children tested.

Communication impairments in children with psychiatric illness, as well as psychiatric disability in children with communication disorders, may often go unrecognized (Alessi, Eisner, & Knight, 1990; Cohen et al., 1993; Love & Thompson, 1988). For example, based on routine screening with standardized language measures, Cohen et al. (1993) identified unsuspected language impairment in 34 percent of a sample of almost 400 children with psychiatric illness. More subtle linguistic deficits were identified in a previously unidentified group. Associated psychiatric illness identified in this study centered primarily on attention deficit/hyperactivity disorder (AD/HD) and disruptive behavior disorders.

This association between communication disorders and psychiatric disorders is far greater than would be expected from estimates of prevalence for childhood speech and language disorders in the general population. These range from less than 1 percent to more than 33 percent for speech, and from 1 percent to 17 percent for language. (For reviews see Beitchman et al., 1986a, and Cantwell & Baker, 1977, 1991b.)

The results of all these studies indicate that children and adolescents with communication disorders are at serious risk for a psychiatric disorder. They also indicate that communication problems should be suspected when children or adolescents are referred for mental health services and diagnosed with psychiatric disorders in acute or outpatient mental health facilities. Similar, or even higher, expectations for communication disorders can be associated with classes for children with serious emotional disturbances (SED) in the public school system (Camarata, Hughes, & Ruhl, 1988).

Speech-language specialists must be alert to the risk factors for these disorders, their signs and symptoms, the diagnostic framework used in the mental health field to identify psychiatric disorders, and the types of communication disorders that can be expected in psychiatric illness. The current chapter is intended to provide such a background.

THE CURRENT DIAGNOSTIC FRAMEWORK FOR MENTAL DISORDERS

In common parlance, *emotional disorder, behavioral disturbance, mental illness*, **psychiatric disorder**, and *psychopathology* are all terms with fuzzy boundaries. Frequently, the terms are also used interchangeably. For example, *emotional disorder* may be used to refer to psychopathology in general, whereas *behavioral disturbance* tends not to be considered under mental illness at all. Differences in the meaning and use of *emotional disorder* and related terminology are seen in speech-language pathology, special education, and psychiatry. In special education the term **emotional disorder** is generally used to refer to a **behavioral disorder** (Wagner, 1995; Wagner, Newman, & Shaver, 1993). The more specific meaning of the term *seriously emotionally disturbed* (SED) is discussed by Wagner (1995; Wagner et al., 1993). It derives from the Education for All Handicapped Children Act (P.L. 94-142), enacted in 1975. This legislation required the schools to document an intrapsychic problem in order to provide special education services for a group of children who generally exhibit behavior disorders. Of interest is the fact that the emphasis on intrapsychic problems in this piece of legislation forced further changes in federal legislation, impacting the classification of autism. As a result, autism was removed from the category of "seriously emotionally disturbed" and placed into the legal category of "other health impairment." Autism has since become a separate category of disability.

The current legislation under which applicable definitions and procedures are mandated for public schools is the Individuals with Disabilities Education Act as amended in 1997 (IDEA97). In current regulations promulgated by the U.S. Department of Education to govern the implementation of IDEA97, the terminology has changed from "serious emotional disturbance" to "emotional disturbance" to avoid the perjorative connotation of the word "serious" (U.S. Department of Education, 1999, p. 12422). These regulations provide the following definition of emotional disturbance:

Emotional disturbance is defined as follows:

(i) The term means a condition exhibiting one or more of the following characteristics over a long period of time and to a marked degree that adversely affects a child's educational performance:

(A) An inability to learn that cannot be explained by intellectual, sensory, or health factors.

(B) An inability to build or maintain satisfactory interpersonal relationships with peers and teachers.

(C) Inappropriate types of behavior or feelings under normal circumstances.

(D) A general pervasive mood of unhappiness or depression.

(E) A tendency to develop physical symptoms or fears associated with personal or school problems.

(ii) The term includes schizophrenia. The term does not apply to children who are socially maladjusted, unless it is determined that they have an emotional disturbance. (U.S. Department of Education, 1999, p. 12422)

Under the current federal regulatory guidelines, children with behavior problems affecting their educational performance continue to be eligible for special educational services within the category of "emotionally disturbed." The specific terminology used can vary from state to state, however, depending on the respective rules and regulations for implementing IDEA97 within the state. Under the federal Americans with Disabilities Act, all these disorders, including emotional and behavioral disorders as well as autism, are considered developmental disabilities.

When emotional and behavioral disorders are discussed by members of the mental health professions, such as psychiatry, psychology, and social work, they denote two distinct groups of mental disorders. These are classified in the *Diagnostic and Statistical Manual of Mental Disorders, 4th edition (DSM-IV)*, (American Psychiatric Association [APA], 1994). Within that framework an "emotional disorder" denotes more than a developmental lag of emotion, affect, or feeling, and a "behavior disorder," more than just a problem in behavior. Specific diagnostic criteria must be met in order to qualify for any one of the specific diagnoses under these rubrics. Emotional disorders are sometimes also called internalizing disorders, because they cause pain or distress to the individual so diagnosed. Similarly, behavior disorders are also called externalizing disorders, because they cause pain, distress, or discomfort to others.

The Diagnostic Framework of the *DSM-IV*

The *DSM-IV* (APA, 1994) is the descriptive, multiaxial framework used in current mental health practice. The *DSM-IV* uses a **multiaxial coding** system whereby disorders are coded across several axes of conditions, along with identifiable psychosocial and environmental stressors and global functioning. According to the *DSM-IV*, **a mental disorder** is seen as the "manifestation of a behavioral, psychological, or biological dysfunction in the individual" (APA, 1994, pp. xxi, xxii). The *DSM-IV* further defines a mental disorder as "a clinically significant behavioral or psychological syndrome or pattern that occurs in an individual and that is associated with present distress (e.g., painful symptom) or disability (i.e., impairment in one or more important areas of functioning) or with a significantly increased risk of suffering death, pain, disability, or an important loss of freedom" (APA, 1994, p. xxi).

The *DSM-IV* identifies the **essential features** that must be present for the diagnosis of a specific mental disorder to be made. For example, a child with the diagnosis of "separation anxiety disorder" (an emotional disorder) or "conduct disorder" (a disruptive behavior disorder) must meet the *essential* characteristics for these diagnoses, as they are listed in the *DSM-IV*. Additional commonly **associated features**, also listed in *DSM-IV*, may also be present. When the clinical conditions of a specific mental disorder are met, the psychiatric diagnosis, together with other possible medical conditions as well as identifiable psychosocial and environmental stressors and a rating of global functioning, are coded on the five separate axes according to the *DSM-IV* multiaxial system. Information coded on all of these axes is then considered in the process of treatment and intervention. It is also not unusual that an individual meets the criteria for more than one mental illness. An example would be a child who meets the criteria for diagnosis of both autism and Tourette's syndrome.

In addition to behavioral disorders and emotional disorders, the *DSM-IV* classifies all other mental disorders that can occur in children and adolescents. These consist of two types: those usually first diagnosed in infancy, childhood, or adolescence, and those more commonly diagnosed in late adolescence or adulthood.

Disorders First Diagnosed in Childhood and Adolescence

The major disorders of childhood and adolescence included in the first category include pervasive developmental disorders (autism, Asperger's disorder, Rett's disorder, and childhood disintegrative disorders; see Watson & Ozonoff, Chapter 4 of this volume), AD/HD (see Giddan & Milling, Chapter 3 of this volume), disruptive behavior disorders (oppositional defiant disorder and conduct disorder), emotional disorders (e.g., anxiety disorders, adjustment disorders, posttraumatic stress disorder, and selective mutism), tic disorders (e.g., Tourette's syndrome, transient tic disorder), mental retardation, communication disorders, and learning disorders, as well as enuresis and encopresis. A further group of problems, which do not constitute diagnoses in themselves but may characterize interpersonal and family conflict (such as a parent-child problem), are also listed (APA, 1994).

Disorders Diagnosed in Late Adolescence and Adulthood

Disorders more generally diagnosed in late adolescence and adulthood but also seen in children include the schizophrenias and psychoses; mood disorders, such as dysthymic disorder, depression, and bipolar disorder; personality disorders, such as schizotypal and schizoid personality disorder (Baltaxe, Russell, d'Angiola, & Simmons, 1995; Baltaxe & Simmons, 1987, 1992a, 1995; Gualtieri et al., 1983) and substance use disorders (APA, 1994).

Almost all mental disorders first diagnosed in infancy, childhood, and adolescence carry a very significant risk for some type of communication deficit or include some type of language dysfunction as part of their essential features (Baltaxe & Simmons, 1988a, 1988b, 1992a, 1992b; Cantwell & Baker, 1987b, 1991b; Trautman et al., 1990). When adult-type disorders, such as schizophrenia or psychosis, occur in the mid-childhood years, prepuberty, or early adolescence, the prevalence of communication disorders also tends to be quite high (Baltaxe, in press; Baltaxe et al., 1995; Baltaxe & Simmons, 1990, 1991, 1995).

Prevalence of Psychiatric Disorders

The prevalence of psychiatric disorders in the general population varies with type of disorder, age, and gender, as well as with **comorbidity** (association) with other psychiatric or medical conditions. AD/HD, disruptive behavior disorders, and emotional disorders are the most common psychiatric disorders of childhood and adolescence in the general population. However, prevalence rates depend on the type of behavioral disorder or emotional disorder. Prevalence in these disorders also varies based on age, gender, and comorbidity with other disorders, as well as with ethnic constitution. For example, prevalence estimates in the general population for AD/HD, based on large-scale epidemiological studies, have ranged between 2.2 percent and 9.9 percent. Baumeister, Canino, and Bird (1994) and Szatmari (1992) provide even somewhat higher estimates for AD/HD. For oppositional defiant disorder, estimates range from 5.7 percent to 9.5 percent, and for conduct disorder, from 1.5 percent and 9.5 percent (Anderson, Williams, McGee, & Silva, 1987; Bird, Gould, Yagert, Staghezza, & Canino, 1989; Costello, Costello, Edelbrock, et al., 1988; Velez, Johnson, & Cohen, 1988). Other disorders occur at a lesser frequency. For example, according to the American Psychiatric Association (APA, 1992), depression probably exists in about 5 percent of children and adolescents in the general population, although estimates vary from between 1.8 percent (Anderson et al., 1987) to 5.9 percent (Bird et al., 1989), and schizophrenia with onset in childhood is rare.

AD/HD, disruptive behavior disorders, and emotional disorders are the psychiatric illnesses most likely seen in children and adolescents with speech and language disorders in community speech and language clinics and school settings, as well as in mental health settings such as psychiatric inpatient and outpatient services (Baltaxe & Simmons, 1988a, 1990, 1992b; Beitchman, 1985a; Beitchman et al., 1986a; Camarata et al., 1988; Cantwell & Baker, 1991b). However, mental illnesses such as schizophrenia, psychosis, mood disorder, and personality disorder also carry a significant risk of communication disorder (Baltaxe et al., 1995; Baltaxe & Simmons, 1995; Weber & Baltaxe, 1995).

COMMUNICATION DISORDERS AND PSYCHIATRIC DISORDERS WITHIN THE *DSM-IV* FRAMEWORK

Communication disorders within the *DSM-IV* framework, and in association with psychiatric disorders, can occur in a number of ways. They also can take a variety of forms. Disorders range from isolated problems in speech, language, and abstract language to problems in auditory processing and social communication and to combinations thereof. Neurological types of speech-language problems, such as dysarthria and apraxia, may also be present. Profiles of language disabilities can include delay, deviance, and combinations of the two. Social communication in psychiatric disorders takes on a separate and special significance in that specific problems in social communication can characterize specific types of mental disorders, and thus play a major role in the **differential diagnosis** of individual mental disorders.

Following is a schema that characterizes the relationships between psychiatric disorder and communication disorders within the *DSM-IV* (APA, 1994).

- *Communication Disorders:* Communication disorders themselves are also considered mental disorders within the *DSM-IV* framework. Separate and essential criteria must be present in order to make a diagnosis of expressive language disorder, mixed receptive-expressive language disorder, phonological disorder, stuttering, or communication disorder not otherwise specified (NOS). Separate criteria must also be met for the learning disabilities such as reading disorder, mathematics disorder, disorder of written expression, and learning disorder not otherwise specified (NOS).

- *Diagnostic Features:* The diagnosis of some specific mental disorders cannot be made without the presence of specific features of disordered communication or language delay. Such features are among the inherent or essential characteristics of the disorder. Examples are autistic disorder and Asperger's disorder, as well as pervasive developmental disorder-NOS.

- *Co-Occurrence:* A communication disorder may co-occur with another psychiatric or mental disorder without obvious ties between the two types of disorders. An example would be the presence of a speech and language disorder in a child diagnosed with a behavior disorder (such as oppositional defiant disorder) or an emotional disorder (such as a reactive attachment disorder of childhood or separation anxiety disorder). Language disorders with and without speech disorders commonly occur.

- *Associated Characteristics:* A communication disorder may constitute an associated characteristic in a mental disorder. For example, language delay may be part of the cognitive characteristics of mental retardation. Language delay or disordered communication are also expected features of selective mutism.

- *Underlying Processes:* Underlying processing deficits commonly associated with communication disorders may also be characteristic of a psychiatric disorder. Examples are auditory language-processing deficits associated with language disorders, as well as with AD/HD and schizophrenia.

- *Essential Characteristics:* Characteristics of disordered communication may constitute an essential aspect of the presence of a thought disorder in schizophrenia and psychosis. The presence of "incoherence" in speech production may be considered among the problems at the grammatical level, whereas other features of a thought disorder, such as derailment, circumstantiality and tangentiality, are translatable into deficits in social communication.

- *Deficits in Social Communication:* Deficits in social communication play a special role in the diagnosis of psychiatric disorders. Deficits in social communication frequently parade in disguise as part of the essential criteria for the diagnosis of a particular psychiatric disorder. Such deficits are readily recognized by the mental health professional following *DSM-IV* criteria, where such deficits are identified by their behavioral concomitants and not necessarily outlined in their linguistic form. For example, the pattern of negativistic, hostile, and defiant behavior that can be seen in oppositional defiant disorder, and that includes losing one's temper, arguing with adults, and refusing to comply with the requests of others, easily translates into the violation of expected and acceptable interpersonal rules of social conduct and communication. The indiscriminate sociability and excessive familiarity with relative strangers seen in reactive attachment disorder translates into a different set of violations of socially acceptable rules, involving both verbal and nonverbal communication. A child with excessive anxiety concerning separation from home or from significant others will evidence yet another set of social communication behaviors outside the normal range. These may include, for example, excessive perseveration on a topic that is causing fear, distress, or anxiety.

SIGNS AND SYMPTOMS OF PSYCHIATRIC DISORDERS, AND THEIR ASSESSMENT

Because psychiatric disabilities in youngsters with communication disorders as well as communication disorders in children with psychiatric illnesses often may go unrecognized (Alessi et al.,1990; Cohen et al., 1993; Love & Thompson, 1988), alertness on the part of all professionals to the signs and symptoms of a possible mental disorder may be of utmost importance to a youngster's overall well-being and treatment.

Psychiatric illness in children must be considered a serious condition that may affect several areas of development and functioning in the child's life. These areas may include emotional, social, and intellectual development and abilities, as well as the development and use of linguistic skills. A careful medical, family, school, and social history, along with direct observation and personal interaction with the child and a mental status examination conducted by a psychiatrist or other mental health professional, are necessary to diagnose a possible mental illness. The diagnostic process should include questions addressing the child's overall functioning and development, as well as development in specific areas (e.g., motor, cognitive, and language), past and present emotional state, language skills, thought processes, school and play behaviors and performance, eating and sleeping patterns, friendships, peer and family relationships, and family history for specific disorders.

A child suspected of having a major psychiatric disorder may display signs and symptoms that are indicative of specific psychiatric conditions. Such signs and symptoms include failure to look or smile at parents or others; lack of, or restricted, facial expression, facial expression and body language that is incongruous with what the child communicates; odd ways of speaking; odd or repetitive movements; lack of interest in, or awareness of, other people; strange and unusual actions or appearance; intense anxiety and panic in response to a change in surroundings; or breaking of rules and disregard for other people's rights and property.

In young children, signs and symptoms of a psychiatric disorder may also include avoidance of, or withdrawal from, specific people or situations; refusal to go to sleep or take part in activities that are normal for the child's age; refusal to go to school; failing at school or a drop in grades; and excessive worrying. Other red flags may include:

- sadness
- clinging behavior
- lack of stranger anxiety
- perseveration on activities or topics
- constant hyperactivity
- fidgeting
- constant movement
- persistent nightmares
- apparent lack of following verbal directions
- persistent disobedience or aggression
- provocative opposition to authority figures

- frequent and unexplainable temper tantrums
- lying
- stealing
- cruelty to animals

These symptoms may also be present or persist into preadolescence. At that time, red flags may include:

- marked change in school performance
- dropping out of school
- abuse of alcohol and/or drugs
- inability to cope with problems and daily activities
- frequent outbursts of anger
- marked changes in sleeping and/or eating habits
- moodiness and mood swings
- many complaints of physical ailments
- consistent aggressive and nonaggressive violation of the rights of others
- opposition to authority
- truancy
- theft
- vandalism
- intense fear of becoming obese with no relationship to actual body weight
- depression, as evidenced by sustained, prolonged, negative mood and attitude, often accompanied by poor appetite, difficulty sleeping, or thoughts of death.

Since there are many different kinds of psychiatric disorders, the specific diagnosis will depend on the combination of symptoms, in conjunction with other history and with family and observational information.

Although no one of these characteristics is symptomatic of any one particular disorder, a constellation of specific behaviors indicates a need for mental health assessment. For example, a child who often does not listen or appear to follow through on instructions from others, has difficulty playing quietly, talks excessively, does not appear to finish thoughts, interrupts and intrudes on others, or has difficulty waiting for a turn in a game, may suffer from AD/HD. On the other hand, a child who swears and uses foul language frequently, argues with adults, and often loses her or his temper may have oppositional defiant disorder, which is a behavior disorder. A child who steals, fights, sets fires, and is cruel to animals may be appropriately diagnosed with conduct disorder. If a child's facial expression is incongruent with what is said, body posture is rigid, and social communication is disturbed and she or he demonstrates, deterioration of function and hallucinations, schizophrenia may be present; and if a child is fearful, has somatic complaints, such as headaches and stomach complaints, and is withdrawn, an anxiety disorder may be present. For a child who has insufficient eye contact, flat prosody, short sentences, and does not initiate conversation, the differential diagnosis must include the confirmation or exclusion of depression and the pervasive developmental disorders. The symptom picture can be complicated because mental disorders can occur in combination and in this way present a challenge to treatment, particularly when psychopharmacological intervention is at issue.

ETIOLOGY OF PSYCHIATRIC DISORDERS AND COMMUNICATION DISORDERS

The reasons for the unusually high co-occurrence between communication disorders and psychopathology are currently unclear. The relationship appears to be complex, however. Several cause-and-effect relationships have been considered by individual investigators (Baltaxe & Simmons, 1988a; Cantwell & Baker, 1977; Prizant, Audet, Burke, Hummel, Maher, & Theodore, 1990). One proposal argues that early communication difficulties may lead to secondary psychiatric problems. Language plays an important role in all aspects of a child's development, including concept formation, play, reasoning, problem solving, academic achievement, the acquisition of interpersonal skills, and the development of a self-image. Language also plays a role in the child's self-regulation of behavior and her or his control and manipulation of the behavior of others. Prizant et al. (1988) suggested that children with language disorders often do not develop the communicative competence needed for mutual regulation and self-regulation. Competence in self-regulation allows a child to use language to modulate her or his internal emotional states and level of arousal. It therefore is reasonable to maintain that language development that is delayed, impaired, or arrested may be among the most disruptive factors in a child's development.

Another proposal suggests that prenatal medical, social, and family history may include risk factors for both communication disorders and psychiatric disorders. Several commonalities and generalizations can be identified regarding the possible risk factors for the development of psychopathology, impaired communication, or both. These will be discussed further.

It is less likely that psychiatric disorders will lead to secondary communication disorders, although this may be true for a small number of psychiatric disorders. An example would be schizophrenia, where disordered language behavior may be part of the unfolding of the schizophrenic syndrome (Baltaxe & Simmons, 1995; Weber & Baltaxe, 1995).

A somewhat different relationship between a communication disorder and a psychiatric disorder was suggested by Prizant et al. (1990), who proposed a transactional model whereby communication development and emotional development continually affect and modify each other. A continued detrimental mutual effect can therefore also be expected when deficits are present in one or the other of these developmental areas.

Formulations as to the etiology of psychiatric disorders range from environmental-social to biological, and a combination of the two. Several risk factors for the development of psychiatric disorders have long been known to exist. These include lower IQ, developmental delays, organicity and central nervous system dysfunction, as well as other medical conditions and environmental hazards. Known risk factors also include psychosocial stressors, adverse family conditions, familial mental illness and genetic predisposition, and gender. Similar risk factors have also been discussed in relation to communication disorders (Baker & Cantwell, 1987b; Baltaxe & Simmons, 1988a, 1992a, 1992b; Beitchman, 1985b; Beitchman et al., 1990; Prizant et al., 1990; Theodore, Maher, & Prizant, 1990). However, as was proposed earlier, the presence of a communication disorder may, in itself, be a risk factor for development of a psychiatric disorder.

Intelligence

Epidemiological and other investigations have shown that psychiatric disorders as well as communication disorders are more frequent in children and adolescents with lower IQ scores than in those with higher IQ scores (Rutter, 1971; Rutter, Tizard, & Whitmore, 1970). This trend tends to be greatest in the lowest-IQ groups, although it can be found throughout the IQ distributions. Mental retardation is a common comorbidity factor in children with pervasive developmental disorders such as autism, Rett's disorder, and disintegrative psychosis. A general deterioration in cognitive function and language abilities can also be expected with the development of some psychiatric disorders, such as the psychoses and the schizophrenias, and, in some instances, autism (APA, 1994; Baltaxe & Simmons, 1983, 1992a, 1995). A somewhat lowered IQ score (especially verbal IQ) can also be a risk factor for AD/HD and the disruptive behavior disorders, although for the most part, IQ level does not show any connection to specific psychiatric syndromes (Rogeness, 1994; Shaffer, 1986).

Developmental Delays and Abnormalities

Delays or abnormalities in all areas of development and behavior, including language, are frequently linked to an increased incidence of perinatal complications, central nervous system dysfunction, and such medical conditions as encephalitis, neoplasms, prenatal trauma, and seizure disorders (Baltaxe & Simmons, 1995). Such delays and abnormalities, as well as the presence of organic factors such as metabolic disease, may also play a role in the development of psychiatric disorders. For example, Baltaxe and Simmons (1992a, 1995) found that developmental language delays or disturbances were present in 80 percent of a sample of 20 children with prepubertal onset schizophrenia, as well as in children diagnosed with prepubertal onset of schizotypal personality disorder.

McGee, Partridge, Williams, et al. (1991) suggested that early language delays and hyperactivity may be a possible risk for the development of AD/HD in early life, and Baumeister et al. (1994) noted that preschool behavior problems constitute a strong risk factor for antisocial disruptive disorders at age 11. Our own studies have shown that two-thirds of children with disruptive behavior disorders also have a communication disorder. A significant number of these children also have a documented history of language delay (Baltaxe & Simmons, 1990).

Organic Factors and Central Nervous System Dysfunction

With respect to organic factors, Wilcox and Nasrallah (1987) reported an increased incidence of head trauma before the age of 10 for individuals with early onset schizophrenia. O'Callaghan, Larkin, and Waddington (1990) noted that an excess of obstetric complications appeared to characterize the histories of patients with schizophrenia. Based on our own experience, previous head trauma is a common finding in the histories of other psychiatric disorders as well.

Steinberg (1985) noted that chronic brain syndromes affecting central nervous function may also place children and adolescents at greater risk for psychiatric disorder. Seizure disorders have long been known to be associated with psychiatric disorders as well as communication disorders. Shaffer (1986) noted that the risk for psychiatric disorder was four times greater in children suffering from uncomplicated idiopathic epilepsy and five times greater in children with structural abnormality than in no afflicted controls. Children with both structural damage and epilepsy had an even higher prevalence of disturbance. In an inpatient sample of 600 children with both language disorders and psychiatric disorders, Baltaxe and Simmons (1992b; Baltaxe, in press) found that approximately one-third of the children also had seizure disorders or other evidence of organicity. A high incidence of seizure disorders also has been reported for children and adolescents diagnosed with psychoses and schizophrenias (Graham, 1986; Shaffer,1986; Slater, Beard, & Clithero, 1963) and documented for autism (Volkmar & Cohen, 1994; Volkmar & Nelson, 1990).

Exposure to toxic substances may also affect a child's brain and behavior and can produce psychiatric symptoms. Thus, children with lead exposure may appear hyperactive, inattentive, and irritable. They may also have problems with language, learning, and growth, and they may be susceptible to hearing loss (Bellinger, Stiles, & Needleman, 1992; Needleman, 1995).

Other Medical Conditions

Hagerman and Falkenstein (1987) associated high frequencies of otitis media in childhood with the later onset of hyperactivity. Hindley, Hill,

McGuigan, and Kitson (1994), in their study of youngsters who were deaf and hearing impaired, found the prevalence of psychiatric disorder to be close to or more than half (42% to 60%). Earlier studies had also pointed to the high prevalence rate of psychiatric disorder in children who were deaf and hearing impaired (Fundudis et al., 1979; Rutter et al., 1970). It is known that recurring otitis media and hearing impairment frequently are also associated with language delays or disturbances.

Psychosocial Stressors and Adverse Family Conditions

A high incidence of **psychosocial stressors**, such as turbulent family conditions, has been associated with children who have both a communication disorder and psychiatric disorder (Baltaxe, in press; Baltaxe & Simmons, 1988b, 1991, 1992a; Beitchman et al., 1986a). Cantwell and Baker (1991b) reported the presence of significant psychosocial stressors in almost two-thirds (65%) of the children in their sample, who were both psychiatrically ill and communication disordered. Difficulties in parent-child relations as an indicator of psychosocial stress were also prominent in the Baltaxe and Simmons (1988a, 1990, 1991, 1992b) studies. Esser, Schmidt, and Woerner (1990) found that in addition to hyperkinetic symptoms, several other factors, including adverse family relations, learning disability at age 8, and the number of stressful life events experienced in the preceding 5 years, predict conduct disorder at age 13. Additionally, low socioeconomic status, physical and sexual abuse, and other stressful life events may contribute to the development of mental illness.

Familial Mental Illness and Genetic Predisposition

Familial mental illness has also been shown to be associated with the presence of psychiatric symptoms as well as communication difficulties in the offspring. For example, Wolff, Narayan, and Moyes (1988) suggested that schizophrenia is common in the mothers and fathers of children with autism. The risk for increased mental illness in the offspring is particularly strong if the parent's illness is manic-depressive illness, major depression, schizophrenia, alcoholism, or other drug abuse. If both parents are mentally ill, the risk for psychiatric illness in the offspring is even greater. In the case of parental mental illness, some of the risk for the offspring may accrue from the parents' behavior or moods and a concomitant inconsistent, unpredictable family environment; however, it is generally assumed that the primary risk for psychiatric disorder is inherited. Other studies have also shown familial genetic factors. Evidence for genetic factors in autism is discussed in Watson and Ozonoff (Chapter 4 of this volume). Convincing and consistent data also indicate that genetic etiological factors are at work in the development of AD/HD (Castellanos & Rapoport, 1992). All these disorders are significantly associated with disordered communication. It is not clear, however, to what degree genetic predisposition also plays a specific role with respect to language dysfunction.

Gender

Differential vulnerabilities to communication disorders for males and females have long been known to exist. Many studies have demonstrated that a greater number of males than females have developmental communication deficits (Hull, Mielke, Timmons, & Willeford, 1971; Ludlow & Cooper, 1983; Neils & Aram, 1986; Stewart, 1981; Stewart & Spells, 1983). Reported male-to-female ratios in these studies have varied, ranging from 1.7:1 to 4.1:1 (Hier & Kaplan, 1980; Milisen, 1971). As noted in Rescorla and Lee (Chapter 1 of this volume), however, a recent prevalence study of over 7,000 kindergarten-age children found a male-to-female ratio for specific language impairment (SLI) of only 1.33:1 (Tomblin, Records, Buckwalter, Zhang, Smith, & O'Brien, 1997). Similar to the preponderance of findings regarding gender factors in communication disorders, greater male vulnerability also exists for most psychiatric disorders of childhood and adolescence (APA, 1994; Earls, 1987; Gould, Wunsch-Hitzig, & Dohrenwend, 1980). The reported male-to-female ratios for vulnerability in psychiatric disorders have also varied, depending on the study and psychiatric disorder examined (Anderson et al., 1987; Crowther, Bond, & Rolff, 1981; Rutter, Cox, Tupling, Berger, & Yule, 1975), but most psychiatric disorders are male dominated.

When communication disorders occur in children and adolescents with psychiatric disorders, male prevalence also appears to increase (Baltaxe & Simmons, 1992b; Chess & Rosenberg, 1974). However, it is not clear to what extent the gender role is affected by the interaction of the two types of disorders because communication disorders in children and adolescents with psychiatric disorders often go unreported. When gender ratios are included in studies of children with both communication disorders and psychiatric disorders, the male-to-female ratio is reported to be close to 3:1 (Baltaxe & Simmons, 1988a; Chess & Rosenberg, 1974; Gualtieri et al.,1983). However, in some cases the male-to-female ratio is even higher (Camarata et al., 1988; Trautman et al., 1990). Variables that have been shown to play a role in the gender ratio are type of psychiatric disorder (Anderson et al., 1987; Costello et al., 1988), type of communication disorder (Stewart, 1981), age of child (Baltaxe & Simmons, 1992b; Cantwell & Baker, 1991b; Offord et al., 1987), and the criteria used in the identification of a communication disorder (Beitchman et al., 1986a). General population studies have found a higher incidence of AD/HD and behavior disorders in boys than in girls (Crowther et al., 1981; Offord et al., 1987). Cantwell and Baker (1991b) reported a greater incidence of behavior disorders for boys in their sample, with more than twice as many boys so identified than girls, whereas for emotional disorders (anxiety disorders in particular), almost three times as many girls as boys were so identified.

The reasons for the greater male vulnerability to developmental communication disorders as well as to psychiatric disorders is currently not well understood. However, the question of genetically predisposing factors and hormonal differences contributing to the higher frequency of these disorders in males during development has been raised (Beitchman et al., 1986a; Earls, 1987; Graham, 1986; Ludlow & Cooper, 1983; Ounsted, Moar, & Scott, 1986).

Whereas earlier studies of children with both communication disorders and psychiatric disorders noted a general male prevalence, those studies did not focus on other differences that may exist between males and females. These include possible differences with respect to specific types of communication disorders, differences in the pattern and severity of communication disorders, and differences due to other diagnostic or medical factors associated with each gender.

Baltaxe and Simmons (1992b) examined the variables related to gender in 600 children and adolescents who had both a psychiatric disorder and a communication disorder. As predicted, males showed a greater incidence of communication disorders than females, at a ratio of 3:1. Although the same types of speech and language deficits were identified in male and female children, in all the language areas tested, including receptive and expressive vocabulary, syntax, abstract language, and auditory language processing, significantly more females than males were impaired. No such gender differences were found for the areas of speech, which included articulation, voice, fluency, and prosody. Earlier studies had found language rather than speech to represent a more severe and serious communication problem (Baltaxe & Simmons, 1988a, 1991; Cantwell & Baker, 1987a, 1987b). Analysis further showed that significantly more males had pure speech disorders, that is, they were only impaired in the areas of speech, such as articulation, voice, or fluency, whereas significantly more females had pure language disorders, that is, deficits in vocabulary, grammar, and abstract language. The female children also showed a greater severity of language problems. In all the language areas tested, significantly more females than males showed global impairment.

With respect to psychiatric disorders, significantly more females had emotional disorders (such as anxiety disorders and adjustment disorders), whereas significantly more males had disruptive behavior disorders and mood disorders. In addition, a greater proportion of females were diagnosed with mental retardation, seizure disorders, and organic brain disorders, but analysis showed that severity of language disorder in the female children was not predicted by either psychiatric or medical diagnosis.

The findings of greater vulnerability but lesser severity in males and lower vulnerability but greater severity in females parallels gender distributional patterns in other developmental, psychiatric, and physical disorders such as autism, AD/HD, stuttering, reading disability, Down syndrome, and cerebral palsy. These results are consistent with the hypothesis of a differential genetic loading for these disorders in males and females (Baltaxe & Simmons, 1992b).

Risk Factors for Psychiatric Disorder Based on Communication Disorder

The results of the studies mentioned here demonstrate that communication disorders of all types co-occur with psychiatric disorders. These studies have overwhelmingly indicated that delays and disturbances of language, rather than speech, appear to carry a greater risk for psychiatric disorder. Language problems tend to persist into adolescence. At least one follow-up study has demonstrated that young children diagnosed with a language disorder may be at increased risk for the development of a psychiatric disorder in adolescence (Baker & Cantwell, 1987a, 1987b). Although research studies clearly show that linguistic deficits and psychiatric disorder are associated (Baltaxe & Simmons, 1988a, 1990; Beitchman et al., 1986a; Cantwell & Baker, 1991b), the cause-and-effect relationships between psychiatric disorders and communication disorders is not at all clear (Baltaxe & Simmons, 1988a, 1990). It is likely that some of the risk factors enumerated here underlie both the development of communication deficits and that of psychiatric disorders. Cantwell and Baker (1977) and Rutter and Martin (1972) postulated that early language dysfunction may lead to impaired social relations and that these social deficits are etiologically important to the development of later psychopathology. As previously indicated, children with all types of disorders, especially those involving the brain, are at risk for the development of social and emotional problems. Beitchman (1985b, p. 801) reported that children with language impairments, at least those with receptive deficits, lack both an "effective internalized map of their environment" and also the "ability to generalize from the individual item to the whole class of items." Because of this lack of generalization, "the world is often confusing and unmanageable." Beitchman described these children as showing a wide range of behavior problems. However, even though it has been proposed that communication disturbances may lead to psychiatric disturbances, it is likely that in many instances linguistic impairment in itself may not be sufficient to cause a psychiatric disturbance. The risk factors identified previously also play a role.

In some instances, it also is plausible that the emergence of a psychiatric disorder may bring about the emergence of some sort of a communication problem (Baltaxe & Simmons, 1988a, 1990). This may be the case in the schizophrenias and the psychoses. In addition, there may be a mutual interactive effect between communication disorder and psychiatric disorder as suggested by Prizant et al. (1990).

SPECIFIC COMMUNICATION DISORDERS AND PSYCHIATRIC DISORDERS

Only a few early studies have focused on the presence of psychiatric symptoms in specific types of communication disorders, whereas later studies have focused on the range of psychiatric disorders associated with communication disorders in general before further investigating specific subgroups. A review of these studies shows a focus on several types of communication disorders, with more general descriptions of a variety of psychiatric symptomatology.

Phonological Disorders

The presence of psychiatric disorders in youngsters with phonological disorders was studied by several investigators. In a sample of 70 first graders with articulation impairments, Fitzsimons (1958) found more behavior and emotional disorders than in a matched control group. More anxious behavior was found by Trapp and Evan (1960) in 54 youngsters between 8 and 10 years of age with articulation impairments, especially in those with more severe articulation impairments. Similarly, Solomon (1961) found significantly more psychiatric disturbances in 49 first graders with impaired articulation than in a matched control group. A high incidence of emotional disorders was identified by Butler (1965) in her young age group of 5- to 8-year-old children. Maladjustment was identified by Sheridan and Peckham (1973) in close to 50 percent of their subjects in a large study of 7-year-olds. Manipulative, noncompliant, overly sensitive, and immature behaviors, together with delayed psychosocial development, were found in a study by Shriberg, Kwiatkowski, Best, et al. (1986), who reviewed the therapy records of 114 children with phonological disorders. A review of the psychiatric signs and symptoms in this population indicates that emotional as well as behavioral disorders were present in this group of studies.

Voice Disorders

Studies have also linked voice disorders with psychiatric symptomatology. For example, Duncan (1947) identified a significant increase in maladjustment in a study of hoarse speakers compared to normally speaking controls. On the other hand, no such relationship was found by Muma, Leader, and Webb (1968) in high-school age adolescents with a harsh, nasal, hoarse, or breathy voice. It is not clear whether behavior or emotional disorders, or both, were involved. Our own studies indicate the presence of voice disorders in a significant number of children and adolescents diagnosed with a psychiatric disorder, although voice disorders occurred rarely in isolation as the only communication deficit (Baltaxe, in press; Baltaxe & Simmons, 1990, 1992b).

Stuttering

Attention has also been given to the psychiatric symptomatology of stuttering at various stages. Associated psychiatric symptoms included emotional problems, such as anxiety and oversensitivity (Glasner, 1949), anxiety and fears

(Wyatt, 1958), fear of speaking in public (Bubenickova, 1977), and psychodynamic difficulties (Gemilli, 1982). On the other hand, Blood and Seiden (1981) used a questionnaire and surveyed elementary school speech pathologists with 1,660 stutterers as clients who suggested that emotional problems were rare in these patients. It is almost certain that age and the continued presence of dysfluency play a role in the development of possible psychiatric symptomatology. Stuttering also falls into the realm of psychiatric treatment. When interpreting the symptoms reported in this group of studies, it seems clear that stuttering is associated more with emotional than behavioral disorders.

Based on our own investigations, all types of psychiatric disorders are highly associated with a variety of other dysfluencies, which include, in particular, reformulations of the speaker's own utterances.

Cleft Palate

Psychiatric pathology in children with cleft palates has received relatively much attention. Difficulties including tantrums, poor concentration, and learning difficulties were identified by Schweckendiek and Danzer (1970) in their study of 200 youngsters aged 7 to 14 with cleft palate. Significantly more behavior problems and problems with bed-wetting were found by McWilliams and Musgrave (1972), in particular in children who also had articulation difficulties. Parallel findings were identified by Simonds and Heimburger (1978), who found psychiatric problems more likely in those youngsters with cleft palate who also had articulation difficulty. Problems with self-concept were found by Kapp (1979). Children with cleft palate also were less happy and less satisfied with their appearance than controls. Shyness and dissatisfaction were identified as problems in children with cleft palate by Spriesterbach (1973), and self-concern and self-doubt, by Harper and Richman (1978). On the other hand, Ruess (1965), in a comparison of youngsters with cleft palate and their typically developing siblings, found no indication of psychiatric disorder. Overall, these studies suggest that both behavioral disorder and emotional disorder are associated with cleft palate speech.

Dyspraxia of Speech

Only one study has focused on children with dyspraxia and the possibility of psychosocial behaviors (Ferry, Hall, & Hicks, 1975). Behavior problems were identified in half of 60 subjects in addition to depressive and autistic symptoms in a significant number of the children. Our own clinical experience and research have shown that dyspraxia is a common problem in children with psychiatric disorders. In our study of communication disorders in 400 consecutive admissions, oral peripheral examination indicated that 17 percent of the children with communication impairments had structural problems, and 41 percent had functional problems including dyspraxia of speech (Baltaxe & Simmons, 1990).

Language

An early study of children with language disorders by Griffiths (1969) identified poor emotional adjustment in about one-half, and poor social adjustment in about one-fourth of the children. Some sort of behavioral or emotional problem was identified by Caceres (1971) in four-fifths of a small sample. Common problems with quasi-obsessional activities, attachments to odd objects, ritualistic activities, and resistance to change were identified in a group of 23 children with dysphasia studied by Bartak and Rutter (1975), who also identified significant behavior problems in more than half of a subgroup of children with speech/language disorders. Significantly greater psychiatric disturbances in children with delayed language compared to normal controls was also identified by Fundudis et al. (1979). Frequent problems in social relations, concentration or attention, shyness, fears, and poor self-concept were identified by Baumgartner (1980) in a sample of youngsters with communication disorders in special schools in Bavaria, Germany. Aram and Nation (1980) found significantly more schizoid, immature, obsessive-compulsive, hostile, and withdrawn characteristics in a sample of 20 teenagers with language disorders compared to a control group of typically developing adolescents. Behavior problems were also identified by McGee, Williams, and Feehan (1992) in 3-year-olds with language delays compared to typically developing controls, and significantly higher mean total psychiatric symptoms and internalizing disorder scores were identified by the same authors in a group of 4-year-olds compared to their normal controls.

The psychiatric descriptors associated with language problems indicate that language disorders can be associated with a variety of psychiatric conditions, in addition to behavioral and emotional disorders.

THE BROAD ASSOCIATION BETWEEN COMMUNICATION DISORDERS AND PSYCHIATRIC DISORDERS

The studies discussed previously used a variety of approaches, which included the use of different protocols involving different types of formal and informal inventories and questionnaires as well as chart review. Different types of criteria were also used for the identification of control groups. The studies focused primarily on the early and middle childhood years, with some excursions into the later years. Because of the looseness and ambiguities of the psychiatric descriptors in studies it is difficult to identify the full range of psychiatric diagnoses seen in these samples. It seems clear, however, that behavioral and emotional disorders play a major role in the children's problems. It is also difficult to identify the specific nature of the communication characteristics. These shortcomings have been remedied in more recent, large-scale studies, which have, consequently, provided more specific information on the relationship between disordered communication and psychiatric disorders. These studies also confirm the central place of behavioral and emotional problems and the prominent position of AD/HD in the relationship.

Community-based Studies

The largest study of psychopathology in children with communication disorders carried out in community speech settings was conducted by Cantwell, Baker, and colleagues between 1977 and 1992 (Baker & Cantwell, 1985, 1987a, 1987b; Cantwell & Baker, 1980, 1985, 1987a, 1987b, 1991a, 1991b, 1992). The study examined 600 children between the ages of 1 year, 7 months (1; 7), and 15 years, 9 months (15; 9); using standardized testing for speech and language deficits and following the criteria of the *Diagnostic Statistical Manual of Mental Disorders, 3rd edition*, and *3rd edition revised* (American Psychiatric Association [APA], 1980, 1987). Male children made up 69 percent of their sample. They found that half the children with communication disorders had a diagnosable psychiatric disorder, with the following distribution: behavior disorders were the most frequent in occurrence (26%), with AD/HD the second most common (19%) and oppositional and/or conduct disorders present in an additional 7 percent of the children studied. Emotional disorders were present in 20 percent of the children, and 4 percent also had an affective or mood disorder (Baker & Cantwell, 1985; Cantwell & Baker, 1991a, 1991b). Less than 2 percent of the children had a diagnosis of pervasive developmental disorder, whereas 6 percent also had a diagnosis of mental retardation. Thus, two groups of mental disorders—AD/HD-disruptive behavior disorder and emotional disorder—occurred at the highest rate. They also occurred at a significantly higher rate than in the general population (Szatmari, 1992). Therefore, of the variety of possible psychiatric disorders, the range of those seen in the children in this large study was rather restricted.

Cantwell, Baker, and colleagues also showed that the presence of a language disorder placed children at particular risk for psychiatric disorder. About half of the children with concurrent speech and language disorders and two-thirds of the children with only a language disorder also had a diagnosable psychiatric disorder. In contrast, this was true for only one-third of the children with only a speech disorder. In addition, more severe behavior problems (short attention span, restlessness, fidgeting, impulsivity) and developmental problems were more common in the group of children with language disorders. The severity of psychiatric symptomatology also varied with the presence of a language or speech disorder. Children with language disorders showed the most serious psychiatric impairment, whereas children with speech disorders alone had the least severe symptoms of psychiatric disorder. Speech disorders tended to be associated more with emotional disorders than with behavior disorders in these studies.

The second community-based, large-scale study of psychopathology in children with communication disorders derived from an epidemiological study of 1,655 aged 5 and children living in Canada by Beitchman and colleagues (Beitchman, 1985b; Beitchman et al., 1986b, 1988, 1989a, 1989b, 1990). The overall incidence of speech and language problems in their sample was 19 percent. A breakdown of their study showed that 27 percent of the children had speech problems only, 44 percent had language problems only, and 29 percent had combined speech-language problems. Psychiatric disorders were identified in about half (49%) of the group with communication disorders. These findings parallel those by Cantwell and Baker, as described previously. Similarly, Beitchman and colleagues found that behavior disorders, in particular AD/HD, were the most frequently occurring psychiatric disorders in their preschool group, with a prevalence rate of 30 percent. The behavioral disturbance was greatest when the language delay was most severe. Emotional disorders occurred at a rate of 13 percent compared to only 2 percent in the rest of this large sample.

The results of these studies support the hypothesis that children with language disorders are particularly at risk for psychiatric disorders. This language risk factor is also supported by several follow-up studies of children with language disorders. Lerner, Inui, Trupin, et al. (1985) followed a group of children initially assessed as preschoolers for more than a decade after initial assessment. They found that speech/language delay at age 5 was a strong predictor for psychiatric illness at follow-up. In a follow-up study of a large subgroup of their subjects, Baker and Cantwell (1987b) and Cantwell and Baker (1991b) found a significant increase of psychiatric disorders, from 50 percent to 60 percent, 4 to 5 years after their initial assessment. The majority of the subjects were diagnosed with disruptive behavior disorders, which increased from an initial 26 percent to 45 percent on follow-up. AD/HD occurred with the greatest frequency (38 percent). In addition, 18 percent of the subjects also had some type of emotional disorder (4 percent had a mood disorder and 14 percent, an anxiety disorder). The emergence of a psychiatric disorder in initially healthy children appeared to be related to whether a language disorder was present at initial evaluation.

Hospital-based Studies

The number of studies carried out in hospital settings is still limited (Alessi et al., 1990; Chess & Rosenberg, 1974; Grinnell, Scott-Hartnett, & Larson-Glasier, 1983; Gualtieri et al., 1983; Loomis & Alessi, 1988; Love & Thompson, 1988; Trautman et al., 1990). These studies are generally also small scale, except for those by Baltaxe and Simmons (discussed subsequently). As noted earlier, these studies support the even higher association between psychiatric disorders and speech-language disorders. They also highlight the central role of language in children and adolescents with psychopathology. For example, Grinnell et al. (1983) studied 80 adolescents and preadolescents without hearing impairment in a psychiatric hospital. Of this group, 80 percent had significant language pathology, including combined receptive and expressive language problems, as well as pure receptive or expressive problems. Gualtieri et al. (1983) found that 24 of the 26 children they studied had serious communication problems that were not readily detected through psychological testing.

Communication disorders identified in children with previously diagnosed psychiatric disorders can range from the subtle and difficult to identify (Cohen et al., 1993) to more marked impairments in one, several, or all areas of communication (Baltaxe & Simmons, 1990, 1992b). Language deficits are generally more pervasive and severe than deficits in speech. Speech disorders more commonly emerge in the younger ages, whereas language disorders are present in all age groups. The severity and pervasiveness of general language disability have also been correlated with the severity and pervasiveness of psychiatric disorder in some of the previously mentioned studies. Thus, it may be postulated that children with a more severe and pervasive language disability are at risk for a more severe and pervasive psychiatric disorder (Baltaxe & Simmons, 1992b). These studies also found that although disruptive behavior disorders, AD/HD, and emotional disorders are still the most common psychiatric disorders, the range of reported psychiatric disorders associated with communication disorders has increased considerably in hospital settings.

Our own studies carried out between 1988 and 1996 (Baltaxe, in press; Baltaxe et al., 1995; Baltaxe & Simmons, 1988a, 1990, 1991, 1992a, 1992b, 1995) confirm the increased incidence of communication disorders when children and adolescents who are psychiatrically ill are studied as the index group. They further underline the fact that when communication disorders occur, language disorders rather than speech disorders are more prevalent, and social communication is usually highly affected as well. The range of psychiatric disorders co-occurring with communication disorders is also increased. For example, Baltaxe and Simmons (1990) and Baltaxe (in press) examined 400 children and adolescents (60% male, 40% female) between the ages of 2 and 22 years (mean = 9; 3; S.D. = 4; 10) admitted consecutively to the child and adolescent inpatient services for acute psychiatric care. Of this sample, 67 percent had a communication disability. Significantly more males than females were affected (75 percent of males compared to 57 percent of females). Psychiatric discharge diagnoses covered a wide range of disorders: developmental disorders, including mental retardation and the pervasive developmental disorders; disruptive behavior disorders, including AD/HD; emotional disorders; parent-child problems; personality disorders; schizophrenia and psychoses; and mood disorders. The likelihood of presence of a communication disorder varied with the type of psychiatric disorder. Not unexpectedly, 99 percent of children with developmental disorders had communication impairment, along with 66 percent of the children with disruptive behavior disorders and 63 percent of the children with emotional disorders. Language disorders also occurred at a rate of 63 percent among children with parent-child problems, family circumstances, and psychosocial stress problems, and at a rate of 59 percent among children with personality disorders, particularly in the categories of schizoid, borderline, and obsessive compulsive personality disorder. In addition, 58 percent of children and adolescents diagnosed with schizophrenia and psychosis were communication disordered, as were 40 percent of the youngsters diagnosed with mood disorders, such as depression, and 91 percent of the children with organically based mental disorders and movement (e.g., tic and Tourette's) disorders.

The type of communication disorder was examined using formal testing and standardized measures. Of the children in this sample with communication disorders, 87 percent had language problems with or without additional speech problems, whereas only 13 percent had pure speech problems. More than one-third of the group with language disorders was globally impaired in all receptive and expressive language areas (receptive and expressive vocabulary, grammar, and abstract language, as well as auditory language processing). Expressive language impairments without receptive impairments were identified in 11 percent of the sample, and receptive impairments without expressive impairment in only 4 percent of the sample. The language areas identified as most commonly impaired were auditory language processing (65%) and abstract language function (receptive, 67%; expressive 72%). Between one-half and two-thirds of children in the sample were also impaired in receptive and expressive vocabulary and grammar. Among children and adolescents with speech disorders, operationally defined as including articulation, fluency, voice, and prosody, 51 percent had articulation deficits. Fluency and prosody each were impaired in about two-fifths of the group, and voice in about one-fifth. Social communication was also very significantly affected.

Except for autism, deficits in social communication have not been extensively studied (Baltaxe, 1993). Deficits in social communication occurred in a wide range of areas in our sample. These included providing irrelevant information to the listener, not distinguishing between old and new information syntactically, inappropriate topic initiation and switch, inappropriate turn taking (e.g., overlapping with and interrupting the speaker, refusal to yield the floor, or lack of response), inappropriate use of register (e.g., using formal language in a conversational setting), and use of body language, facial expressions, or prosodic features that are incongruent with the content of what is said.

The deficits in social communication also included those specific features that are diagnostic for individual psychiatric disorders. For example, the child with schizotypal personality disorder, schizophrenia, or psychosis may not be able to use or interpret the required prosodic signals to communicate or evoke certain emotions in the listener. Children and adolescents with these disorders may also have difficulties with the use or interpretation of secondary or derived meanings, with abstract language, and with taking the listener's perspective, thus creating serious social communication disorders. The child with reactive attachment disorder (an emotional disorder) may not differentiate her or his social use of language, regardless of whether the listener is a familiar person or a stranger. The child's verbal and nonverbal behaviors may thus be overfamiliar and inappropriate for strangers. On the other hand, a child with an anxiety disorder (i.e., a different emotional disorder) may shrink from social contact with strangers, and her or his pragmatics will reflect this as well, whereas a child with a behavior disorder, such as a conduct disorder, may violate the principles of politeness in a social situation.

When communication disorders in children who are psychiatrically ill are studied in outpatient and inpatient hospital settings, the association between communication disorders and psychiatric disorders is generally even higher than in community speech-language clinics and school settings. Importantly, the range of psychiatric disorders associated with communication disorders also widens and the psychiatric disorder may be more severe. However, disruptive behavior disorders, AD/HD, and emotional disorders are still the most frequent, even in hospital settings. Findings from hospital studies further underline the fact that when communication disorders occur, language, rather than speech, disorders are more prevalent, and social communication is usually highly affected as well. The range of psychiatric disorders co-occurring with communication disorders is also increased.

In addition to mental retardation and the pervasive developmental disorders, the distribution of psychiatric diagnoses in Baltaxe and Simmons's (1991) sample of hospitalized children and adolescents diagnosed with both psychiatric disorders and communication disorders included the following: disruptive behavior disorders including ADHD (35%, N = 209), emotional disorders (19%, N = 111), schizophrenias (14%, N = 85), mood disorders (13%, N = 76), parent-child problems (11%, N = 71), family psychosocial stress (10%, N = 69), and personality disorders (9%, N = 54). All the children had some kind of a speech-language disorder, and most also had deficits in social communication. Children with combined speech and language disorders accounted for nearly three-fourths of the sample with communication disorders. Only 7 percent of the sample had pure speech disorders, and 19 percent had pure language disorders. Language disorders were significantly more global and pervasive, affecting all areas of language. Speech disorders occurred more in isolation; for example, an articulation problem generally occurred without another area of speech being involved. The pattern of language disorders in this study mimicked that of the study (Baltaxe, in press) involving 400 subjects, with speech disorders, especially articulation impairment, being more limited to the younger ages.

INTERVENTION AND PROGNOSIS

When a child has both a communication disorder and a psychiatric disorder, it seems clear that both disorders require attention and intervention. It is also clear that the cooperation and exchange of information between the treating mental health professional and the treating communication disorders specialist will benefit the child, not only with respect to diagnostic identification but also with respect to optimal intervention for both types of disorders. The coexistence of communication disorders and psychiatric disorders thus underscores the need for **interdisciplinary** and **transdisciplinary** training and cooperation between mental health professionals and communication disorders specialists. *Interdisciplinary* refers to professionals collaborating across disciplines to assess and intervene with a child. In contrast, *transdisciplinary* refers to collaboration in planning and interpreting assessment and intervention, which is typically provided by one professional. These types of interactions call for each discipline to develop at least a rudimentary understanding of the other disciplines' realms of knowledge and tools. Clinical experience has shown that the diagnosis and treatment of one or both types of disorders in a child will depend on referral patterns, that is, what type of services are sought first, speech-language services or medical/psychiatric services. However, it also will depend on the training and sophistication of the professionals involved in evaluating and treating the child, as well as the existing biases of the discipline that is first consulted. Ignoring either the psychiatric disorder or the communication disorder in treatment could have far-reaching negative consequences, such as an impact on the child's self-concept, school achievement, and interpersonal relations, as well as her or his self-regulation and regulation of the behavior of others. Because of the possible consequences of these two disorders interacting with each other, nontreatment could also contribute to the development, persistence, or worsening of one or both types of conditions (Baker & Cantwell, 1987b; Prizant et al., 1990). Both major psychiatric disorders and communication disorders often last a long time and may be life-long. However, when children with such disorders begin treatment early, their skills, abilities, and adjustment to the demands of daily living will typically improve. Comprehensive treatment may include psychotherapy, medication, special schools or hospitals, special school programs and therapy programs (e.g., speech and language therapy, social skills training, and behavior programs), and active involvement of the family.

The best possible assessment takes place within an interdisciplinary framework with professionals from relevant disciplines communicating with each other within a team. The interdisciplinary process should involve psychiatry, psychology, regular education, special education, speech-language pathology, social work, and the family. Useful tools in the process of differential diagnosis include a variety of parent and teacher observational rating scales suitable to the age of the child, such as the Achenbach Behavioral Rating Scale for Parents and Teachers (Achenbach, 1991), sentence completion tests, the Goodenough Draw a Person Test (Harris, 1963), the Thematic Apperception Test (Murray, 1971), the Rorschach Test (Exner, 1993; Rapoport, Gill, & Schafer, 1968; Rorschach, 1942), the Bender Gestalt Test (Koppitz, 1964), and the Developmental Test of Visual Motor Integration (VMI), (Beery & Buktenica, 1989), in addition to the assessment of cognitive, linguistic and reading, writing, and mathematics skills. The speech-language pathologist plays an important role on the interdisciplinary team or as a consultant to individual mental health professionals. Expected input on her or his part to the interdisciplinary team will include comments stemming from chart review, parental interview, informal observations, and formal testing relating to language behaviors. It is her or his duty to identify typical speech and language behaviors as well as possible specific deficits, such as pragmatic features, auditory processing problems and other speech and language features, level of speech and language development, abnormal features, indications of organicity, and strengths and weaknesses seen in language behaviors. Further, the speech-language pathologist must effectively share her or his findings with the team. The speech-language pathologist's contributions are important from both a diagnostic and an intervention perspective. Specific language behaviors often corroborate a specific psychiatric diagnosis. Thus, the specific pragmatic deficits seen in an adolescent suspected of being schizophrenic may corroborate the presence of a thought disorder. A specific linguistic profile, which might include abnormal prosodic features, comprehension problems, and specific pragmatic deficits, may corroborate a diagnosis of autism. Auditory language processing, slight word-finding difficulties, and pragmatic deficits, as well as reading and writing difficulties, may be expected for some children with AD/HD. The information on speech and language behaviors contributed by the speech-language pathologist on the interdisciplinary team complements and/or supports that provided by the other professions, and it may provide the basis for additional referrals, such as for neurological or audiological evaluations. Such information also assists in school placement and the determination of services needed. If the speech-language pathologist is a member of the interdisciplinary team, collaboration in intervention is also possible. Medication and/or behavior management may play a role with respect to speech language intervention, as may the sequencing of these approaches. Whether functioning as members of the interdisciplinary team or as consultants, the more knowledgeable speech-language pathologists are with respect to psychiatric disorders, the more valuable they can be to others. In other settings, knowledgeable speech-language pathologists can act as a catalyst in further addressing possible emotional, behavior, and mental health problems in the children and adolescents for whom they provide service.

CASE STUDY: DAVID

David is a handsome boy, aged 7; 4, who was hospitalized for temper tantrums and severe noncompliant behaviors. He was referred for speech and language assessment because of immature articulation.

David is an only child. He lives at home with his mother and stepfather. He was the product of a pregnancy remarkable for fetal distress at 42 weeks of gestation and an induced delivery. His mother reportedly did not receive prenatal care until the 8th month of pregnancy. David's Apgar scores were normal.

David's medical history is remarkable for multiple episodes of recurrent otitis media since birth. Reported developmental milestones were within normal limits: David walked at 10 months and spoke his first word at 1 year of age. David is reported to have displayed "acting out" behavior from an early age. This included throwing severe temper tantrums, hitting, and kicking, and demonstrating other forms of noncompliant behaviors. When he was 3 years old he was enrolled in preschool, but he was asked to leave because of noncompliant behaviors and fear he might injure other children. He completed public kindergarten and first grade, but recently was placed into a special classroom for the severely emotional disturbed.

Results of psychological testing placed David in the high-average range of intellectual functioning overall. Test behavior during speech and language assessment showed David to be cooperative and fully participating in all aspects of the assessment on three of the five occasions when he was seen for assessment in a one-to-one structured or semistructured situation. On two other occasions David had difficulty with making the transition from his other activities on the ward.

Hearing screening indicated David's hearing to be within normal limits bilaterally. The following are the results of his speech/language assessment: oral motor examination and diadokokinesis were within normal limits. With respect to articulation, David consistently substituted /w/ for /l/ and /r/ in all positions. He simplified consonant clusters in some positions inconsistently. His voice, prosody, and fluency were within normal limits.

David scored within the high-average range on receptive and expressive vocabulary, as tested by the Peabody Picture Vocabulary Test–III (Dunn & Dunn, 1997) and the Expressive One Word Picture Vocabulary Test–R (Gardner, 1983). His language profile, established by using the Clinical Evaluation of Language Fundamentals–3 (Semel, Wiig, & Secord, 1995), showed a receptive language score within the normal range, although he performed 2 SDs below the mean for his chronological age on the subtest of oral directions. In contrast, his expressive language score was 1.5 SDs below the mean, with particular difficulties in formulated sentences and word structure. David also scored more than 1.5 SDs below the mean on abstract language skills and metalinguistic competence in semantics, syntax, and pragmatics on the Test of Language Competence-Exp.–Level 1 (Wiig & Secord, 1988); he had particular difficulty with the ambiguous sentence subtest. David performed poorly in auditory language processing, as identified through the Test of Auditory Perceptual Skills subtests of auditory number, sentence, and word memory (Gardner, 1996). On the other hand, David performed within normal limits on the Test of Problem Solving (Zachman, Barrett, Huisingh, Orman, & Blagden, 1991), which was administered to evaluate his problem-solving and reasoning abilities. A 30-minute language sample collected in a semistructured interview showed simple sentence structure characteristic of a younger age child. Morphology, except for irregular plurals and past tenses, was within normal limits (Miller, 1981). Eye contact and turntaking were appropriate.

Summarizing the test results, David was identified with an articulation problem, auditory language-processing and expressive language deficits, and deficits in some areas of abstract language function. Although David had been observed to have "immature" articulation prior to the speech-language evaluation, the more serious deficits in expressive language, auditory language processing, and abstract language function, as well the role of these problems in social communication, had not been identified by either his school or the referring psychiatrist. Unsuspected language problems are often present in children identified with a psychiatric disorder. Recommendations included placement in a special educational classroom, individual language therapy, participation in a social communication group to learn acceptable ways of communicating, parent training to cope with ways to deal with David's temper tantrums, and individual psychotherapy for David on an outpatient basis, with periodic team follow-up.

CASE STUDY: LISA

Lisa is a fit, well-groomed, 14-year-old Asian-American female who was hospitalized for possible anxiety and depressive disorder and posttraumatic stress disorder. She was referred for speech and language evaluation because of obvious problems in speech and language.

Lisa lives with her mother and two brothers in an apartment in a suburb of Los Angeles. English is spoken at home. There is a recent history of severe psychological stressors, including sexual abuse. Her developmental history was unremarkable until the age of 9. She was reported to be an average student. At age 9, she contacted viral encephalitis and subsequently developed a grand mal seizure. Lisa was placed on medication for seizures and is currently seizure free. Her mother describes her as having been a quiet but friendly girl prior to the encephalitis. Subsequent to the encephalitis and seizure, Lisa also developed a language disturbance. She is currently in a special day class where speech and language services have been provided.

Lisa's overall behavior and level of function have deteriorated within the past three months. She refuses to go to school and withdraws from social contact. She also has made overtures to slitting her wrist, and razor marks are visible. She has been given to crying spells, but also has had some temper tantrums. Lisa insisted on bringing a toy teddy bear to the speech/language testing session. She perseverated on this topic throughout testing. Lisa's eye contact was inappropriate, being either absent or too long in duration. Moreover, her use of eye contact was not attributable to cultural differences, being clearly divergent from the patterns of eye contact used by her mother and brothers.

Receptive and expressive vocabulary were tested using the Peabody Picture Vocabulary Test–III (Dunn & Dunn, 1997) and the Expressive One Word Test-Upper Extension (Gardner, 1983). Lisa obtained an age equivalence of 5;5 on receptive vocabulary function and an age equivalent of 5;2 on expressive vocabulary function. Lisa had difficulty with naming, instead producing circumlocutions and phonemic and semantic paraphasias. The language profile provided by testing with the Clinical Evaluation of Language Fundamentals–3

(Semel, Wiig, & Secord, 1995) indicated that all areas tested were more than 2 SDs below the mean. Lisa's language sample was characterized by short sentences, omissions of grammatical markers and function words, and errors in syntax. Lisa's auditory language processing, as tested through the Test of Word Sequences of the Detroit Test of Learning Aptitude-3 (Hammill, 1995), also was more than 2 SDs below the mean for her age. With respect to social communication, Lisa evidenced poor turn-taking skills in that she either did not wait for her turn or did not answer at all. She did not initiate conversation. Her utterances were short, and she perseverated on topics. Her affect was flat, body posture rigid, and eye contact poor. Lisa was unable to perform adequately on oral motor examination. Diadokokinesis was poor, with a noticeable slowing of rate and transpositions of syllables. Lisa's articulatory pattern was inconsistent, with fluctuating errors in speech production. Her rate of speech at times was slowed, and her prosody was affected by the slowing of her rate of speech. Her voice appeared to be normal. Lisa's fluency was impaired in that she made false starts and self-repairs of misnaming.

Lisa's composite speech/language/communication profile showed both "delay" and "deviance" in speech, language, and communication. It was the profile of a youngster evidencing organicity, in this case, an acquired aphasia due to encephalitis and seizure disorder. However, verbal and nonverbal social communication characteristics, as well as prosody, may also be affected by the presence of an anxiety disorder and a depressive disorder. Children with a depressive disorder may not be interested in communicating. Lack of interest or shyness and anxiety may occasion poor turn-taking skills, poor topic development, and unwillingness to take the listener's perspective. This, in turn, can affect the child's ability to differentiate between new and old information and provide adequate information to the listener. A sad mood may affect the melody of speech, as well as nonverbal communication including eye contact, facial expression, and body posturing in accordance with conversation. Youngsters with an organic, physical disorder or with a high score in psychological stressors are five times as likely to develop a psychiatric disorder than children without either history. Children with an acquired aphasia may also be acutely aware of their deficits and develop depressive symptoms. Our recommendation for Lisa was to place her into a classroom for children with severe verbal disorders. Medication for depression and psychological counseling and follow-up were also indicated.

SUMMARY

When examining the association between psychiatric disorders and communication disorders, there are several bits of information that may assist the professional in forming expectations when she or he suspects a youngster to have a mental health problem or psychiatric disorder. These include frequency of occurrence of specific type of psychiatric disorder in the population at large and frequency of a particular language disorder associated with psychiatric disorder.

There is a timetable for the emergence of specific psychiatric disorders. Different psychiatric disorders emerge at different times during life. Thus, pervasive developmental disorders are present at birth or close to birth and mental retardation is apparent before the age of 18, whereas AD/HD and disruptive behavior disorders emerge in mid-childhood and personality disorders and schizophrenias, as a general rule, can be expected to emerge in adolescence or adulthood (they may also occur in preadolescence).

There may be a diagnostic change in symptoms of the psychiatric disorder over time. Thus, the presenting symptoms for AD/HD vary with age of child. In young children, hyperactivity symptoms may include excessive running or climbing, whereas older children may display extremely restless and fidgety behaviors, particularly in group situations. They may also be poorly organized and not goal directed. For some individuals with autism, the symptom picture may change later in life due to the development of seizure activity.

Consideration must also be given to the possible coexistence of other psychiatric disorders in the same individual. The symptom picture may indicate comorbidity and may impact the communication disorder as well. High comorbidity has been shown, for example, among AD/HD and the disruptive behavior disorders. Also, consideration must be given to the differential diagnosis of related disorders. For example, the category of disorders that has been loosely termed *social communication spectrum disorders* includes autism, pervasive developmental disorder–not otherwise specified, schizotypal personality disorder, schizophrenia, and psychosis. Care must be taken in determining the appropriate diagnosis on the part of the psychiatrist or other mental health professional, which makes careful history taking and observations mandatory in addition to formal testing. A detailed analysis of existing communication disorders in the child will aid in the diagnosis.

Knowledge of the frequencies of specific communication disorders across psychiatric disorders in general and/or specific pragmatic disorders is also desirable. For psychiatric disorders, a high frequency of deficits is expected for the communication areas of pragmatics, abstract language, auditory processing, and expressive and receptive language.

There are age-related variables of communication disorders in psychiatric disorders. Speech variables across different psychiatric disorders show an age effect, whereas pragmatics, receptive and expressive language, and auditory processing are very significantly impaired across all age groups with psychiatric disorder.

There are gender-related variables in communication disorders, in psychiatric disorders, and in the co-occurrence of psychiatric and communication disorders. More males than females generally show both communication disorders and psychiatric disorders, but, when impaired, females show more pervasive and severe impairments than males.

To serve their young clients optimally, all professionals should be aware and knowledgeable of the signs and symptoms of a possible psychiatric disorder in the child with a communication disorder. This is important for the development of a comprehensive treatment plan, which may include referral to, and consultation with, a mental health professional so that treatment can be extended to ameliorate the psychiatric signs and symptoms as well as the communication deficits. In addition, all professionals need to be aware of the increased likeihood of co-occurring communication deficits in order for speech-language pathologists and audiologists to begin treatment in the communication areas.

References

Achenbach, T. M. (1991). *Child Behavior Checklist*. Burlington: University of Vermont, Dept of Psychiatry.

Affolder, F., Brubaker, R., & Bischofberger, W. (1974). Comparative studies of normal and language disturbed children based on performance profiles. *Acta Otolanryngologia, 323*(Suppl.), 1–32.

Alessi, N. E., Eisner, S. J., & Knight, C. (1990). *The association of language disturbances with cognitive and motoric impairments in psychiatrically hospitalized children*. Poster session presented at the meeting of the Society for Research in Child and Adolescent Psychopathology, Costa Mesa, Calif.

Alessi, N. E., & Loomis, S. (1988, October). *The frequency and severity of language disturbances in depressed children*. Paper presented at the 35th annual meeting of the American Academy of Child and Adolescent Psychiatry, Seattle.

American Psychiatric Association. (1980). *Diagnostic and statistical manual of mental disorders* (3rd ed.). Washington, D.C.: Author.

American Psychiatric Association. (1987). *Diagnostic and statistical manual of mental disorders* (3rd ed. rev.). Washington, D.C.: Author.

American Psychiatric Association. (1992). *Depression in childhood* (leaflet). Washington, D.C.: Author.

American Psychiatric Association. (1994). *Diagnostic and statistical manual of mental disorders* (4th ed.). Washington, D.C.: Author.

Anderson, J. C., Williams, S., McGee, R., & Silva, P. A. (1987). *DSM–III* disorders in preadolescent children. *Archives of General Psychiatry, 44*, 69–76.

Aram, D. M., & Nation, J. E. (1980). Preschool language disorders and subsequent language and academic difficulties. *Journal of Communication Disorders, 13*, 159–170.

Baker, L., & Cantwell, D. P. (1985). Psychiatric and learning disorders in children with communication disorders: A critical review. In K. D. Gadow (Ed.), *Advances in learning and behavioral disabilities* (pp. 4–32). Greenwich, Conn.: JAI Publishers.

Baker, L., & Cantwell, D. P. (1987a). Comparison of well, emotionally disordered, and behaviorally disordered children with linguistic problems. *Journal of the American Academy of Child and Adolescent Psychiatry, 26*, 190–196.

Baker, L., & Cantwell, D. P. (1987b). A prospective psychiatric follow-up of children with speech/language disorders. *Journal of American Child and Adolescent Psychiatry, 26,* 546–553.

Baltaxe, C. (1993). Pragmatic language disorders in children with social communication disorders and their treatment. (American-Speech Language-Hearing Association), *Neurophysiology and Neurogenic Speech and Language Disorders,* 3(1), 2–9.

Baltaxe, C. (in press). Prevalence of communication disorders in 400 children and adolescents with psychiatric disorders: A descriptive study. *Journal of Orthopsychiatry.*

Baltaxe, C., Russell, A., d'Angiola, N., & Simmons, J. Q. (1995). Discourse cohesion in the verbal interactions of individuals diagnosed with autistic disorder or schizotypal personality disorder. *Australian and New Zealand Journal of Communication Disorders,* 20(2), 79–96.

Baltaxe, C., & Simmons, J. Q. (1983). Communication deficits in adolescent and adult autistics. *Seminars in Speech and Language,* 4(1), 27–41.

Baltaxe, C., & Simmons, J. Q. (1987). Communication deficits in the adolescent with autism, schizophrenia, and language-learning disabilities. In T. L. Layton (Ed.), *Language and treatment of autistic and developmentally disordered children* (pp. 155–180). Springfield, Ill.: Thomas.

Baltaxe, C., & Simmons, J. Q. (1988a). Communication deficits in preschool children with psychiatric disorders. *Seminars in Language,* 9(1), 81–91.

Baltaxe, C., & Simmons, J. Q. (1988b). Pragmatic deficits in emotionally disturbed children and adolescents. In J. Schiefelbusch & L. Lloyd (Eds.), *Language perspectives: Acquisition, retardation, and intervention* (pp. 223–253). Austin, Tex.: Pro-Ed.

Baltaxe, C., & Simmons, J. Q. (1990). The differential diagnosis of communication disorders in child and adolescent psychopathology. *Topics in Language Disorders,* 10(4), 17–31.

Baltaxe, C., & Simmons, J. Q. (1991). *Communication disorders in children and adolescents with psychiatric disorders: Age related variables.* Paper presented at the Annual Meeting American Academy of Child and Adolescent Psychiatry, San Francisco.

Baltaxe, C., & Simmons, J. Q. (1992a). A comparison of language issues in high-functioning autism and related disorders with onset in childhood and adolescence. In E. Schopler & G. Mesibov (Eds.), *High-functioning individuals with autism* (pp. 201–225). New York: Plenum.

Baltaxe, C., & Simmons, J. Q. (1992b) Gender-related vulnerability to communication disorders in children and adolescents with psychiatric disorders. *Brain Dysfunction,* 5, 239–252.

Baltaxe, C., & Simmons, J. Q. (1995). Speech and language disorders in children and adolescents with schizophrenia. *Schizophrenia Bulletin,* 21(4), 125–140.

Bartak, L., & Rutter, M. (1975). Language and cognition in autistic and "dysphasic" children. In N. O'Connor (Ed.), *Language, cognitive deficit and retardation* (pp. 193–202). London: Butterworths.

Baumeister, J. J., Canino, G., & Bird, H. (1994). Epidemiology of disruptive behavior disorders. *Child and adolescent psychiatric clinics of North America*, 3(2), 177–194.

Baumgartner, S. (1980). The social behavior of speech disordered children as viewed by parents. *International Journal of Rehabilitative Research*, 3, 82–84.

Beery, K., & Buktenica, N. (1989). *Developmental Test of Visual Motor Integration*. Cleveland: Modern Curriculum Press.

Beitchman, J. H. (1985a). Childhood schizophrenia: A review and comparison with adult-onset schizophrenia. *Psychiatric Clinics of North America*, 8, 793–814.

Beitchman, J. H. (1985b). Speech and language impairment and psychiatric risk: Toward a model of neurodevelopmental immaturity. *Psychiatric Clinics of North America*, 8, 721–735.

Beitchman, J. H., Hood, J., & Inglis, A. (1990). Psychiatric risk in children with speech and language disorders. *Journal of Abnormal Child Psychology*, 18(3), 283–296.

Beitchman, J. H., Hood, J., Rochon, J., & Peterson, M. (1989a). Empirical classification of speech/language impairment in children, I: Identification of speech/language categories. *Journal of American Academy of Child and Adolescent Psychiatry*, 28, 112–117.

Beitchman, J. H., Hood, J., Rochon, J., & Peterson, M. (1989b). Empirical classification of speech/language impairment in children, II: Behavioral characteristics. *Journal of American Academy of Child and Adolescent Psychiatry*, 28, 118–123.

Beitchman, J. H., Nair, R., Clegg, M., Ferguson, B., & Patel, P. (1986a). Prevalence of psychiatric disorders in children with speech and language disorders. *Journal of the American Academy of Child Psychiatry*, 25, 528–535.

Beitchman, J. H., Nair, R., Clegg, M., Ferguson, B., & Patel, P. (1986b). Prevalence of speech and language disorders in 5-year-old kindergarten children in the Ottawa-Carleton region. *Journal of Speech and Hearing Disorders*, 51, 98–110.

Beitchman, J. H., Peterson, M., & Clegg, M. (1988). Speech and language impairment and psychiatric disorder: The relevance of family demographic variables. *Child Psychiatry and Human Development*, 18, 191–207.

Bellinger, D., Stiles, K., & Needleman, H. (1992). Low level lead exposure, intelligence and academic achievement: A long term follow-up study. *Pediatrics* 90(6), 855–861.

Bird, H. R., Gould, M. S., Yagert, T., Staghezza, R., & Canino, R. (1989). Risk factors for maladjustment in Puerto Rican children. *Journal of American Child and Adolescent Psychiatry*, 28, 847–850.

Blood, G. W., & Seiden, R. (1981). The concomitant problems of young stutterers. *Journal of Speech and Hearing Disorders*, 46, 31–33.

Bubenickova, M. (1977). The stuttering child's relation to school. *Psychologia a Patopsychologia Dietata*, 12, 535–545.

Butler, K. G. (1965). The Bender Gestalt Visual Motor Test as a diagnostic instrument with children exhibiting articulation disorders. *Asha, 7*, 380–381.

Caceres, V. A. (1971). Retardo del lenguaje verbal [Verbal language delay]. *Revista de Neuropsiquiatria, 34*, 210–226.

Camarata, S., Hughes, C., & Ruhl, K. (1988). Mild/moderate behaviorally disordered students: A population at risk for language disorders. *Language Speech and Hearing Services in the Schools, 19*, 191–200.

Cantwell, D. P., & Baker, L. (1977). Psychiatric disorder in children with speech and language retardation: A critical review. *Archives of General Psychiatry, 34*, 583–591.

Cantwell, D. P., & Baker, L. (1980). Psychiatric and behavioral characteristics of children with communication disorders. *Journal of Pediatric Psychology, 5*, 161–178.

Cantwell, D. P., & Baker, L. (1985). Psychiatric and learning disorders in children with speech and language disorders: A descriptive analysis. *Advances in Learning and Behavioral Disabilities, 4*, 29–47.

Cantwell, D. P., & Baker, L. (1987a). Clinical significance of childhood communication disorders: Perspectives from a longitudinal study. *Journal of Child Neurology, 2*, 257–264.

Cantwell, D. P., & Baker, L. (1987b). Prevalence and type of psychiatric disorder and developmental disorders in three speech and language groups. *Journal of Communicative Disorders, 20*, 151–160.

Cantwell, D. P., & Baker, L. (1991a). Association between attention deficit-hyperactivity disorder and learning disorders. *Journal of Learning Disabilities, 24*(2), 88–95.

Cantwell, D. P., & Baker, L. (1991b). *Psychiatric and developmental disorders in children with communication disorder.* Washington, D.C.: American Psychiatric Press.

Cantwell, D. P., & Baker, L. (1992). Attention deficit disorder with and without hyperactivity: A review and comparison of matched groups. *Journal of the American Academy of Child and Adolescent Psychiatry, 31*(3), 432–438.

Castellanos, F., & Rapoport, J. (1992). Etiology of attention-deficit hyperactivity disorder. *Child and Adolescent Psychiatric Clinics of North America, 1*, 373–384.

Chess, S., & Rosenberg, M. (1974). Clinical differentiation among children with initial language complaints. *Journal of Autism and Childhood Schizophrenia, 4*, 99–109.

Cohen, N. J., Davine, M., Horodesky, N., Lipsett, L., & Isaacson, L. (1993). Unsuspected language impairment in psychiatrically disturbed children: Prevalence and language and behavioral characteristics. *Journal of the American Academy of Child and Adolescent Psychiatry, 33*(3), 595–603.

Costello, E. J., Costello, A. J., Edelbrock, C., et al. (1988). Psychiatric disorders in pediatric primary care: Prevalence and risk factors. *Archives of General Psychiatry, 45*, 1107–1116.

Crowther, J. H., Bond. L. A., & Rolf, J. E. (1981). The incidence, prevalence, and severity of behavior disorders among preschool-aged children in day care. *Journal of Abnormal Child Psychiatry, 9,* 23–42.

Dunn, L. M., & Dunn, L. M. (1997). *Peabody Picture Vocabulary Test–III.* Circle Pines, Minn.: American Guidance Service.

Duncan, M. H. (1947). Personality adjustment techniques in voice therapy. *Journal of Speech Disorders, 12,* 161–167.

Earls, F. (1987). Sex differences in psychiatric disorders: Origins and developmental influences. *Psychiatric Development, 5,* 1–23.

Esser, G., Schmidt, M., & Woerner, W. (1990). Epidemiology and course of psychiatric disorders in school-age children: Results of a longitudinal study. *Journal of Child Psychology and Psychiatry, 31,* 243.

Exner, J. E. (1993). *The Rorschach: A comprehensive system* (3rd ed.). New York: Wiley.

Ferry, P. C., Hall, S. M., & Hicks, J. L. (1975). Dilapidated speech: Developmental verbal dyspraxia. *Developmental Medical Child Neurology, 17,* 749–756.

Fitzsimons, R. (1958). Developmental, psychosocial, and educational factors in children with nonorganic articulation problems. *Child Development, 29,* 481–489.

Fundudis, T., Kolvin, I., & Garside, R. (1979). *Speech retarded and deaf children: Their psychological development.* New York: Academic.

Gardner, M. F. (1983). *Expressive One Word Picture Vocabulary Test.* Novato, Calif.: Academic.

Gardner, M. F. (1996). *Test of Auditory Perceptual Skills–Revised.* San Francisco: Children's Hospital of San Francisco.

Gemilli, R. J. (1982). Classification of child stuttering, I: Transient developmental, neurogenic acquired, and persistent child stuttering. *Child Psychiatry and Human Development, 12,* 220–253.

Glasner, P. J. (1949). Personality characteristics and emotional problems of stutterers under the age of five. *Journal of Speech and Hearing Disorders, 14,* 135–138.

Gould, M. S., Wunsch-Hitzig, R., & Dohrenwend, B. P. (1980). Formulation of hypotheses about the prevalence, treatment, and prognostic significance of psychiatric disorders in children in the United States. In B. P. Dohrenwend, M. B. Dohrenwend, & M. S. Gould (Eds.), *Mental illness in the United States: Epidemiological estimates* (pp. 9–44). New York: Praeger.

Graham, P. (1986). *Child psychiatry: A developmental approach.* Oxford, U.K.: Oxford Medical Publications.

Griffiths, C. P. S. (1969). A follow-up study of children with disorders of speech. *British Journal of Disordered Communication, 4,* 46–56.

Grinnell, S. W., Scott-Hartnett, D., & Larson-Glasier, J. L. (1983). Language disorders [Letter to the editor]. *Journal of the American Academy of Child Psychiatry, 22,* 580–581.

Gualtieri, C. T., Koriath, U., Van Bourgondien, M., & Saleeby, N. (1983). Language disorders in children referred for psychiatric services. *Journal of the American Academy of Child Psychiatry, 22,* 165–171.

Hagerman, R. J., & Falkenstein, A. R. (1987). An association between recurrent otitis media in infancy and later hyperactivity. *Clinical Pediatrics, 26,* 253–257.

Hammill, D. (1995). *Detroit Test of Learning Aptitude–3.* Austin,Tex.: Pro-Ed.

Harper, D. C., & Richman, L. C. (1978). Personality profiles of physically impaired adolescents. *Journal of Clinical Psychology, 34,* 636–642.

Harris, D. (1963). *Children's drawings as measures of intellectual maturity.* New York: Harcourt Brace.

Hier, D. B., & Kaplan, J. (1980). Are sex differences in cerebral organization clinically significant? *Behavioral Brain Science, 3,* 238–239.

Hindley, P. A., Hill, P. D., McGuigan, S., & Kitson, N. (1994). Psychiatric disorder in deaf and hearing impaired children and young people: A prevalence study. *Journal of Child Psychology and Psychiatry and Allied Disciplines, 35*(4), 917–934.

Hull, F. M., Mielke, P. W., Jr., Timmons, R. J., & Willeford, P. A. (1971). The national speech and hearing survey: Preliminary results. *Asha, 13,* 501–509.

The Individuals with Disabilities Education Act Amendments of 1997 (IDEA97), P.L. No. 105–17. U.S.C. Secs. 1400–1485.

Kapp, K. (1979). Self-concept of the cleft lip and/or palate child. *Cleft Palate Journal, 16,* 171–176.

Koppitz, E. (1964). *The Bender Gestalt Test for Young Children.* New York: Grune & Stratton.

Lerner, J. A., Inui, T. S., Trupin, E. W., et al. (1985). Preschool behavior can predict future psychiatric disorders. *Journal of the American Academy of Child Psychiatry, 24,* 42-48.

Loomis, S., & Alessi, N. E. (1988, October). *Speech/language disorders in a group of child psychiatric inpatients.* Paper presented at the 35th annual meeting of the American Academy of Child and Adolescent Psychiatry, Seattle.

Love, A. J., & Thompson, M. G. (1988). Language disorders and attention deficit disorders in young children referred for psychiatric services: Analysis of prevalence and a conceptual synthesis. *American Journal of Orthopsychiatry, 58,* 52–64.

Ludlow, C., & Cooper, J. (1983). *Genetic aspects of speech and language disorders.* New York: Academic.

McGee, R., Partridge, F., Williams, S., et al. (1991). A twelve year follow-up of preschool hyperactive children. *Journal of the American Academy of Child and Adolescent Psychiatry, 30,* 224.

McGee, R., Williams, S., & Feehan, M. (1992). Attention deficit disorder and age of onset of problem behaviors. *Journal of Abnormal Child Psychiatry, 20*(5), 487–502.

McWilliams, B. J., & Musgrave, R. H. (1972). Psychological implications of articulation disorders in cleft palate children. *Cleft Palate Journal, 9,* 294–303.

Milisen, R. (1971). The incidence of speech disorders. In L. Travis (Ed.), *Handbook of speech pathology and audiology* (pp. 619–633). Englewood Cliffs, N.J.: Prentice-Hall.

Miller, J. (1981). *Assessing language production in children: Experimental procedures*. Baltimore: University Park Press.

Muma, J. R., Leader, R. L., & Webb, C. E. (1968). Adolescent voice quality aberrations: Personality and social status. *Journal of Speech and Hearing Research, 11*, 576–582.

Murray, H. (1971). *Thematic Apperception Test*. Cambridge, Mass.: Harvard University Press.

Needleman, H. (1995, March). *Childhood lead poisoning*. Paper presented at Johns Hopkins Conference on Neurodevelopmental Disabilities, Baltimore.

Neils, J., & Aram, D. M. (1986). Family history of children with developmental language disorders. *Perceptual Motor Skills, 63*, 655–658.

O'Callaghan, E., Larkin, C., & Waddington, J. L. (1990). Obstetric complications in schizophrenia and the validity of maternal recall. *Psychological Medicine, 20*(1), 89–94.

Offord, D. R., Boyle, M. H., Szatmari, P., Rae-Grant, N. I., Links, P. S., Cadman, D. T., Byles, J. A., Crawford, J. W., Byrne, C., Thomas, H., & Woodward, C. A. (1987). Ontario child health study. II. Six-month prevalence of disorder and raters of service utilization. *Archives of General Psychiatry, 44*, 69–76.

Ounsted, M., Moar, V. A., & Scott, A. (1986). Factors affecting development: Similarities and differences among children who were small, average, and large for gestational age at birth. *Acta Paediatrica Scandanavica, 75*, 261–266.

Prizant, B., Audet, L., Burke, G., Hummel, L., Maher, S., & Theodore, G. (1988). *Serving children and adolescents with communication disorders and emotional/behavioral disorders*. Paper presented at the annual convention of the American Speech-Language-Hearing Association, Boston.

Prizant, B., Audet, L., Burke, G., Hummel, L., Maher, S., & Theodore., G. (1990). Communication disorders and emotional/behavioral disorders in children and adolescents. *Journal of Speech and Hearing Disorders, 55*, 179–192.

Rapoport, D., Gill, M., & Schafer, R. (1968). *Diagnostic psychological testing* (rev. ed.). New York: International Universities.

Rogeness, G. A. (1994). Biologic findings in conduct disorder. *Child and Adolescent Psychiatric Clinics of North America, 3*(2), 217–284.

Rorschach, H. (1942). *Psychodiagnostics: A diagnostic test based on perception* (P. Lenkau & B. Kronenburg, trans.). New York: Grune & Stratton.

Ruess, A. L. (1965). A comparative study of cleft palate children and their siblings. *Journal of Clinical Psychology, 21*, 354–360.

Rutter, M. (1971). Psychiatry. In J. Wortis (Ed.), *Mental retardation: An annual review* (Vol. 3, pp. 186–221). New York: Grune & Stratton.

Rutter, M., Cox, A., Tupling, C., Berger, S., & Yule, R. (1975). Attainment and adjustment in two geographical areas, I: The prevalence of psychiatric disorder. *British Journal of Psychiatry, 126*, 493–509.

Rutter, M., & Martin, J. (Eds.). (1972). *The child with delayed speech.* London: Heinemann.

Rutter, M., Tizard, J., & Whitmore, K. (1970). *Education, health, and behavior.* London: Longman.

Schweckendiek, W., & Danzer, C. (1970). Psychological studies in patients with clefts. *Cleft Palate Journal, 7,* 533–539.

Semel, E., Wiig, E., & Secord, W. (1987). *Clinical Evaluation of Language Fundamentals–Revised.* San Antonio: Psychological Corporation.

Semel, E., Wiig, E., & Secord, W. (1995). *Clinical Evaluation of Language Fundamentals–3.* San Antonio: Psychological Corporation.

Shaffer, D. (1986). Brain damage. In M. Rutter & L. Hersov (Eds.), *Child and adolescent psychiatry: Modern approaches* (pp. 129–151). Oxford, U.K.: Blackwell Scientific Publications.

Sheridan, M. D., & Peckham, C. S. (1973). Hearing and speech at seven. *Special Education, 62,* 16–20.

Shriberg, L., Kwiatkowski, J., Best, S., et al. (1986). Characteristics of children with phonologic disorders of unknown origin. *Journal of Speech and Hearing Disorders, 51,* 140–161.

Simonds, J. F., & Heimburger, R. E. (1978). Psychiatric evaluation of youth with cleft lip-palate matched with a control group. *Cleft Palate Journal, 15,* 193–201.

Slater, E., Beard, A. W., & Clithero, E. (1963). The schizophrenia-like psychoses of epilepsy. *British Journal of Psychiatry, 109,* 95–105.

Solomon, A. I. (1961). Personality and behavior patterns of children with functional defects of articulation. *Child Development, 32,* 731–737.

Spriesterbach, D. C. (1973). *Psychosocial aspects of "the cleft palate problem"* (Vol. 1). Iowa City: University of Iowa Press.

Steinberg, D. (1985). Psychotic and other disorders in adolescence. In M. Rutter & L. Hersov (Eds.), *Children and adolescent psychiatry: Modern approaches* (pp. 567–583). Oxford, U.K.: Blackwell Scientific Publications.

Stevenson, J. E., & Richman, N. (1976). The prevalence of language delay in a population of three-year-old children and its association with general retardation. *Developmental Medical Child Neurology, 18,* 431–441.

Stevenson, J. E., & Richman, N. (1978). Behavior, language and development in three-year-old children. *Journal of Autism and Childhood Schizophrenia, 8,* 299–313.

Stewart, J. M. (1981). Multidimensional scaling analysis of communicative disorders by race and sex in a mid-south public school system. *Journal of Communicative Disorders, 14,* 467–483.

Stewart, J. M., & Spells, V. R. (1983). Learning disabilities with communicative disorders as related disorders: A two year study. *Journal of Communicative Disorders, 16,* 345–355.

Szatmari, P. (1992). The epidemiology of attention-deficit hyperactivity disorders. *Child and Adolescent Psychiatric Clinics of North America, 1*(2), 361–372.

Theodore, G., Maher, S., & Prizant, B. (1990). Early assessment and intervention with emotional and behavioral disorders and communication disorders. *Topics in Language Disorders, 10*(4), 42–56.

Tomblin, J. B., Records, N. L., Buckwalter, P., Zhang, X., Smith, E., & O'Brien, M. (1997). Prevalence of specific language impairment in kindergarten children. *Journal of Speech, Language, and Hearing Research, 40,* 1245–60.

Trapp, E. P., & Evan, J. (1960). Functional articulatory defect and performance on a non-verbal task. *Journal of Speech and Hearing Disorders, 25,* 176–180.

Trautman, J., Giddan, J. J., & Jurs, S. (1990). Language risk factors in emotionally disturbed children within a school and day treatment program. *Journal of Child Communication Disorders, 13,* 123–133.

U.S. Department of Education. (1999). Assistance to states for the education of children with disabilities and the early intervention program for infants and toddlers with disabilities: Final regulations. *Federal Register, 64*(48), 12405–12454.

Velez, C. N., Johnson, J., & Cohen, P. (1988). The children in the community project: A longitudinal analysis of selected risk factors for childhood psychopathology. *Journal of the American Academy of Child and Adolescent Psychiatry, 28,* 861–864.

Volkmar, F. R., & Cohen, D. (1994). Autism: Current concepts. *Child and Adolescent Psychiatric Clinics of North America, 3*(1), 43–52.

Volkmar, F. R., & Nelson, D. S. (1990). Seizure disorders in autism. *Journal of the American Academy of Child and Adolescent Psychiatry, 29*(1), 127–129.

Wagner, M. (1995). *Outcomes for youth with serious emotional disturbance in secondary school and early adulthood. The Future of Children (Critical Issues for Children and Youths),* 5(2), Menlo Park, Calif.: David and Lucille Packard Foundation.

Wagner, M., Newman, L., & Shaver, B. (1993). *The national longitudinal transition study of special education students: Sample characteristics and procedures.* Menlo Park, Calif.: SRI International.

Weber, E., & Baltaxe, C. (1995). Self-initiated repair in the talk of a catatonic schizophrenic patient. *Rocky Mountain Journal of Communication Disorders, 11*(3), 22–28.

Wiig, E., & Secord, W. (1988). *Test of Language Competence.* San Antonio, Tex.: Psychological Corporation.

Wilcox, J., & Nasrallah, H. (1987). Childhood head trauma and psychosis. *Psychiatry Research, 21,* 303–306.

Wolff, S., Narayan, S., & Moyes, B. (1988). Personality characteristics of parents of autistic children: A controlled study. *Journal of Child Psychology and Psychiatry, 29,* 143–153.

Wyatt, G. L. (1958). Mother-child relationship and stuttering in children. *Dissertation Abstracts, 19,* 881.

Zachman, L., Barrett, M., Huisingh, R., Orman, J., & Blagden, C. (1991). *Test of Problem Solving.* East Moline, Ill.: LinguiSystems.

Attention Deficit/ Hyperactivity Disorder in Young Children

Jane J. Giddan, MA, CCC-SLP
Medical College of Ohio
Toledo
and
Leonard Milling, Ph.D.
Medical College of Ohio
Toledo

Key Terms

behavioral disinhibition
behavior modification
cognitive-behavioral strategies
distractibility

hyperactivity
impulsivity
inattention
psychostimulants

Overview

What is the most common behavior problem for which school-age children are referred to medical, mental health, and allied health professionals? Undoubtedly, many professionals would argue that the answer to this question is attention deficit/hyperactivity disorder (AD/HD), a pattern of excessive impulsivity, overactivity and inattention. Not only is AD/HD a frequently encountered problem in school and clinical settings that serve children, it has also been the subject of an enormous amount of research and scholarly writing. For example, more than 700 empirical studies of AD/HD have been published since 1990 alone. Moreover, a number of important books (R. Barkley, 1990; R. A. Barkley, 1981; Ross & Ross, 1982) and monographs (Conners & Wells, 1986; Hinshaw, 1994) have appeared that extensively analyze the vast scientific literature on this disorder. It is not possible in the relatively short space of this chapter to review comprehensively the empirical literature on AD/HD. Rather, we attempt to offer an overview of current knowledge about AD/HD with a special emphasis on the communication features that may be of particular interest to many readers of this volume.

DEFINITION AND CLASSIFICATION

Through the years, the problem that is now commonly referred to as **hyperactivity** has been described as a defect in moral control (Still, 1902), minimal brain dysfunction (Strauss & Lehtinen, 1947), hyperactive child syndrome (Chess, 1940; Laufer & Denhoff, 1957), Hyperkinetic Reaction of Childhood (American Psychiatric Association [APA] 1968), Attention Deficit Disorder (APA, 1980), Attention Deficit Hyperactivity Disorder (APA, 1987), and most recently, Attention Deficit/Hyperactivity Disorder (APA, 1994). As currently conceptualized, youngsters with AD/HD are thought to evidence three main symptoms—inattention, overactivity, and impulsivity (Barkley, 1990; Hinshaw, 1994).

The first primary symptom of AD/HD is chronic **inattention**. Compared to other youngsters, children with AD/HD are thought to have difficulty sustaining attention (Douglas, 1983), especially to tasks that are not intrinsically interesting or that do not incorporate immediate reinforcements or consequences for persistence and completion (Barkley, 1990). According to some professionals, these children are easily distracted by extraneous stimuli (APA, 1994), although there is not a consensus on this feature (Barkley, 1990). Perhaps as a consequence of inattention, these youngsters tend to be careless and disorganized. They are often forgetful and lose things easily. They have difficulty following through, particularly on schoolwork, homework, and chores. These children often appear to be daydreaming and act as if they are not listening even when spoken to directly (APA, 1994).

The second primary symptom of AD/HD is chronic overactivity that includes elevated motor and verbal behavior. Youngsters with AD/HD tend to exhibit excessive motor activity (Halperin, Matier, Bedi, Sharma, & Newcorn, 1992; Porrino et al., 1983), which may be particularly evident in structured situations (Luk, 1985; Roberts, 1990; Routh & Schroeder, 1976). Accordingly, these children talk immoderately, fidget, squirm, and have difficulty staying seated or playing quietly. They are commonly described as "always on the go" or as "driven by a motor" (APA, 1994).

The third primary symptom of AD/HD is chronic **impulsivity**. By impulsivity, we mean an inability to delay responding in reaction to situational demands. Youngsters with AD/HD have been found to respond more quickly and inaccurately to tasks (Barkley, DuPaul, & McMurray, 1990; Brown & Wynne, 1977; Milich & Kramer, 1985) and to suffer from an inability to delay gratification (Rapport, Tucker, DuPaul, Merlo, & Stoner, 1986). Thus, these children are more likely to blurt out answers, to interrupt others, and to experience difficulty awaiting their turn (APA, 1994).

Although disagreements continue about the nature of the main symptoms of AD/HD, there appears to be growing recognition that at least some of the conflict is a function of the multidimensional nature of inattention, overactivity, and impulsivity (Barkley, 1990; Hinshaw, 1994; Milich & Kramer, 1985). That is, the specific aspects or dimensions of the constructs that characterize AD/HD have not yet been fully specified. Studies of how the three main sets of AD/HD symptoms cluster together have shown that there are two, rather than three, primary dimensions (Bauermeister, Alegria, Bird, Rubio-Stipec, & Canino, 1992; Lahey et al., 1988). One dimension includes the symptoms of inattention, while the other dimension consists of the referents of overactivity and impulsivity. To characterize this second dimension, Barkley (1990) has invoked the overarching term, **behavioral disinhibition**. A more detailed discussion of what is meant by behavioral disinhibition follows in the section of this chapter on theories of etiology. It is important to distinguish between descriptive factors and causal factors. For example, Barkley appears to have questioned whether inattention might not be a descriptive symptom of AD/HD that is secondary to (i.e., caused by) impulsivity.

The *Diagnostic and Statistical Manual of Mental Disorders, 4th Edition (DSM-IV)* (APA, 1994), describes the basic criteria for AD/HD (Table 3-1). There are several patterns of AD/HD. Attention-Deficit/Hyperactivity Disorder, Combined Type is diagnosed if both criteria A and B are met. The label Attention-Deficit/Hyperactivity Disorder, Predominantly Inattentive Type, is applied if the symptoms of hyperactivity-impulsivity are not present,

Table 3-1. Diagnostic Criteria for Attention Deficit/Hyperactivity Disorder

A. Six or more developmentally inappropriate symptoms of inattention of at least six months duration.
B. Six or more developmentally inappropriate symptoms of hyperactivity-impulsivity of at least six months duration.
C. Some symptoms present before age 7 years.
D. Clinically significant impairment in social, academic or occupational functioning, some of which is evident in two or more settings (e.g., school and home).
E. The symptoms are not due to Pervasive Developmental Disorder, Schizophrenia, or other Psychotic Disorder and are not better accounted for by some other mental disorder.

(Reprinted with permission from the *Diagnostic and statistical manual of mental health disorders [4th edition].* American Psychiatric Association [1994]. Washington, D.C.).

whereas Attention-Deficit/Hyperactivity Disorder, Predominantly Hyperactive-Impulsive Type is utilized if the symptoms of inattention are not evident. Finally, Attention Deficit/Hyperactivity Disorder Not Otherwise Specified is diagnosed when the symptoms of inattention or hyperactivity-impulsivity are present but do not meet the criteria for the other types of AD/HD enumerated previously.

ONSET AND PROGNOSIS

In order to establish a diagnosis of AD/HD as specified by *DSM-IV*, at least some of the symptoms of impulsivity, overactivity, and inattention must have been present before age 7. Indeed, several studies have shown that the mean age of onset of AD/HD symptoms is between 3 and 4 (Barkley, Fisher, Edelbrock, & Smallish, 1990). Certainly, by shortly after the beginning of first grade, the behavior of most children with AD/HD has come to the attention of teachers and parents because the school environment is particularly taxing for youngsters who have difficulty sitting still, following directions, staying on-task, and delaying gratification (Barkley, 1990). Like children who are developing typically, youngsters with AD/HD will show improvements in their impulse control, activity level, and attention skills as they age. However, the trajectory of their development in these key areas will be lower than that of their counterparts who are not hyperactive.

Previously, it was believed that the prognosis of AD/HD was benign and that most children would "outgrow" the disorder. However, empirical research has proven this bit of clinical lore to be inaccurate. Recent prospective studies have shown that over two-thirds of children diagnosed with AD/HD continue to meet the diagnostic criteria for this disorder in their mid to late teens (Barkley, Fischer, et al., 1990; Brown & Borden, 1986; Gittelman, Mannuzza, Shenker, & Bonagura, 1985; Klein & Mannuzza, 1991; Mannuzza et al., 1991; Thorley, 1984). Sadly, less than a third of youngsters with AD/HD experience a remission of symptoms by the time they reach early adulthood. There have been few studies of the course of AD/HD into adulthood, but the little existing evidence suggests that 50 to 65 percent of the individuals who were diagnosed with AD/HD in childhood continue to have problems with impulsivity, overactivity, and inattention as adults (Gittelman et al., 1985; Klein & Mannuzza, 1991). It is somewhat dismaying to note that at least 20 to 45 percent of children with AD/HD will have problems with antisocial behavior as adults, with about 25 percent meeting the criteria for Antisocial Personality Disorder.

PREVALENCE

It is estimated that from 3 to 5 percent of school-age children meet the criteria for AD/HD (APA, 1994). Similar figures have been reported for school-age children in Canada (Szatmari, Offord, & Boyle, 1989), New Zealand

(Anderson, Williams, McGee, & Silva, 1987), Puerto Rico (Bird et al., 1988), Japan (Kanbayashi, Nakata, Fuji, Kita, & Wada, 1994), and Italy (O'Leary, Vivian, & Nisi, 1985). There is some evidence that the prevalence of AD/HD is somewhat greater among youngsters from lower socioeconomic backgrounds (Taylor, 1986; Trites, 1979). AD/HD is much more common among males than females, with ratios ranging from 4:1 to 9:1 (APA, 1994). However, the proportion of boys to girls tends to be greater in clinical samples, where males are overrepresented, than in samples drawn from the general population (Szatmari et al., 1989).

THEORIES OF ETIOLOGY

A variety of theories of etiology have been proposed to explain the development and maintenance of AD/HD. Many of these theories are mutually compatible in that (1) there may be a variety of etiological pathways to AD/HD, (2) the theories explain different AD/HD symptoms, and (3) the theories conceptualize AD/HD at different levels of abstraction (e.g., molecular, neurological explanations versus motor, behavioral explanations).

Neurological Dysfunction

Researchers and clinicians alike have long proposed neurological involvement in AD/HD, although the precise neurological structures or functions were never pinpointed. However, Barkley (1990) recently concluded that several lines of evidence point toward dysfunction in the pathways between the prefrontal cortex, particularly the striatum, and the limbic system (Heilman, Voeller, & Nadeau, 1991; Lou, Henriksen, & Bruhn, 1984; Lou, Henriksen, Bruhn, Borner, & Nielsen, 1989; Zametkin & Rapoport, 1986). First, cerebral spinal fluid studies indicate a dopamine deficiency in the brains of children with AD/HD (Raskin, Shaywitz, Shaywitz, Anderson, & Cohen, 1984). The prefrontal cortex is known to be particularly rich in dopamine in children who are developing typically. Second, some research has revealed decreased blood flow in the striatum and other prefrontal areas of the brains of youngsters with AD/HD (Lou et al., 1984, 1989). Finally, neuropsychological studies of frontal lobe functioning in children with AD/HD have yielded diminished scores on measures associated with the inhibition of behavior (Grodzinsky, 1990; Korkman & Pesonen, 1994; Mariani, 1990). In short, these various lines of research provide promising evidence that AD/HD is associated with dopamine depletion in the prefrontal cortex.

Genetic Transmission

Evidence in support of a genetic predisposition to AD/HD comes from three areas of research. First, Hauser et al. (1993) reported a distinct genetic anomaly that directly accounts for a small portion of the total cases of AD/HD. Second, several studies have shown a greater than expected prevalence of AD/HD among the biological relatives of children with AD/HD (Biederman et al., 1986; Deutsch et al., 1982; Faraone, Biederman, & Milberger, 1994; Safer, 1973; Schachar & Wachsmuth, 1990). These studies are noteworthy because they employed pure samples of youngsters with AD/HD rather than samples evidencing both hyperactive and conduct disordered behavior, thereby safeguarding against the possibility that the obtained results could reflect the heritability of aggression rather than AD/HD. Third, a number of studies have shown greater concordance of AD/HD among identical twins than among fraternal twins (Goodman & Stevenson, 1989; Lopez, 1965; Stevenson, 1992). Together, these sources of evidence suggest that genetic factors play a significant role in the transmission of AD/HD, although for most cases of the disorder, this genetic predisposition is likely to interact with other risk factors in a complex manner rather than presenting as a clear-cut genetic anomaly.

Prenatal and Perinatal Factors

Numerous prenatal and perinatal factors, including mother's age at conception, pregnancy and birth complications, as well as low birth weight, have been mentioned in connection with AD/HD, but epidemiological research generally has not found these influences to be strongly associated with the disorder (Goodman & Stevenson, 1989; Werner et al., 1968). Thus, it is unlikely that these prenatal and perinatal factors will be implicated in more than a small percentage of cases of AD/HD. The possible exceptions to this pattern are maternal cigarette smoking (Denson, Nanson, & McWatters, 1975; Nichols & Chen, 1981; Streissguth et al., 1984) and alcohol consumption (Bennett, Wolin, & Reiss, 1988; Shaywitz, Cohen, & Shaywitz, 1994; Streissguth et al., 1984). However, it is unclear whether the associations between maternal cigarette smoking/alcohol consumption and offspring with AD/HD indicate causality or simply correlation. Research indicates that adolescents with AD/HD are more likely to smoke cigarettes and consume alcohol. A noncausal correlation between cigarette smoking/alcohol consumption and AD/HD could arise because AD/HD is transmitted across generations genetically, giving rise to increased cigarette smoking and alcohol consumption in each generation of individuals with AD/HD.

Behavioral Disinhibition

Utilizing the principles of operant conditioning, Barkley (1990) conceptualized AD/HD as a deficiency in the regulation and inhibition of behavior. Specifically, Barkley indicated, "that the problem may rest in several deficits; (1) decreased control by partial schedules of behavioral consequences; (2)

rapid habituation or satiation to behavioral consequences, leading to rapid extinction of responding; and (3) diminished regulation of behavior by rules" (p. 70). Barkley's first point is that children with AD/HD are less likely to perform a behavior when only some of its occurrences are rewarded (i.e., partial reinforcement schedule) than when every occurrence of the behavior is rewarded (i.e., continuous reinforcement schedule). Unfortunately for youngsters with AD/HD, most naturalistic adaptive behaviors are rewarded on a partial, rather than a continuous, schedule of reinforcement.

Barkley's second point is that reinforcers (and punishments) lose their salience more quickly for children with AD/HD than for other children. This causes youngsters with AD/HD to stop performing a learned behavior sooner than other youngsters. For example, compared to other children, a youngster with AD/HD would more rapidly lose interest in earning candy pieces for each minute that he or she did homework.

Barkley's third point is that in comparison to other children, children with AD/HD are less able to control their behavior using "rules" (i.e., self-statements, beliefs, expectancies, or other linguistic cues indicating that if a behavior is performed, it is likely to be followed by a particular consequence). Rather, the behavior of children with AD/HD is more likely to be controlled by the immediate consequences for the behavior. So, for example, when asked to sit at a desk and do homework, a child with AD/HD is less likely to be influenced by the "rule" that "if I do my homework now, I will be able to watch TV after dinner" and more likely to be influenced by the questionable, but more immediate, pleasure of an activity such as playing with a pencil on the desktop.

Coercion Theory

Coercion theory explicates an unfortunate process that can develop when the behavior of an aggressor comes into conflict with the standards of a limit-setting agent (Patterson, 1982). If the limit-setting agent elects to placate the aggressor by relaxing the standards rather than enforcing them, it increases the likelihood that in the future, the aggressor will continue, and even escalate, the aggressive behavior. This is because the aggressor receives the immediate reward of attaining the goal of the aggressive behavior (i.e., positive reinforcement) and, at the same time, the limit-setting agent receives the immediate reward of escaping from conflict with the aggressor (i.e., negative reinforcement). Although coercion theory cannot explain the development of AD/HD symptoms, it does help us to understand how these behaviors are maintained and can even escalate. The impulsive and overactive behaviors of youngsters with AD/HD certainly provide parents and teachers with many opportunities to set limits. Inevitably, it is very tempting for some parents and teachers to give in to the seemingly relentless demands and transgressions of the youngsters with AD/HD in their care. Unfortunately, over the long run, this is bound to exacerbate rather than reduce existing behavior problems.

CLINICAL ASSESSMENT

Ideally, the assessment of AD/HD should yield a comprehensive biopsy-chosocial formulation that incorporates a combination of self-report, parent report, teacher report, clinician report, and laboratory measures. These measures should sample the child's functioning in the home, school, peer, cognitive, affective, and medical domains.

Rating Scales

Rating scales are perhaps the most common assessment tool, and of these, the *Child Behavior Checklist* (CBCL), (Achenbach, 1991) provides a particularly well-constructed and well-normed measure of the symptoms of AD/HD, as well as a broad array of other symptoms clusters. Another advantage of the CBCL is that there are comparable versions for parents and teachers (as well as an analogous self-report measure for adolescents).

Structured or Unstructured Clinical Interviews

Clinical interviews with the child's parents are very important. In particular, parent interviews should be utilized to gather information about family, medical, and developmental history, including such risk factors as: (a) family history of AD/HD; (b) low parental academic achievement; (c) maternal health problems, smoking, and alcohol consumption during pregnancy; (d) only one parent in the home; (e) poor health and developmental delays during infancy; and (f) excessive activity level and demandingness during infancy (Barkley, 1990). Information provided by the parents should be supplemented by a telephone interview with the child's teacher.

A clinical interview with the youngster is probably a standard element of every child assessment. However, clinicians should keep the following caveats in mind. First, youngsters are likely to underreport symptoms when asked about their attention, level of motor activity, and impulse control problems. Second, the behavior of the child during the actual interview can be misleading. For many youngsters with AD/HD, the novelty and one-to-one attention of a clinical interview is sufficient to elicit behavior that is far more appropriate than their usual demeanor.

Standardized Measures of Cognitive Functioning

Standardized cognitive measures are often employed in the assessment of AD/HD. In particular, measures of intellectual functioning such as the Wechsler Intelligence Scales for Children-III (WISC-III), (Wechsler, 1991), and academic achievement such as the Wechsler Individual Achievement

Test (Wechsler, 1992) are typical mainstays of an overall assessment of cognitive functioning. However, these instruments will not be helpful in ruling out a diagnosis of AD/HD, and in particular, Barkley and his colleagues recommend against using Kaufman's (1975) freedom from distractibility factor on the WISC as a basis for measuring attention or diagnosing AD/HD (Anastopolous, Spisto, & Maher, 1994; Barkley, 1990). Compared to intellectual and achievement tests, neuropsychological measures of frontal lobe functioning might be more valuable in assessing the cognitive capacity of youngsters with AD/HD, but this is a luxury that is not available to most clinicians.

Continuous Performance Tests

One of the continuous performance tests developed to test AD/HD, the Gordon Diagnostic System (GDS), (Gordon, 1983) is said to have adequate psychometric and normative properties for use in clinical settings (Barkley, 1990). The GDS is classified as a continuous performance test that measures vigilance. On the GDS, the child must press a button each time a particular numerical sequence appears on the screen. The test is scored for errors of omission (i.e., neglecting to push the button when the appropriate sequence appears) and errors of commission (i.e., pushing the button when the wrong sequence of numbers has appeared). Omission errors are thought to reflect inattention, whereas commission errors are said to indicate both inattention and impulsivity.

Sociometric Measures

Several peer sociometric measures and direct observation systems have been employed in the assessment of AD/HD. However, their use is typically confined to research studies of this disorder. Some clinicians find it helpful to make informal observations of the child's behavior in naturalistic settings such as the classroom or playground.

Medical Evaluation

The child should receive a thorough pediatric medical examination. The purposes of the medical examination are to rule out medical conditions that may mimic the symptoms of AD/HD, to identify medical conditions that can co-occur with AD/HD, and determine whether there are conditions that contraindicate the use of certain medications (e.g., high blood pressure, cardiac difficulties, tic disorders, Tourette's syndrome). It may also be necessary to evaluate the need for referrals to specialists, such as psychiatrists, neurologists, or neuropsychologists.

Speech and Language Assessment

Speech and language assessment is critical, but often omitted. It is warranted for children with AD/HD, especially those who are having difficulty in school or are in special education placements, because linguistic delay is easily overlooked and may underlie some of their behaviors and learning difficulties (Giddan, 1991).

Speech-language pathologists have a wide array of tests and measures to evaluate the articulation, receptive and expressive language, listening skills, fluency, and vocal quality of these children, but adaptations must be made to manage the behaviors of AD/HD in evaluation sessions. Whether or not the child's behavior has been stabilized with medication and/or behavioral programming, strategies for assessment include using multiple, brief testing sessions and the creative application of frequent, interesting rewards to maintain involvement in the assessment tasks. Periodic hearing screenings are also useful. Recurrent otitis media may hamper listening ability for children who already have difficulty sustaining auditory and visual attention. Careful observation of communication across a variety of settings and communication partners can help determine the child's range of pragmatic skills and can offer broader samples of conversation and narratives for linguistic analysis. In addition, the speech-language pathologist can help determine whether language deficits are contributing factors to any social deficits that are exhibited.

COMMUNICATION FEATURES

Children with AD/HD complicated by comorbid speech and language delay are in "double jeopardy" for future problems with learning, socialization, and self-esteem. Ornoy, Uriel, and Tannenbaum (1993) found that overactivity, inattention, and disorders of language development in 2- to 4-year-olds predicted AD/HD in later school years for 80 percent of their sample.

Young children often cry, scream, or even throw tantrums at times when they lack the language to express their needs or share their feelings. Irritated caregivers may, in turn, react negatively by ignoring or punishing these nonverbal requests or demands. Often, when these active youngsters do not comprehend warnings, reprimands, and instructions, they are thought to be naughty or "bad" kids who "won't listen," and are subject to punishment or rejection. This negative spiral accelerates as these children continue to experience failures in social interactions with their parents and others. Their misbehaviors become reinforced as the way to get attention.

Children with AD/HD often act before they consider their actions or their impact on others. For those with linguistic deficits, there tends to be a concomitant immaturity or even an absence of the internalized self-talk needed to guide one's behavior (Berk & Landau, 1993). Problems of behavioral self-regulation then become quite evident in school settings where continued linguistic delays are also likely to be precursors to learning disabilities (Baker & Cantwell, 1992).

Contrasting features of communication style have been noted in children with AD/HD. On one hand, they seem overly talkative (Sandler et al., 1993). They may overwhelm the listener by speaking very quickly and saying more than is required in the situation. On the other hand, when they are responsible for sharing specific information, they may say too little, demonstrating difficulties in coherent reporting. They may mispronounce words or sound dysfluent, with excessive pauses or fillers (Barkley, 1990).

Pragmatics and Social Skills Deficits

Pragmatic deficits are inherent in the definition of AD/HD (APA, 1994). The items in Table 3-2 are listed as diagnostic criteria in DSM-IV and reflect impulsive behaviors in social situations that interfere with communication.

Impulsive behavior in social situations frequently involves unmonitored comments or other tactless reactions expressed at inappropriate times. These behaviors are annoying to peers, unproductive in play situations, and detrimental to social acceptance. Children with AD/HD misjudge or do not take into account the cues implicit in the situation, or else they fail to recognize, or may even distort, the nonverbal language of those around them. They have limited empathy, so they do not appreciate the impact of their actions on others, just as they do not appreciate the reactions of others. They fail to attend to the nonverbal cues from facial expression, body language, and vocal inflection, and they are limited in their capacity to share the mood of others or to put themselves in the shoes of another. They are intrusive in conversation, may shift topics abruptly, and disregard customary turn-taking rules of conversation (Baltaxe & Simmons, 1988a, 1988b; Humphries, Koltun, Malone, & Roberts, 1994). They may seem overly talkative (Sandler et al., 1993) and disorganized because they lack the planning, editing, and self-monitoring required to communicate successfully.

The pragmatic effects of impulsivity, high activity, and subsequent inattention render children with AD/HD awkward, if not inappropriate, at school or home. Clumsiness in ordinary discourse causes them to be rebuffed by

Table 3-2.   Pragmatic Features Derived from *DSM-IV* Diagnostic Criteria

- Often does not seem to listen when spoken to directly.
- Is often easily distracted by extraneous stimuli.
- Often talks excessively.
- Often blurts out answers before question has been completed.
- Often has difficulty awaiting turn.
- Often interrupts or intrudes on others (e.g., butts into conversation or games).

peers (Whalen & Henker, 1985), and sometimes painfully fooled or deceived by others; curiously, they appear to be very naive about relationships.

Comorbid Speech and Language Deficits

In more intensive special education, mental health, and psychiatric settings, we tend to see children who have both emotional and language problems. In mental health settings, the co-occurrence of communication and behavioral symptomatology is often considerable. Among preschoolers in Toronto family mental health clinics, 73 percent of the children were identified as AD/HD. Nearly 65 percent of them scored low on language measures (Love & Thompson, 1988).

In a special education program for children with severe behavior disorders, one-third were identified as AD/HD; 54 percent of that group had speech and language deficits (Trautman, Giddan, & Jurs, 1990). Similarly, in a psychiatric inpatient preadolescent unit, 67 percent of the children diagnosed as AD/HD were identified with communication problems (Giddan, Milling, & Campbell, 1996).

In an urban private psychiatric practice, 19 percent of 135 children identified with speech and language problems were labeled "hyperactive" (Chess & Rosenberg, 1974). Of child psychiatric inpatients who were of low socioeconomic status, 50 percent of those with language problems were designated as attention deficit disordered (Gualtieri, Koriath, Van Bourgondien, & Saleeby, 1983).

It is easy to see how speech and language delay, in combination with the inherent pragmatic deficits in AD/HD, can cause havoc with critical processes affecting communication efforts, social adjustment, and mental health. As children with linguistic delays are rejected by peers, they lose opportunities to develop social skills and social relationships. Self-esteem and self-image are affected, and isolation, loneliness, and depression can follow. Baker and Cantwell (1992) detected the greatest risk for negative outcomes among children with AD/HD with combined speech and language impairment; they found the least difficulty among those with articulation problems alone.

Central Auditory Processing

The identification and investigation of listening problems among individuals with AD/HD has stimulated a plethora of studies concerning central auditory processing disorder (CAPD.) The overlap of the characteristics of AD/HD and CAPD have led to questions about their distinctiveness (Keith & Engineer, 1991; Keller, 1992), as well as to conclusions about their comorbidity (Riccio, Hynd, Cohen, Hall, & Molt, 1994).

The confusion was exacerbated by the report of the American Speech-Language and Hearing Association (ASHA, 1992) Ad Hoc Committee of

CAPD, which added "possible" **distractibility** and "inattentiveness" to its definition, along with "potential difficulties in reading, spelling, written language and memory." The overlap of CAPD with both AD/HD and learning disabilities is clearly suggested. The committee report (ASHA, 1992) defines CAPD as "limitations in the ongoing transmission, analysis, organization, transformation, elaboration, storage, retrieval and use of information contained in audible signals" (p. 2).

McPherson and Davies (1995) suggest that immaturity of the neural system affects binaural processing in children with AD/HD. They believe binaural processing to be essential for "sound localizations, noise suppression, fusion of auditory signals, ability to identify a target sound in the presence of noise . . . and to attend to speech" (p. 47).

Studies that have tested children with AD/HD on measures of central auditory processing have found deficits in these areas (Keith & Engineer, 1991; Ludlow, Dudahy, Bassich & Brown, 1983). Conversely, when children with CAPD were examined for AD/HD, it was found that 50 percent met those diagnostic criteria (Gascon, Johnson, & Burd, 1986; Riccio et al., 1994). Some researchers have even suggested that it is the AD/HD that causes poor central auditory processing test performance (Gascon et al., 1986) and that CAPD as a discrete entity is rare.

The relationship of AD/HD and CAPD remains unclear and needs continued study. Some of the children who failed CAPD measures did not meet the criteria for AD/HD (Riccio et al., 1994), demonstrating that these symptom sets or disorders do not always coexist. Stimulant medication used to reduce symptoms of hyperactivity and inattention has also improved central auditory-processing performance (Gascon et al., 1986). Finally, children who meet the criteria for AD/HD have difficulty on measures of central auditory processing, even if they have normal language and reading skills (Gascon et al., 1986; Ludlow et al., 1983).

Learning Disabilities

In the search for mediating processes that might be associated with both learning disabilities and attention deficit disorder, Cantwell and Baker (1991) pointed to speech and language disorders. Their studies of 600 children in a speech and language clinic setting led them to two conclusions: first, AD/HD is quite common among the types of psychiatric problems of children who also have speech and language disorders, and second, the prevalence of learning disorders is higher in the children with behavior disorders who have comorbid speech and language disorders. They hypothesized an association between the psychiatric disorders and the learning disorders found in children with language impairment.

August and Garfinkel (1989) identified a "cognitive" subtype of AD/HD characterized by significant academic underachievement with skill deficits related to the encoding and retrieval of linguistic information. Shaywitz, Fletcher, and Shaywitz (1995) referred to a cognitive-inattentive type of AD/HD with similar characteristics. They suggested that learning disabilities tend to lie in this domain, with phonologically based language difficulties affecting both speaking and writing.

There is indeed an overlap between AD/HD and the symptoms and problems characteristic of a learning disability (LD). Baker and Cantwell (1992) reported that 40 percent of children with AD/HD in their study had learning problems. These learning problems can reflect early linguistic weakness (Cantwell & Baker, 1991; Shaywitz et al., 1995) as well as the types of information-processing problems and disorganized thinking (Barkley, 1990) that characterize this group.

TREATMENT

A variety of options are available for the treatment of children with AD/HD, ranging from pharmacological to behavioral and cognitive-behavioral interventions. The following sections provide an overview of these options.

Pharmacological Treatment

The medications of choice for AD/HD are the **psychostimulants** methylphenidate (Ritalin), dextroamphetamine (Dexedrine), and pemoline (Cylert). A full 70 to 80 percent of children with AD/HD respond positively to these medicines (Barkley, 1990), showing improvements in attention span and reductions in impulsive and disruptive behaviors. Children with AD/HD taking stimulant medications have been shown to sustain better attention to assigned tasks and to experience diminished extraneous restlessness and motor activity. Reductions are seen in aggressiveness and noncompliance, accompanied by improved responsiveness to parental commands and better social interactions (Barkley, 1990).

Stimulants seem to act on underaroused areas in the frontal lobe and limbic system (Barkley, 1990, p. 576). Studies have shown that stimulant medications increase blood flow activity in the areas that underlie aspects of response inhibition, inattention, and sensitivity to reinforcement (Barkley, 1990).

Side effects of stimulants include decreased appetite, insomnia, weight loss, and irritability. Ritalin may temporarily slow growth in some children, but they regain expected height when the medicine is periodically stopped (Barkley, 1990). Sleep problems can be addressed by shifting the last dose of the day to an earlier hour. The drug can have adverse effects in children with a history of psychosis, hypertension, or seizures. In cases where tics or twitches are observed, medication should be changed, as Ritalin can unmask an underlying Tourette's syndrome.

Barkley administered Ritalin to preschoolers (1988) and found that even at low doses (.5 mg), behaviors were positively affected, and consequently, conflicts with parents were reduced. In older children (Hinshaw, Whalen, & Henker, 1984), the combination of Ritalin plus cognitive behavioral intervention enhanced cooperation and other appropriate social interactions.

It can be reassuring for families to know that the long-term use of these medications is not considered addicting (*Physician's Desk Reference*, 1995), nor is their use likely to lead to addiction to other drugs. This is fortunate, as about one-third of individuals with AD/HD will continue to be candidates for psychostimulants into their adult years (Barkley, 1990).

Clonidine (Catapres), a medication developed for the treatment of high blood pressure, is often used in combination with Ritalin. It can reduce aggression and anger and is helpful in managing sleep schedules, but its positive effects may not be seen for 2 to 4 months.

The tricyclic antidepressants imipramine (Tofranil) and desipramine (Norpramin) are alternate medicines frequently used for children who do not respond to Ritalin or who experience troubling side effects from it. They are slower-acting than stimulants, with side effects that can include dry mouth and increases in blood pressure and heart rate. Baseline electrocardiogram (EKG), pulse, and blood pressure measures are necessary. These medicines may increase the risk of seizures, especially for individuals in whom there has been previous neurological insult (Dulcan, 1992).

The tricyclic antidepressants are useful for children who have AD/HD plus anxiety or depression, although it takes several weeks to obtain therapeutic effects. The newer selective serotonin reuptake inhibitors (SSRIs), like fluoxetine (Prozac) and sertraline (Zoloft), are also available for treating the comorbid depression and anxiety; research is just beginning on their effectiveness.

Many people wonder if Ritalin and the other medications may be overprescribed. From our point of view, the issue is not that Ritalin is overprescribed but rather that AD/HD may be overdiagnosed. Our review suggests that Ritalin is clearly the treatment of choice (Pelham et al., 1993) for children who truly have AD/HD. The problem is distinguishing those with AD/HD from children with other disruptive disorders like oppositional defiant disorder and conduct disorder, where psychostimulants have a less clear impact.

Behavioral Interventions

Variously referred to as **behavior modification**, applied behavior analysis, behavior management, or contingency management, the behavioral intervention approach is based on the principles of operant conditioning. A behavioral intervention for children with AD/HD is usually implemented through operating a contingency management program in the classroom or by training parents in the principles and methods of contingency management. Whether at home or in school, the typical behavioral program utilizes a combination of positive reinforcement, response cost, and time-out periods. The positive reinforcement component of such a program is intended to provide immediate, systematic rewards for desirable behaviors such as compliance, on-task behaviors, or completing homework. The response cost component involves the immediate, systematic loss of rewards for undesirable behaviors such as defiance, off-task behavior, or failing to complete chores. The time-out component entails removing access to rewards for inappropriate behavior, such as secluding a child so that he or she will not receive social attention for disruptive behavior.

A relatively large empirical literature on the use of contingency management in the classroom has shown these programs to be very useful in promoting on task-behavior and improved academic performance in youngsters with AD/HD, as well as in decreasing their disinhibited and disorderly behavior (Pelham et al., 1993; Robinson, Newby, & Ganzell, 1981). Also, some literature has demonstrated the efficacy of parent training in contingency management at home (Bidder, Gray, & Newcombe, 1978; Dubey, O'Leary, & Kaufman, 1983; Firestone, Kelly, Goodman, & Davey, 1981; O'Leary, Pelham, Rosenbaum, & Price, 1976; Pisterman et al., 1989; Pollard, Ward, & Barkley, 1983). Unfortunately, there is little, if any, evidence that the benefits of contingency management generalize to situations where the program is not in place or continue after the program has ended (Hinshaw, 1994).

The combination of contingency management programming with stimulant medication does not appear to have a benefit greater than either intervention by itself (Firestone et al., 1981; Pollard et al., 1983; Wolraich, Drummond, Saloman, O'Brien, & Sivage, 1978). Furthermore, although increased academic productivity and diminished disruptive behavior have been found with behavior management techniques, the gains are not as strong as from stimulant medication alone (Pelham et al., 1993). Although stimulants may be the preferred treatment for many youngsters with AD/HD (Abikoff & Gittelman, 1984), contingency management can still be of benefit during the late afternoon and evening, when the effects of medication may have worn off, or during weekends and vacations, when medication might not be used.

Cognitive-Behavioral Interventions

Cognitive-behavioral strategies emphasize training the child with AD/HD in adaptive cognitive skills such as self-monitoring, self-reinforcement, and self-instruction. Self-monitoring involves having the child keep track of his or her own target behaviors. In self-reinforcement, the child tracks personal target behaviors and obtains rewards contingent on performance of those behaviors. Self-instruction involves having the professional use verbal directives to guide the child's behavior. Later, the child is taught to utilize external and internal speech to regulate his or her own actions. While there are some data suggesting the utility of self-monitoring and self-reinforcement (Barkley, 1989), there is little evidence that self-instruction training is of benefit to youngsters with AD/HD (Abikoff & Gittelman, 1985; Hinshaw & Erhardt, 1993). Considered along with the research on contingency management, what seems clear is that systematic reinforcements, delivered either by oneself or by others, are of benefit to children with AD/HD; however, the gains do not generalize across time or place to situations where the program is not actively implemented (Barkley, 1989).

COMMUNICATION INTERVENTION WITH CHILDREN WITH AD/HD

To work effectively with children with AD/HD in speech and language treatment settings, professionals need to understand the principles of behavioral management. These children require, above all, consistency of program structure and routine to help them organize themselves in time, in space, and, perhaps most importantly, in function. They need schedules and accompanying aids for organizing themselves and their tasks throughout the day. In therapy they can be given responsibility for determining the order of activities from a small set of possible tasks. The sequence can then be posted in pictures or print for them to follow. Motor activities are useful as a break between events. Because children with AD/HD can be expected invariably to touch or manipulate objects around them, activities should be designed to include holding or handling objects as well as some degree of physical movement.

Incorporating incentives from an existing classroom reward system can be effective initially, while the clinician decides with the child what might prove reinforcing in their future encounters. Table 3-3 summarizes some more specific recommendations.

Professionals will find intervention efforts optimized after prescribed medications have taken effect, but the activity levels of children with AD/HD may still vary with the time of day. To avoid unproductive reactions to a child's rapid rate of speech, high activity level, and sudden attentional shifts, one must consciously assume a slower, calmer demeanor; exert control over the pace of activities; and offer ample time for the consideration of responses.

In initially short sessions, the professional can set the pattern of rewards for participation; then, session length can gradually be expanded. Behavioral messages like, "We don't do that here," or "Are you making a good choice or a bad choice?" can help refocus a child who is beginning to behave inappropriately.

If a child expresses an emotionally laden verbal assault or epithet, rather than reacting to the words, it is useful to reflect aloud what has been said and felt: "It sounds like _____ made you mad." Only then can the child reconsider the message and its impact.

Table 3-3.   Intervention Strategies for Children with AD/HD and Speech-Language Problems

1. Incorporate a team effort to help understand the complexity of issues.
2. Use standard procedures to remediate the speech and language disorders. Give specific attention to:
   a. Articulation
   b. Semantics
   c. Syntax
   d. Pragmatics
3. Use specific procedures to manage the behavioral component:
   a. Intervene after medication has taken effect.
   b. Schedule relatively short sessions.
   c. Integrate with classroom (or milieu) reward system or contract.
   d. Provide frequent positive rewards—social, tangible, or edible.
   e. Offer positive individualized attention, which is often rewarding in and of itself.
   f. Avoid matching the rapid pace of AD/HD child.
   g. Remain calm, steady and consistent.
   h. Reflect what the child says, rather than reacting to it.
   i. Develop vocabulary to address negative or inappropriate behaviors such as, "We don't do that here" or "Are you making a good choice or a bad choice?"
   j. Return a child who is out of control to the classroom. "You can come back another time when you're settled down."

The professional should know how to get assistance should behaviors escalate and become difficult to control safely in a therapy or classroom setting. The child who is then taken to another location or to a time-out spot should know that he or she can return to the therapy setting in the future and will become eligible to earn rewards provided he or she can follow the rules and maintain better control.

Pragmatic interventions can focus on social skills development (McGinnis & Goldstein, 1984), with role-playing of greetings, overtures to play, phone calls, and topical conversations. Scripts can be used to assign roles and to guide appropriate responses. It is essential that all material is utilized to some degree in real life settings if there is to be any carry-over of this learning.

The pragmatic framework described by Baltaxe (1993) is useful for delineating these problematic behaviors. It offers a structured way for children to help identify their own areas of difficulty and to keep track of progress as they begin to take responsibility for their own behavior. The framework focuses on the components of a social interaction shown in Table 3-4.

Criticism from adults (Barkley, 1990), rejection by peers, and failure in academic, athletic, and social arenas (Whalen & Henker, 1985) can all lead to sadness, frustration, disappointment, and anger. If a language deficit is comorbid with AD/HD, there is likely to be difficulty in identifying, describing, and sharing these emotions. Speech-language pathologists as well as counselors, psychotherapists, and special education teachers have developed ways to teach the language of feelings (Giddan, Bade, Rickenberg, & Ryley, 1995).

Table 3-4.   Pragmatic Framework

Speaker component
- mental state

Message and its function
- referential
- conative
- denotative

Message code
- non-verbal
- verbal

Linguistic or extra linguistic context or setting
Listener variable

Reprinted by permission from Baltaxe, C. (1993). Pragmatic disorders in children with social communication disorders and their treatment. Newsletter, Special Interest Divisions, Division 2. Neurophysiology and Neurogenic Speech and Language Disorders. Rockville, MD: American Speech-Language-Hearing Association, 3 (1), 2-9.

In speech-language therapy settings, the expansion of this abstract "emotion" vocabulary can be linked to play with toy animals or people, with feelings labeled verbally and then written on assigned pages in a notebook. It is most instructive to name each feeling that is generated through play as it occurs and then to describe the characteristics of that emotional experience to the child.

Intervention for CAPD when it coincides with AD/HD in children involves optimizing listening conditions with the aid of suggestions from the audiologist (Keith, 1986). The list of strategies in Table 3-5 is a compilation of auditory skills measures recommended for school settings.

Good use can be made of tape recordings at home and at school. The child with AD/HD can be guided through daily home routines by a recording of his mother's voice reminding him or her what task comes next and rewarding him or her with verbal praise. At school the teacher's instructions for the day or for specific activities can also be taped for later reference.

The following case study shows how a multidisciplinary team approach can be effective in treating the child whose AD/HD is exacerbated by linguistic and learning deficits.

CASE STUDY: ROCKY

This is the story of Rocky—a boy on the move. Small for his age, muscular, with a round face and big expressive eyes, he had a quick smile and was very friendly to adults. However, Rocky was extremely impulsive and distractible, and he lacked self-control. While in kindergarten, he was referred to a class for children with severe behavioral handicaps (SBH) after having moved through the first few months of the school year like a cyclone. Rocky's kinder-

Table 3-5.   Interventions to Enhance Listening

1. Seek classroom placement to avoid settings that are noisy or reverberant.
2. Provide the child preferential seating near the place where the teacher spends most of his/her time giving auditory instructions, and away from distracting auditory and visual "noise."
3. Teach children to use visual information (look and listen).
4. Encourage teachers to gain the child's attention before giving auditory instruction.
5. Check the child's comprehension of auditory information.
6. Rephrase and restate important information to provide auditory redundancy.
7. Use FM sound amplification systems to enhance the speech to noise ratio for the child.
8. Teach listening skills, including when to listen for meaning rather than exact repetition.
9. Give the child time to think and to respond to auditory instructions or questions.
10. Use attention devices such as calling the child's name, saying "listen" and "are you ready" before giving assignments.
11. Limit the amount of information in each instruction.
12. Allow a "buddy system" that the child can use to check on homework assignments or other instructions.
13. Counsel teachers and parents regarding the child's auditory needs.

garten class teacher wondered if his molded plastic seat might actually be tilted, because he constantly slid off it and onto the floor. He was disorganized, had difficulty waiting his turn, was easily frustrated, and was always ready to fight. Rocky worried about crises and tragedies at home involving his family members. The multidisciplinary treatment team was concerned about the possibility that he might have an anxiety or mood disorder. His home life was poorly organized indeed, and in somewhat of a turmoil. Rocky's mother moved quickly, talked fast, and seemed to be rather agitated. She provided little structure, and there were few predictable routines for Rocky and his sister.

A complete diagnostic evaluation at age 5;10 revealed poor performance in many areas. Rocky's language skills were delayed. His Expressive One Word Picture Vocabulary Test (Gardner, 1990) was scored at age 4;5. The Peabody Picture Vocabulary Test–Revised (Dunn & Dunn, 1981) standard score was 64 (age equivalent of 3;6). On the Clinical Evaluation of Language Functions Screening Test (Semel & Wiig, 1980), he earned a 1st percentile rank for language processing and a 10th percentile rank for language production. Rocky had a frontal and lateral lisp, he spoke quickly and loudly, and his voice was husky. He failed his pure tone hearing screening and, upon further audiological evaluation, was found to have a previously undiagnosed 4000 Hz hearing loss in both ears. He performed at a prekindergarten level in math readiness and letter matching. Severe problems with visual perceptual skills and motor planning prevented him from assembling even a three-piece paper snowman.

Rocky's communication deficits were apparent whenever he tried to describe or explain anything. He spoke in short bursts, and used his hands to aid his descriptions, as he did not know the prepositions needed to designate location or adjectives of quality or quantity. Lacking words to describe how he felt, he would instead vigorously rub his hands together as he spoke about a fire at his house or his lost cat.

It was apparent that Rocky engaged in no self-talk. He acted on impulse, responding to what caught his eye, without any mediation from an inner voice to help him plan or carry out the steps of his activities.

Rocky's social skills were poor. He teased and insulted other children, did not know how to engage others in play, and continually violated the boundaries of others. However, he was charming to adults. He related in an animated, lively way and had a warm smile, to which people responded positively.

Rocky's program was coordinated by a multidisciplinary team that included the special education teacher, a psychologist, a psychiatrist, a speech-language pathologist, an occupational therapist, and Rocky's family.

His classroom was structured according to behavioral guidelines, with predictable reward schedules and clear consequences for behaviors. All students were encouraged to make "good choices" throughout the day as they tried to take responsibility for their own behaviors. Individualized teaching in each academic skill area began at a point where Rocky could experience some successes. His teacher taught him ways to organize his materials and required only short units of work, which were followed by opportunities to move about. She intervened with "life-space interviews" (Wood & Long, 1990) to help him process and better understand relevant events at times when Rocky began to lose control. Life-space interviews are designed to use classroom conflicts as opportunities for the student to gain insight into his or her own behavior and assume some responsibility for changing self-defeating behavior patterns.

The speech-language pathologist worked with Rocky on articulation, language concepts, and conversational skills, at first individually, later in a small group setting, and finally within the classroom. The occupational therapist addressed Rocky's eye-hand coordination problems. All of the multidisciplinary team members developed home programs to help Rocky's mother create some structure in her setting with schedules and reward charts. Medication was prescribed by the psychiatrist, and over time, the prescription was changed from Ritalin to Clonidine because of concerns about Rocky's growth. As the years went on, whenever Rocky failed to take his medication, his impulsivity and other inappropriate behaviors increased markedly, he performed very poorly in school, and he frequently got into trouble due to his behavior. When he took the Clonidine he would become organized again and at least maintain himself at school, although he was never a good student. In spite of years of intervention, Rocky remains a boy at risk. As an adolescent he is easily led into trouble and still has difficulty using judgment and forethought before acting.

SUMMARY

Attention deficit/hyperactivity disorder, AD/HD, comes to the attention of educators, counselors, physicians, psychologists, psychiatrists, and speech-language pathologists across many settings. In schools, private practices, and mental health clinics, such children experience motor disinhibition and problems maintaining attention to tasks and thus need multidisciplinary evaluation and treatment. Biological, psychological, and social aspects of their disorder, as well as the complicating comorbid conditions, must be addressed. Clearly, language and learning deficits can exacerbate their problems at school, at home, and in all social situations with parents, peers, and siblings.

As research into AD/HD continues and the definition becomes more refined, we will likely see a stronger distinction made between children who display performance symptoms of behavioral disinhibition with impulsivity and hyperactivity and those who show cognitive inattention with slow processing of information and disorganization. Professionals might expect to see CAPD to be identified more in the latter group, while the more severe combined speech and language disorders might be found in the former. We look forward to these and other evolving developments in the study of AD/HD.

References

Abikoff, H., & Gittelman, R. (1984). Does behavior therapy normalize the classroom behavior of hyperactive children? *Archives of General Psychiatry, 41,* 449–454.

Abikoff, H., & Gittelman, R. (1985). Hyperactive children treated with stimulants: Is cognitive training a useful adjunct? *Archives of General Psychiatry, 42,* 953–961.

Achenbach, T. M. (1991). *Manual for the Child Behavior Checklist/4-18 and 1991 Profile.* Burlington: University of Vermont Medical School, Department of Psychiatry.

American Psychiatric Association. (1968). *Diagnostic and statistical manual of mental disorders* (2nd ed.). Washington, D.C.: Author.

American Psychiatric Association. (1980). *Diagnostic and statistical manual of mental disorders* (3rd ed.). Washington, D.C.: Author.

American Psychiatric Association. (1987). *Diagnostic and statistical manual of mental disorders* (3rd ed., rev.). Washington, D.C.: Author.

American Psychiatric Association. (1994). *Diagnostic and statistical manual of mental disorders* (4th ed.). Washington, D.C.: Author.

American Speech-Language and Hearing Association (ASHA). (1992). *Issues in central auditory processing disorders: A report from the ASHA Ad Hoc Committee on Central Auditory Processing.* Washington, D.C.: Author.

Anastopolous, A. D., Spisto, M. A., & Maher, M. C. (1994). The WISC-III freedom from distractibility factor: Its utility in identifying children with attention deficit hyperactivity disorder. *Psychological Assessment, 6,* 368–371.

Anderson, J. C., Williams, S. M., McGee, R. O., & Silva, P. A. (1987). *DSM-III* disorders in preadolescent children. *Archives of General Psychiatry, 44,* 69–76.

August, G. J., & Garfinkel, B. D. (1989). Behavioral and cognitive subtype of ADHD. *Journal of the American Academy of Child and Adolescent Psychiatry, 28,* 739–748.

Baker, L., & Cantwell, D. P. (1992). Attention deficit disorder and speech/language disorders. *Comprehensive Mental Health Care, 2,* 3–16.

Baltaxe, C. (1993). Pragmatic disorders in children with social communication disorders and their treatment. *Neurophysiology and Neurogenic Speech and Language Disorders,* Newsletter, Special Interest Divisions, Division 2. Rockville, Md.: American Speech-Language-Hearing Association, 3(1), 2–9.

Baltaxe, C., & Simmons, J. Q. (1988a). Communication deficits in preschool children with psychiatric disorders. *Seminars in Speech and Language, 9,* 81–91.

Baltaxe, C., & Simmons, J. Q. (1988b). Pragmatic deficits in emotionally disturbed children and adolescents. In R. Schiefelbusch & L. Lloyd (Eds.), *Language perspectives: Acquisition, retardation, and intervention* (2nd ed.). Austin, Tex.: Pro-Ed.

Barkley, R. (1981). *Hyperactive children: A handbook for diagnosis and treatment.* New York: Guilford.

Barkley, R. (1989). Attention deficit-hyperactivity disorder. In E. J. Marsh & R. A. Barkley (Eds.), *Treatment of childhood disorders* (pp. 39–72). New York: Guilford.

Barkley, R. (1990). *Attention deficit hyperactivity disorder: A handbook for diagnosis and treatment.* New York: Guilford.

Barkley, R., DuPaul, G. J., & McMurray, M. D. (1990). Attention deficit disorder with and without hyperactivity: Clinical response to three dose levels of methylphenidate. *Pediatrics, 87,* 519–531.

Barkley, R., Fischer, M., Edelbrock, C. S., & Smallish, L. (1990). The adolescent outcome of hyperactive children diagnosed by research criteria: I. An 8 year prospective follow-up study. *Journal of the American Academy of Child and Adolescent Psychiatry, 29,* 546–557.

Bauermeister, J. J., Alegria, M., Bird, H., Rubio-Stipec, M., & Canino, G. (1992). Are attentional-hyperactivity deficits unidimensional or multidimensional syndromes? Empirical findings from a community survey. *Journal of the American Academy of Child and Adolescent Psychiatry, 31,* 423–431.

Bennett, L. A., Wolin, S. J., & Reiss, D. (1988). Cognitive, behavioral, emotional problems among school-age children of alcoholic parents. *American Journal of Psychiatry, 145,* 185–190.

Berk, L. E., & Landau, S. (1993). Private speech of learning disabled and normally achieving children in classroom academic and laboratory contexts. *Child Development, 64,* 556–571.

Bidder, R. T., Gray, O. P., & Newcombe, R. (1978). Behavioural treatment of hyperactive children. *Archives of Disease in Childhood, 53,* 574–579.

Biederman, J., Munir, K., Knee, D., Habelow, W., Armentano, M., Autor, S., Hoge, S. K., & Waternaux, C. (1986). A family study of patients with attention deficit disorder and normal controls. *Journal of Psychiatric Research, 20,* 263–274.

Bird, H. R., Canino, G., Rubio-Stipec, M., Gould, M. S., Ribera, J., Sesman, M., Woodbury, M., Huertas-Goldman, S., Pagan, A., Sanchez-Lacay, A., & Moscoso, M. (1988). Estimates of the prevalence of childhood maladjustment in a community survey in Puerto Rico. *Archives of General Psychiatry, 45,* 1120–1126.

Brown, R. T., & Borden, K. A. (1986). Hyperactivity at adolescence: Some misconceptions and new directions. *Journal of Clinical Child Psychology, 15,* 194–209.

Brown, R. T., & Wynne, M. E. (1977). Reflection-impulsivity of normal and behavior-disordered children. *Journal of Clinical Child Psychology, 11,* 262–267.

Cantwell, D. P. & Baker, L. (1991). Association between attention deficit hyperactivity disorder and learning disorders. *Journal of Learning Disabilities, 24,* 88–94.

Chess, S. (1940). Diagnosis and treatment of the hyperactive child. *New York State Journal of Medicine, 60,* 2379–2385.

Chess, S., & Rosenberg, M. (1974). Clinical differentiation among children with initial language complaints. *Journal of Autism and Childhood Schizophrenia, 4,* 99–109.

Conners, C. K., & Wells, K. C. (1986). *Hyperkinetic children: A neuropsychological approach.* Beverly Hills, Calif.: Sage.

Denson, R., Nanson, J. L., & McWatters, M. A. (1975). Hyperkinesis and maternal smoking. *Canadian Psychiatric Association Journal, 20,* 183–187.

Deutsch, C. K., Swanson, J. M., Bruell, J. H., Cantwell, D. P., Weinberg, F., & Baren, M. (1982). Over-representation of adoptees in children with attention deficit disorder. *Behavioral Genetics, 12,* 231–238.

Douglas, V. I. (1983). Attention and cognitive problems. In M. Rutter (Ed.), *Developmental neuropsychiatry* (pp. 280–329). New York: Guilford.

Dubey, D. R., O'Leary, S. G., & Kaufman, K. F. (1983). Training parents of hyperactive children in child management: A comparative outcome study. *Journal of Abnormal Child Psychology, 11,* 229–246.

Dulcan, M. K. (1992). Information for parents and youth on psychotropic medications. *Journal of Child and Adolescent Psychopharmacology, 2,* 81–101.

Dunn, L. M., & Dunn, L. M. (1981). *Peabody Picture Vocabulary Test, Form L–Revised.* Circle Pines, Minn.: American Guidance Service.

Faraone, S. V., Biederman, J., & Milberger, S. (1994). An exploratory study of ADHD among second-degree relatives of ADHD children. *Biological Psychiatry, 35,* 398–402.

Firestone, P., Kelly, M. J., Goodman, J. T., & Davey, J. (1981). Differential effects of parent training and stimulant medication with hyperactives. *Journal of the American Academy of Child Psychiatry, 20,* 135–147.

Gardner, M. F. (1990). *Expressive One-Word Picture Vocabulary Test–Revised Manual.* Novato, Calif.: Academic.

Gascon, G. G., Johnson, R., & Burd, L. (1986). Central auditory processing and attention deficit disorders. *Journal of Child Neurology, 1,* 27–33.

Giddan, J. J. (1991). Communication issues in attention-deficit hyperactivity disorder. *Child Psychiatry and Human Development, 22,* 45–51.

Giddan, J. J., Bade, K. M., Rickenberg, D., & Ryley, A. T. (1995). Teaching the language of feelings to students with severe emotional and behavioral handicaps. *Language, Speech, and Hearing Services in Schools, 26,* 3–10.

Giddan, J. J., Milling, L., & Campbell, N. B. (1996). Unrecognized language and speech deficits in preadolescent psychiatric inpatients. *American Journal of Orthopsychiatry, 6,* 85–92.

Gittelman, R., Mannuzza, S., Shenker, R., & Bonagura, N. (1985). Hyperactive boys almost grown up. *Archives of General Psychiatry, 42,* 937–946.

Goodman, R., & Stevenson, J. (1989). A twin study of hyperactivity: II. The aetiological role of genes, family relationships, and perinatal adversity. *Journal of Child Psychology and Psychiatry, 30,* 691–709.

Gordon, M. (1983). *The Gordon Diagnostic System.* Boulder, Colo.: Clinical Diagnostic Systems.

Grodzinsky, G. (1990). *Assessing frontal lobe dysfunctioning in 6 to 11 year old boys with attention deficit hyperactivity disorder.* Unpublished doctoral dissertation, Boston College.

Gualtieri, C. T., Koriath, U., Van Bourgondien, M., & Saleeby, N. (1983). Language disorders in children referred for psychiatric services. *Journal of the American Academy of Child Psychiatry, 22,* 165–171.

Halperin, J. M., Matier, K., Bedi, G., Sharma, V., & Newcorn, J. H. (1992). Specificity of inattention, impulsivity, and hyperactivity to the diagnosis of attention-deficit hyperactivity disorder. *Journal of the American Academy of Child and Adolescent Psychiatry, 31,* 190–196.

Hauser, P., Zametkin, A. J., Martinez, P., Vitiello, B., Matochik, J. A., Mixson, A. J., & Weintraub, B. D. (1993). Attention deficit-hyperactivity disorder in people with generalized resistance to thyroid hormone. *New England Journal of Medicine, 328,* 997–1001.

Heilman, K. M., Voeller, K. K. S., & Nadeau, S. E. (1991). A possible pathophysiological substrate of attention deficit hyperactivity disorder. *Journal of Child Neurology, 6,* S76–S81.

Hinshaw, S. P. (1994). *Attention deficits and hyperactivity in children.* Beverly Hills, CA: Sage.

Hinshaw, S. P., & Erhardt, D. (1993). Behavioral treatment. In V. B. Van Hasselt & M. Hersen (Eds.), *Handbook of behavior therapy and pharmacotherapy for children: A comparative analysis* (pp. 233–250). Needham Heights, Mass.: Allyn & Bacon.

Hinshaw, S. P., Whalen, C. K., & Henker, B. (1984). Cognitive-behavioral and pharmacologic interventions for hyperactive boys: Comparative and combined effects. *Journal of Consulting and Clinical Psychology, 52,* 739–749.

Humphries, T., Koltun, H., Malone, M., & Roberts, W. (1994). Teacher-identified oral language difficulties among boys with attention problems. *Developmental and Behavioral Pediatrics, 15,* 92–98.

Kanbayashi, Y., Nakata, Y., Fuji, K., Kita, M., & Wada, K. (1994). ADHD-related behavior among non-referred children: Parents ratings of DSM-III-R symptoms. *Child Psychiatry and Human Development, 25,* 13–29.

Kaufman, A. S. (1975). Factor analysis of the WISC-R at eleven age levels between 6.5 and 16.5 years. *Journal of Consulting and Clinical Psychology, 43,* 135–147.

Keith, R. W. (1986). *SCAN: A screening test for auditory processing disorders.* San Antonio, Tex.: Psychological Corporation.

Keith, R. W., & Engineer, P. (1991). Effects of methylphenidate on the auditory processing abilities of children with attention deficit-hyperactivity disorder. *Journal of Learning Disabilities, 24,* 630–636.

Keller, W. D. (1992). Auditory processing disorder or attention deficit disorder? In J. Katz, N. A. Stecker, & D. Henderson (Eds.), *Central auditory processing: A transdisciplinary view* (pp. 107–114). St. Louis: Mosby Year Book.

Klein, R. G., & Mannuzza, S. (1991). Long-term outcome of hyperactive children: A review. *Journal of the American Academy of Child and Adolescent Psychiatry, 30,* 383–387.

Korkman, M., & Pesonen, A. E. (1994). A comparison of the neuropsychological test profiles of children with attention-deficit/hyperactivity disorder. *Journal of Learning Disabilities, 27,* 383–392.

Lahey, B. B., Piacentini, J. C., McBurnett, K., Stone, P., Hartdagen, S., & Hynd, G. (1988). Psychopathology in the parents of children with conduct disorder and hyperactivity. *Journal of the American Academy of Child and Adolescent Psychiatry, 27,* 163–170.

Laufer, M. W., & Denhoff, E. (1957). Hyperkinetic behavior syndrome in children. *Journal of Pediatrics, 50,* 463–473.

Lopez, R. (1965). Hyperactivity in twins. *Canadian Psychiatric Association Journal, 10,* 421.

Lou, H. C., Henriksen, L., & Bruhn, P. (1984). Focal cerebral hyperfusion in children with dysphasia and/or attention deficit disorder. *Archives of Neurology, 41,* 825–829.

Lou, H. C., Henriksen, L., Bruhn, P., Borner, H., & Nielsen, J. B. (1989). Striatal dysfunction in attention deficit and hyperkinetic disorder. *Archives of Neurology, 46,* 48–52.

Love, A. J. & Thompson, M. G. G. (1988). Language disorders and attention deficit disorders in young children referred for psychiatric services. *American Journal of Orthopsychiatry, 58,* 52–64.

Ludlow, C. L., Cudahy, E. A., Bassich, C., & Brown, G. L. (1983). Auditory processing skills of hyperactive, language impaired and reading disabled boys. In E. Z. Lasky & J. Katz, (Eds.), *Central auditory processing disorders: Problems of speech, language and learning* (pp. 163–184). Baltimore: University Park Press.

Luk, S. (1985). Direct observation studies of hyperactive behaviors. *Journal of the American Academy of Child Psychiatry, 24,* 338–344.

Mannuzza, S., Klein, R. G., Bongura, N., Malloy, P., Giampino, T. L., & Addalli, K. A. (1991). Hyperactive boys almost grown up: V. Replication of psychiatric status. *Archives of General Psychiatry, 48,* 77–83.

Mariani, M. A. (1990). *The nature of neuropsychological functioning in preschool-age children with attention-deficit hyperactivity disorder.* Unpublished doctoral dissertation, Boston College.

McGinnis, E., & Goldstein, A. P. (1984). *Skill-streaming the elementary school child: A guide for teaching prosocial skills.* Champaign, Ill.: Research Press Company.

McPherson, D. L., & Davies, K. (1995). Preliminary observations of binaural hearing in an attention-deficit pediatric population. *Fiziologia Cheloveka, 21,* 47–53.

Milich, R., & Kramer, J. (1985). Reflections on impulsivity: An empirical investigation of impulsivity as a construct. In K. D. Gadow & I. Bialer (Eds.), *Advances in learning and behavioral disabilities* (pp. 283–339). Greenwich, Conn.: JAI Press.

Nichols, P. L., & Chen, T. C. (1981). *Minimal brain dysfunction: A prospective study.* Hillsdale, N.J.: Erlbaum.

O'Leary, K. D., Pelham, W. E., Rosenbaum, A., & Price, G. H. (1976). Behavioral treatment of hyperkinetic children: An experimental evaluation of its usefulness. *Clinical Pediatrics, 15,* 510–515.

O'Leary, K. D., Vivian, D., & Nisi, A. (1985). Hyperactivity in Italy. *Journal of Abnormal Child Psychology, 13,* 485–500.

Ornoy, A., Uriel, L., & Tannenbaum, A. (1993). Inattention, hyperactivity and speech delay at 2.4 years of age as a predictor for ADD-AD/HD syndrome. *Israeli Journal of Psychiatry and Related Sciences, 30,* 155–163.

Patterson, G. R. (1982). *Coercive family process.* Eugene, Ore.: Castilia.

Pelham, W. E., Carlson, C., Sams, S. E., Vallano, G., Dixon, M. J., & Hoza, B. (1993). Separate and combined effects of methylphenidate and behavior modification on the classroom behavior and academic performance of ADHD boys: Group effects and individual differences. *Journal of Consulting and Clinical Psychiatry, 61,* 506–515.

Physicians' Desk Reference. (1995). Montvale, N.J.: Medical Economics.

Pisterman, S. J., McGrath, P., Firestone, P., Goodman, J. T., Webster, I., & Mallory, R. (1989). Outcome of parent mediated treatment of preschoolers with attention deficit disorder. *Journal of Consulting and Clinical Psychology, 57,* 628–635.

Pollard, S., Ward, E. M., & Barkley, R. A. (1983). The effects of parent training and Ritalin on parent-child interactions of hyperactive boys. *Child and Family Therapy, 5,* 51–69.

Porrino, L. J., Rapoport, J. L. Behar, D., Sceery, W., Ismond, D. R., & Bunney, W. E. (1983). A naturalistic assessment of the motor activity of hyperactive boys: I. Comparison with normal controls. *Archives of General Psychiatry, 40,* 681–687.

Rapport, M. D., Tucker, S. B., DuPaul, G. J., Merlo, M., & Stoner, G. (1986). Hyperactivity and frustration: The influence of control over the size of rewards in delaying gratification. *Journal of Abnormal Child Psychology, 14,* 191–204.

Raskin, L. A., Shaywitz, S. E. , Shaywitz, B. A., Anderson, G. M., & Cohen, D. J. (1984). Neurochemical correlates of attention deficit disorder. *Pediatric Clinics of North America, 31,* 387–396.

Riccio, C. A., Hynd, G. W., Cohen, M. J., Hall, J., & Molt, L. (1994). Comorbidity of central auditory processing disorder and attention deficit hyperactivity disorder. *Journal of the American Academy of Child and Adolescent Psychiatry, 33,* 849–857.

Roberts, M. A. (1990). A behavioral observation method for differentiating hyperactive and aggressive boys. *Journal of Abnormal Child Psychology, 18,* 131–142.

Robinson, P. W., Newby, T. J., & Ganzell, S. L. (1981). A token system for a class of underachieving children. *Journal of Applied Behavior Analysis, 14,* 307–315.

Ross, D. M., & Ross, S. A. (1982). *Hyperactivity: Current issues, research and theory.* New York: Wiley.

Routh, D. K., & Schroeder, C. S. (1976). Standardized playroom measures as indices of hyperactivity. *Journal of Abnormal Child Psychology, 4,* 199–207.

Safer, D. J. (1973). A familial factor in minimal brain dysfunction. *Behavior Genetics, 3,* 175–186.

Sandler, A. D., Hooper, S. R., Watson, T. E., Coleman, W. L., Footo, M., & Levine, M. (1993). Talkative children: Verbal fluency as a marker for problematic peer relationships in clinic referred children with attention deficit. *Perceptual and Motor Skills, 76,* 943–951.

Schachar, R., & Wachsmuth, R. (1990). Hyperactivity and parental psychopathology. *Journal of Child Psychology and Psychiatry, 31,* 381–392.

Semel, E., & Wiig, E. H. (1980). *Clinical Evaluation of Language Functions Elementary Screening Test.* San Antonio: Psychological Corporation.

Shaywitz, S. E., Cohen, D. J., & Shaywitz, B. A. (1994). Behavior and learning difficulties in children of normal intelligence born to alcoholic mothers. *Pediatrics, 96,* 978–982.

Shaywitz, B. A., Fletcher, J. M. & Shaywitz, S. E. (1995). Defining and classifying learning disabilities and attention-deficit/hyperactivity disorder. *Journal of Child Neurology, 10,* S50–S57.

Stevenson, J. (1992). Evidence for a genetic etiology of hyperactivity in children. *Behavior Genetics, 22,* 337–343.

Still, G. F. (1902). Some abnormal psychical conditions in children. *Lancet, 1,* 1077–1082.

Strauss, A. A., & Lehtinen, L. E. (1947). *Psychopathology and education of the brain-injured child.* New York: Grune & Stratton.

Streissguth, A. P., Martin, D. C., Barr, H. M., Sandman, B. M., Kirchner, G. L., & Darby, B. L. (1984). Intrauterine alcohol and nicotine exposure: Attention and reaction time in 4-year-old children. *Developmental Psychology, 20,* 533–541.

Szatmari, P., Offord, D. R., & Boyle, M. H. (1989). Ontario Child Health Study: Prevalence of attention deficit disorder with hyperactivity. *Journal of Child Psychology and Psychiatry, 30,* 219–230.

Taylor, E. A. (1986). Childhood hyperactivity. *British Journal of Psychiatry, 149,* 562–573.

Thorley, G., (1984). Review of follow-up and follow-back studies of childhood hyperactivity. *Psychological Bulletin, 96,* 116–132.

Trautman, R. C., Giddan, J. J. & Jurs, S. G. (1990). Language risk factors in emotionally disturbed children within a school and day treatment program. *Journal of Childhood Communication Disorders, 13,* 123–133.

Trites, R. L. (1979). *Hyperactivity in children: Etiology, measurement and treatment implications.* Baltimore: University Park Press.

Wechsler, D. (1991). *Wechsler Intelligence Scale for Children* (3rd ed.). New York: Psychological Corporation.

Wechsler, D. (1992). *Wechsler Individual Achievement Test.* New York: Psychological Corporation.

Weiss, G., & Hechtman, L. (1986). *Hyperactive children grown up: Empirical findings and theoretical considerations.* New York: Guilford.

Werner, E. E., Bierman, J. M., French, F. E., Simonian, K., Connor, A., Smith, R. S., & Campbell, M. (1968). Reproductive and environmental causalities: A report on the 10-year follow-up of the children of the Kaui pregnancy study. *Pediatrics, 42,* 112–127.

Whalen, C. K. & Henker, B. (1985). The social worlds of hyperactive (AD/HD) children. *Child Psychiatry Review, 5,* 447–478.

Wolraich, M., Drummond, T., Saloman, M. K., O'Brien, M. L., & Sivage, C. (1978). Effects of methylphenidate alone and in combination with behavior modification procedures on the behavior and academic performance of hyperactive children. *Journal of Abnormal Child Psychology, 6,* 149–161.

Wood, M., & Long, N. (1990). *Life-space intervention: Talking to children and youth in a crisis.* Austin, Tex.: Pro-Ed.

Zametkin, A. J., & Rapoport, J. L. (1986). The pathophysiology of attention deficit disorder with hyperactivity: A review. In B. Lahey & A. Kazdin (Eds.), *Advances in clinical child psychology* (Vol. 9, pp. 177–216). New York: Plenum.

Pervasive Developmental Disorders in Young Children

Linda R. Watson, Ed.D., CCC-SLP
Clinical Associate Professor
University of North Carolina
Chapel Hill
and
Sally Ozonoff, Ph.D.
Associate Professor
University of Utah
Salt Lake City

Key Terms

Asperger's disorder
autistic disorder
childhood disintegrative disorder
hyperlexia
pervasive developmental disorders
   (PDD)

pervasive development disorder—
   not otherwise specified
   (PDDNOS)
pragmatics
Rett's disorder

Overview

Pervasive developmental disorders (PDD) is a term that came into widespread use with the publication of the 1980 (third) edition of the *Diagnostic and Statistical Manual of Mental Disorders (DSM-III)* by the American Psychiatric Association (APA). It refers to a group of disorders that affect a child's ability to communicate, play, understand, and relate to others. The term was adopted to emphasize the developmental nature of these disorders and to distinguish them from psychoses arising in late childhood to adulthood. These disorders have also been called the "autistic syndromes" (Rutter & Schopler, 1987) or the "autism continuum" (Wing, 1988). The current subtypes of PDD, as presented in the *Diagnostic and Statistical Manual of Mental Disorders, Fourth Edition (DSM-IV)*, (APA, 1994) include **autistic disorder, Asperger's disorder, childhood disintegrative disorder, Rett's disorder**, and **pervasive developmental disorder—not otherwise specified (PDDNOS).**

A common thread across these disorders is that individuals have difficulty with the development of the language and communication skills necessary for smooth social transactions. The specific language and communication characteristics of individuals with PDD and the extent to which these areas are impaired vary greatly from one person to the next. Especially among young children with PDD, it is common to find individuals with little or no verbal communication. At the other extreme, there are also some children with PDD who exhibit syntax and vocabulary within the normal range for their age. Another important point is that the language and communication skills of children with PDD develop and change with age. For instance, a toddler who does not engage in nonverbal joint attention acts may develop the ability to do so by the time she or he is 5; similarly, a child who exhibits frequent echolalia at age 4 may not be echolalic by the time she or he reaches late elementary school.

Our purpose in this chapter is to provide readers who have specific interests in language impairments in young children with an overview of diagnosis and development among children with PDD. We discuss the diagnostic criteria for PDD as well as variations in diagnosis, etiological factors, and cognitive, social, and communication development. We address prognoses for children with PDD. Last, we present information on intervention issues and resources specific to this population.

DIAGNOSIS

There are a number of sources of diagnostic criteria that have been used to classify the pervasive developmental disorders. Currently, the most commonly used diagnostic system is that of the *Diagnostic and Statistical Manual of Mental Disorders, Fourth Edition (DSM-IV)* (APA, 1994). As specified in the DSM-IV, all PDDs involve some difficulty with social relatedness, verbal and nonverbal communication, and developing a typical range of interests and behaviors. In the social domain, the symptoms listed in the *DSM-IV* include impaired use of nonverbal behaviors (e.g., eye contact, facial expression, gestures) to regulate social interaction, failure to develop age-appropriate peer relationships, little spontaneous seeking to share enjoyment or interests with other people, and little social-emotional reciprocity. The symptoms of communicative dysfunction for PDD include delay in, or absence of, spoken language; difficulty initiating or sustaining a conversation, idiosyncratic or repetitive language; echolalia; and deficits in pretend play. In the domain of behaviors and interests, there is often an encompassing preoccupation or un-usual interest that is abnormal in intensity, an inflexible adherence to non-functional routines, stereotyped body movements, and preoccupation with parts of objects (APA, 1994).

Autism, or autistic disorder, as it is called in the *DSM-IV*, is the most pro-totypical and pure form of pervasive developmental disorder. In order to meet criteria for a diagnosis of autistic disorder, an individual must demonstrate at least 6 of the 12 symptoms listed in the *DSM-IV*, with at least 2 coming from the social domain and 1 each from the communication and restricted behav-iors/interests categories. Additionally, at least 1 of the symptoms must have been present before 36 months of age to qualify for this diagnosis (APA, 1994). Table 4-1, on pages 112 and 113, summarizes the *DSM-IV* criteria for a di-agnosis of autism.

What has become increasingly apparent in the last decade is that the symp-toms of autism vary widely in severity and span a continuum, from the clas-sic symptoms described by Kanner (1943) to much milder forms (Wing, 1988). The easily recognized individual with autism is socially remote, has little com-munication ability, and is absorbed in stereotypic behavior. What has been less well recognized is that an individual who is socially outgoing, talkative, and has no stereotyped mannerisms can also meet *DSM-IV* diagnostic criteria for autistic disorder. What does an aloof, mute individual share with an engag-ing, talkative person that makes them both autistic? A core difficulty in peo-ple with autism of all functioning levels appears to be reciprocity. Even individuals mildly affected with autism who are quite interested in others have difficulty with social reciprocity. Their relationships tend to be one-sided and do not involve the same level of mutuality, shared interests, and intimacy ob-served in their peers who are not autistic. They often talk in monologues without giving others a chance to contribute, have difficulty building on com-ments made by others, and, compared to peers, engage in less chatting for pure social purposes. Their interests tend to be idiosyncratic and difficult for others to share, revolving around unusual themes such as vacuum cleaners, automobile hubcap emblems, or venomous snakes.

Higher-functioning versions of autistic disorder must be distinguished from Asperger's disorder, a related PDD in which language abilities are relatively well developed and cognitive functioning falls in the normal range. Although it was described over a half-century ago by Hans Asperger (1944), an Aus-trian pediatrician, Asperger's disorder was not included in the *DSM* until 50 years later, in the manual's fourth edition. The main point of differentiation from higher functioning children with autistic disorder is that those children with Asperger's disorder never exhibit the typical autistic symptom of severe language delay. As specified by the *DSM-IV*, purposeful use of single words must be demonstrated by age 2, and meaningful phrase speech by age 3. Most parents of children with Asperger's disorder are not concerned about their child's language development when the child is very young. To the con-trary, many parents report that language development was precocious, with

Table 4-1.   Diagnostic Features of Autistic Disorder and Asperger's Disorder

Autistic Disorder

I.   Symptoms (total of 6 or more from a, b, & c)
   a. Qualitative impairment in social interaction (at least 2)
   • Marked impairment in use of multiple nonverbal behaviors
   • Failure to develop peer relations appropriate to developmental level
   • Lack of spontaneous seeking to share interests/enjoyment
   • Lack of social or emotional reciprocity
   b. Qualitative impairment in communication (at least 1)
   • Delay in, or total lack of development of spoken language
   • Marked impairment in ability to initiate or sustain conversation (for individuals with adequate speech)
   • Stereotyped, repetitive, or idiosyncratic language
   • Lack of varied, spontaneous imaginative play appropriate to developmental level
   c. Restricted, repetitive and stereotyped patterns of behavior, interests and activities (at least 1)
   • Stereotyped or restricted pattern(s) of interest abnormal in intensity or focus
   • Inflexible adherence to specific, nonfunctional routines or rituals
   • Stereotyped and repetitive motor mannerisms
   • Persistent preoccupation with parts of objects

II.   Additional specifications
   None

III.   Age-related criteria
   Delays or abnormal functioning in at least one of the following areas with onset prior to 3 years of age: social interaction; language as used in social communication; symbolic or imaginative play

IV.   Rule out diagnosis
   Disturbance not better accounted for by Rett's Disorder or Childhood Disintegrative Disorder

Adapted with permission from *Diagnostic and Statistical Manual of Mental Disorders, Fourth Edition*. Copyright 1994, American Psychiatric Association.

the child using adult-like language and vocabulary from an early age. *DSM-IV* criteria do make no explicit mention of other communication oddities (e.g., echolalia, idiosyncratic language, pragmatic impairments) in Asperger's disorder, but they also do not prohibit their presence. In fact, these kinds of atypical communication behaviors are widely reported in individuals with As-

Asperger's Disorder

I. Symptoms
   a. Qualitative impairment in social interactions (at least 2)
      - Marked impairment in use of multiple nonverbal behaviors
      - Failure to develop peer relations appropriate to developmental level
      - Lack of spontaneous seeking to share interests/enjoyment
      - Lack of social or emotional reciprocity
   b. Qualitative impairment of communication
      No symptoms specified for diagnosis

   c. Restricted, repetitive and stereotyped patterns of behavior, interests and activities (at least 1)
      - Stereotyped and restricted patterns of interest abnormal in intensity or focus
      - Inflexible adherence to specific, nonfunctional routines or rituals
      - Stereotyped and repetitive motor mannerisms
      - Persistent preoccupation with parts of objects

II. Additional specifications
      - Disturbance causes clinically significant impairment in social, occupational, or other important areas of functioning
      - No clinically significant general delay in language (e.g., single words used by age 2 years, communicative phrases by 3 years)
      - No clinically significant delay in cognitive development, self-help skills, adaptive behavior (other than social interaction) and curiosity about environment

III. Age-related criteria
      None (appears to have later onset or be recognized later than Autistic Disorder)

IV. Rule out diagnoses
      Criteria are not met for another specific PDD or Schizophrenia

perger's disorder (Asperger, 1944, Klin, 1994; Szatmari, Bremner, & Nagy, 1989; Wing, 1981).

The developers of the *DSM-IV* intended that the disorders within the PDD category be related, but mutually exclusive and nonoverlapping. Thus, a child cannot simultaneously meet criteria for autistic disorder and Asperger's disorder. Consequently, a second critical differentiation between the two disorders is that children with the former demonstrate six or more of the symptoms outlined in the *DSM-IV*, while those in the latter demonstrate five or fewer characteristics.

Rett's disorder and childhood disintegrative disorder represent two severe forms of PDD. Although sharing the basic features of all PDDs—namely, social, communication, and behavioral impairments—these disorders are relatively easily distinguished from autism and Asperger's disorder by their distinctive degenerative courses. Rett's disorder has been described only in females. After a period of normal development until at least 5 months of age, there is a reduction of interest in social interactions and the environment, a loss of previously acquired purposeful hand skills, and development of characteristic stereotyped midline hand movements. Head circumference is normal at birth and for several months afterward, but growth begins to decelerate between 5 and 48 months. Rett's disorder is also characterized by severe motor, communication, and intellectual impairments (APA, 1994; Holm, 1985; Van Acker, 1991).

Similarly, childhood disintegrative disorder involves regression after a period of normal functioning, in this case, at least 2 years of development (but less than 10). Mean age of onset is between 3 and 4 years of age (Volkmar, 1992). This disorder is seen in both males and females, and like autism, it predominates in males (Volkmar, 1992). After the regression, the characteristic features of autism are present, that is, deficits in social relatedness, communication, and behaviors and interests; thus, this disorder has also been called "late onset autism" (Volkmar & Cohen, 1989). In addition, there may be regression in motor and/or toileting skills. Disintegrative disorder is typically associated with severe mental retardation (see also Volkmar & Rutter, 1995).

Finally, according to the *DSM-IV* diagnostic system, if a child exhibits at least two symptoms falling in the social, communication, and behaviors/interests realms (of which at least one symptom is social) but does not meet criteria for any of the four specific PDDs outlined above, she or he is diagnosed with pervasive developmental disorder–not otherwise specified (PDDNOS). This diagnosis is intended to be used when there is late age of onset, atypical symptomatology, or subthreshold number of symptoms. In practice, however, PDDNOS is often misdiagnosed. The *DSM-IV* field trials found that almost half of individuals diagnosed with PDDNOS by clinicians actually met full criteria for autistic disorder (Volkmar et al., 1994). Because, in many regions of the country, services are more difficult to obtain with a diagnosis of PDDNOS than with one of autism, it is critical that the correct diagnosis be made by an experienced diagnostician.

There are a number of associated features that are present in some, but not all, individuals with a PDD. These include abnormalities in eating, drinking, and sleeping; oddities or fluctuations of mood; attentional and activity-level disturbances; aggression; self-injurious behavior; and unusual fears or attachments (APA, 1994). Some children demonstrate odd responses to sensory stimuli, including a high threshold for pain, oversensitivity to sound, and fascination with sensory experiences (e.g., lights and visual patterns). Many children with PDD demonstrate "tactile defensiveness" in which there is an overly negative emotional response to tactile sensations. Although these features are commonly seen and may present great challenges to parents and professionals working with the child, they are not required for a diagnosis since they are not universally present.

Another widely used diagnostic system is that of the International Classification of Diseases (ICD), which is currently in its 10th revision (World Health Organization [WHO], 1992). As mandated by a treaty obligation between the American developers of the *DSM-IV* and WHO, an explicit effort was made to maintain similarity between the *DSM-IV* and ICD-10 (10th revision) systems. Thus, the PDD subtypes, specific diagnostic criteria, coding, and terminology are almost identical in the two systems. ICD-10 criteria are used more frequently in countries outside the United States.

Historically, other methods of defining autism have existed. Perhaps the best known are those of the National Society for Autistic Children (NSAC, 1978) and Rutter's (1978) criteria. The NSAC definition was similar in many ways to the present criteria but emphasized sensory abnormalities more than the *DSM-IV* and ICD-10. Rutter's definition followed closely that of Kanner as outlined in his initial paper (Kanner, 1943). Since the time when autism was first included in the *DSM-III* (APA, 1980) and ICD-9 (WHO, 1977) systems, however, other sources of diagnostic criteria for autism are used very rarely.

There are a number of instruments that have been developed to collect the information used to make *DSM-IV* and ICD-10 diagnoses. The Autism Diagnostic Interview–Revised (ADI-R), (Lord, Rutter, & LeCouteur, 1994) and Autism Diagnostic Schedule–Generic (ADOS-G), (Lord, Rutter, & DiLavore, 1998) have become the gold standards for diagnosing autism in research settings and are gaining in popularity for clinical use as well. The ADI-R is a structured parent interview that collects detailed information about current behavior and early development relevant to autism. For a diagnosis of autism, scores in the three *DSM-IV* ICD-10 domains (social, communication, and restricted/repetitive behaviors) must be above empirically derived thresholds. The ADI-R's companion, the ADOS-G, is a standardized observational assessment that provides several opportunities for social interaction and communication and measures behaviors of particular interest in diagnosing autism, such as social overtures, pretend play, joint attention, imitation, requesting, conversation reciprocity, and verbal and nonverbal communication (e.g., eye contact, gesture, facial expression). The ADOS-G measures the same domains as the ADI-R, providing opportunities for the examiner to directly observe behaviors reported by parents in the interview. Both instruments have high reliability and validity when used by trained examiners (Lord et al., 1989; Lord, et al., 1994).

An assessment tool more widely used in clinical settings is the Childhood Autism Rating Scale (CARS), (Schopler, Reichler, & Renner, 1986). The CARS takes substantially less training to administer than the ADI-R and ADOS-G. It was developed to distinguish children with autism from those with other developmental disabilities or normal functioning. It contains 15 items that measure behavior relevant to autism, including relating to others, communication, sensory functioning, emotional reactions, and resistance to change. Each item is rated on a 1-to-4 scale, with 1 indicating behavior that is age-appropriate and 4 indicating behavior that is highly abnormal for the child's age and characteristic of severe autism. Total scores can range from 15 to 60, with a cutoff of 30 indicating autism. The dimensional nature of this instrument is useful in quantifying the severity of autistic symptoms, with higher scores indicating more severe symptoms. The CARS has been shown to have high reliability and validity as a diagnostic tool (Schopler et al., 1986).

Recent work in the early diagnosis of autism has suggested that it is possible to identify the disorder in children as young as age 2 years with a high degree of reliability (see Stone, 1997). At this young age, however, children may not yet exhibit all the diagnostic features required by the *DSM-IV* criteria for a diagnosis of autism. For instance, because most very young children with autism are nonverbal, abnormal language features such as echolalia and repetitive or idiosyncratic use of language are usually not apparent. Similarly, impairment in peer relationships is not readily apparent because little sophistication in such relationships is expected by this chronological age. A need for sameness and routine is another feature that often is not apparent in very young children but emerges at later developmental ages. Research on appropriate criteria for diagnosis of autism in very young children is continuing and is important to developing more effective early intervention.

ETIOLOGY

Kanner (1943) originally suggested that children with autism were born with "an innate inability to form the usual, biologically provided affective contacts with people" (p. 42). He later suggested, however, that the disorder was not inborn but rather environmentally caused. He and others of his time, particularly those trained in the psychoanalytic tradition predominant in the 1940s and 1950s, believed autism to be the result of inadequate nurturance by emotionally cold, rejecting parents (Bettelheim, 1967). By the 1960s, however, evidence that autism was a biologically based disorder began to accumulate. One theorist who was influential in this paradigm shift was Rimland (1964), who attacked psychogenic theories of autism as "pernicious." Rimland pointed out that these theories had never been subjected to empirical testing, and he discussed evidence suggesting that autism was due instead to a neurological defect.

Since Rimland's initial suggestion, a good deal of research has been focused on understanding the neural substrate(s) of autism. The following information is largely specific to autistic disorder, as very little research has been done on the neurological bases of other PDDs. In subsets of individuals with autism, structural neuroanatomical abnormalities have been documented in the limbic system (Bauman & Kemper, 1985, 1988), cerebellum (Courchesne,

Yeung-Courchesne, Press, Hesselink, & Jernigan, 1988; Ritvo et al., 1986), parietal lobes (Courchesne, Press, & Yeung-Courchesne, 1993), and temporal lobes (Hoon & Reiss, 1992; White & Rosenbloom, 1992). Individuals with autism have also been found to have larger-than-average brain volume (Filipek et al., 1992; Piven, Arndt, Bailey, & Andreasen, 1996). Functional imaging studies have failed to demonstrate consistent patterns in autism, with some finding evidence of global hypermetabolism (Rumsey, Duara, et al., 1985), others finding evidence of specific areas of hypometabolism (George, Costa, Kouris, Ring, & Ell, 1992; Sherman, Nass, & Shapiro, 1984; Zilbovicius et al., 1995), and still others finding no brain metabolic differences in autism relative to controls (Zilbovicius et al., 1992). Small sample size (e.g., George et al., 1992) and different control groups may account for some of the inconsistencies found across studies. Taking an alternate approach, Horwitz and colleagues (Horwitz, Rumsey, Grady, & Rapoport, 1988) examined metabolic patterns across different brain regions, looking for intercorrelations that might reflect "functional loops" that are important to behavior. Control subjects demonstrated large, positive correlations among frontal, parietal, and subcortical regions, which are thought to indicate coordinated neural circuitry. In contrast, individuals with autism demonstrated large negative correlations. Thus, it may not be that the structure or function or individual brain regions are abnormal in autism but rather that the functional coordination among them causes symptoms of the disorder.

Genetic factors also appear to play some role in the development of autism. Evidence for a genetic contribution to the disorder comes from four primary sources (Rutter et al., 1990; Smalley, Asarnow, & Spence, 1988). First, the recurrence rate for autism after the birth of one child with the disorder is approximately 3 percent, a rate that is 60 to 100 times the general population risk. Second, the concordance rate for autism in monozygotic twins is elevated relative to that for dizygotic twins, averaging 64 percent in the former but only 9 percent in the latter when results are aggregated across studies. Third, autism occurs in association with a variety of known genetic abnormalities, including fragile X syndrome (Bailey et al., 1993) and tuberous sclerosis complex (Gillberg, Gillberg, & Ahlsen, 1994; Hunt & Shepherd, 1993). A maternally inherited duplication of the long arm of chromosome 15 recently has been identified in between 1 percent and 4 percent of three separate samples of individuals with autism (Cook et al., 1998; Schroer et al., 1998; Weidmer-Mikhail, Sheldon, & Ghaziuddin, 1998). Fourth, research suggests that a broader phenotype of familial cognitive and social anomalies runs in the families of people with autism. Higher rates of learning disabilities, mental retardation, speech and language disorders, shyness, social awkwardness, and depression have been reported in first-degree relatives of individuals with autism than in family members of controls with other disabilities, such as Down syndrome (Bolton et al., 1994; DeLong, 1994; Fombonne, Bolton, Prior, Jordan, & Rutter, 1997; Piven, Palmer, Jacobi, Childress, & Arndt, 1997). Thus, what appears to be genetically transmitted in these families is not autism per se, but a vulnerability to cognitive, language, and social disorders, with the most severe outcome of the genetic diathesis being autism.

A number of other factors have been proposed to cause autism. There is some evidence that infectious agents, affecting the fetus in utero or the infant in the first years of life, may contribute to development of the disorder (Coleman, 1987). For example, approximately 10 percent of children exposed to the rubella virus in utero develop autism (Chess, Korn, & Fernandez, 1971). Warren (1998) has hypothesized that some cases of autism may result from an inherited immune deficiency that increases susceptibility to viruses or bacteria. Unable to clear pathogens in a timely manner, it is hypothesized that the fetus or young infant is at increased risk for a pathogen damaging the brain directly or triggering an autoimmune reaction that affects brain function. Infections later in life are a very rare factor in the development of autism but have been documented in a few cases, particularly herpes simplex–induced encephalopathies (DeLong, Bean, & Brown, 1981; Gillberg, 1986; I. C. Gillberg, 1991). Metabolic diseases, such as phenylketonuria and purine synthesis disorders, may underlie some cases of autism (Coleman, 1987); however, others have argued that such medical conditions are involved in only a very small proportion of cases (Rutter, Bailey, Bolton, & LeCouteur, 1994).

Finally, a number of pre- and perinatal factors have been associated with autism, including advanced maternal age, bleeding during pregnancy, preeclampsia, anoxia at birth, and other delivery complications (Gillberg & Gillberg, 1983; Tsai, 1987). These factors are not specific to autism, however, and have been found in the histories of individuals with a number of other developmental disabilities as well. In addition, there is some suggestion that these pre- and perinatal factors may be the consequences of autism rather than causative factors in the disorder (Goodman, 1990). Specifically, it has been hypothesized that obstetrical complications indicate that a fetus is already developmentally compromised, perhaps due to genetic factors; thus, in this account the central nervous system insult causing autism is proposed to occur long before the obstetrical complications take place (Bailey et al., 1995; Bolton et al., 1994).

COGNITIVE CHARACTERISTICS

Children with autism, unlike those with mental retardation or other developmental disabilities, demonstrate a wide scatter of skills on cognitive testing. Research has demonstrated a specific neuropsychological profile that includes spared performance on tasks relying on rote, mechanical, or visual-spatial-perceptual processes and deficient performance on tasks requiring higher-order conceptual processes, reasoning, interpretation, integration, or abstraction (Minshew, Goldstein, & Siegel, 1997). This pattern is present across multiple cognitive domains, with dissociations between simple and complex information processing demonstrated in the areas of language, memory, executive function, reading, mathematics, perspective taking, and motor skills

(Klinger & Dawson, 1995; Minshew, Goldstein, Taylor, & Siegel, 1994; Ozonoff & Strayer, 1997; Reed & Peterson, 1990; Rumsey & Hamburger, 1988). Learning, in general, is characterized by difficulty seeing relationships between pieces of information, identifying central patterns or themes, distinguishing relevant from irrelevant information, and deriving meaning. Individuals with autism tend to be detail oriented but have difficulty "seeing the big picture" and can be quite literal in their thinking. Such difficulties are apparent across the autism continuum and are present in even very high-functioning individuals (Grandin, 1995).

Intelligence

The majority of children with autism function intellectually in the mentally handicapped range (i.e., IQ less than 70). An early study by DeMyer and colleagues (DeMyer et al., 1974) examined the distribution of IQ scores among children with autism. They found that almost 50 percent of their sample functioned in the severe-profound range of mental retardation (IQ less than 35); 26 percent, in the moderately handicapped range (IQ equals 35–50); 20 percent, in the mildly retarded range (IQ equals 50–70); and only 6 percent, in the nonretarded range (IQ greater than 70). The low representation of high-functioning cases in this sample is likely a reflection of the era (the early 1970s), during which there was less recognition of mild forms of autism than today, and thus less opportunity for early intervention. A more recent study found that 23 percent of a sample of preschool children with autism demonstrated IQ scores in the moderate range of mental retardation; 48 percent, in the mild range; and 29 percent, in the nonretarded range (Lord & Schopler, 1988); however, children functioning in the severe and profound ranges were not included in this study. Although the results of these two studies are not completely convergent, they are consistent, along with many others (e.g., Freeman, Ritvo, Needleman, & Yokota, 1985; Ritvo et al., 1989), in finding that the majority of individuals with autism (approximately 75 percent) are also mentally handicapped. In general, girls with autism obtain lower scores on tests of intellectual function than boys (Lord & Schopler, 1985).

Numerous studies have demonstrated a particular intellectual pattern characteristic of autism when individuals are tested on standardized measures such as the Wechsler Intelligence Scales (Wechsler, 1974, 1981). A typical pattern is a higher Performance IQ than Verbal IQ and specific intersubtest scatter, with Block Design typically the highest subtest and Comprehension usually the lowest (Lincoln, Allen, & Kilman, 1995). However, there is substantial variability in the intellectual profiles of people with autism, and these patterns are by no means universal (Siegel, Minshew, & Goldstein, 1996). Thus, they should never be used for differential diagnostic purposes. No specific cognitive pattern confirms or rules out a diagnosis of autism.

There are particular concerns about the validity of testing younger, lower-functioning, and nonverbal children with autism. It is critical that care be taken in choosing which intellectual test to administer to the lower-functioning and/or nonverbal individual (Groden & Mann, 1988; Johnson-Martin, 1988; Sparrow, 1997; Watson & Marcus, 1988). It is recommended that tests be used that (1) are appropriate for both mental and chronological age, (2) provide a full range (in the lower direction) of standard scores, (3) measure and score verbal abilities and nonverbal abilities separately, (4) provide an overall index of ability, and (5) have relatively current norms. The intellectual assessment measures currently available that meet most of these criteria are the Differential Abilities Scale (Elliott, 1990), the Mullen Scales of Early Learning (Mullen, 1989, 1992), and the Leiter International Performance Scale–Revised (Leiter, 1979). Finally, it is essential that a measure of adaptive functioning be collected for any children evaluated for an associated mental handicap. A diagnosis of mental retardation relies on both subaverage intellectual functioning (IQ less than 70) and concurrent deficits in adaptive functioning.

IQ scores in individuals with autism appear to be relatively stable over time and development. Correlations of IQ scores from preschool testing with IQ scores from school-age testing are generally significant in children with autism and are similar to values seen in nonhandicapped children (Lord & Schopler, 1988). The older the age at initial assessment, the more stable and predictive are the scores (Lord & Schopler, 1989). Scores can change over time, however, with a proportion of children changing IQ grouping levels (e.g., from moderately to mildly retarded; see Lord & Schopler, 1989; Freeman et al., 1991). Such changes in IQ may become more common as intensive early intervention becomes the norm. Thus, narrowly categorizing intellectual level based on early IQ scores may not be appropriate.

Attention

Many investigations have found attentional abnormalities in individuals with autism. Early studies, for example, suggested that arousal modulating systems were dysfunctional, leading to fluctuations between states of over- and underarousal (Hutt, Hutt, Lee, & Ounsted, 1964; Ornitz & Ritvo, 1968). Later work, using cortical event–related potentials, confirmed that orienting and processing of novel stimuli by persons with autism is reduced (Courchesne, Lincoln, Kilman, & Galambos, 1985; Dawson, Finley, Phillips, & Galpert, 1986). Many individuals with autism appear to have "overfocused" attention. The term *stimulus overselectivity* has been used to describe the tendency of individuals with autism to respond to only a subset of environmental cues during learning situations (Lovaas, Koegel, & Schreibman, 1979).

Consistent with overly focused attention is a deficit in shifting attention. Recently, several researchers have demonstrated that individuals with autism, even those with IQs in the normal range, have difficulty moving their attention from one spatial location to another (Casey, Gordon, Mannheim, & Rumsey, 1993; Courchesne et al., 1994; Wainwright-Sharp & Bryson, 1993). This pattern of attentional dysfunction distinguishes children with autism from those with attention deficit/hyperactivity disorder (AD/HD), another childhood condition involving attention problems. Although children with AD/HD have little difficulty moving attention (Swanson et al., 1991), they demonstrate severe impairment in sustaining attention and controlling impulses (Douglas & Peters, 1979). In contrast, a number of studies have suggested that the ability to sustain attention is a relatively spared function in autism (Buchsbaum et al., 1992; Casey et al., 1993; Garretson, Fein & Waterhouse, 1990).

Executive Functions

Recent research has found widespread executive function impairments in individuals with autism. Executive function is a broadly defined cognitive construct originally used to describe the deficits found in patients with focal frontal lobe lesions. It refers to the many skills required to prepare for and execute complex behavior, including planning, inhibition, mental flexibility, and the mental representation of tasks and goals. Executive dysfunction has been consistently found across different ages and ability levels of people with autism when compared with appropriate controls (for a review, see Ozonoff, 1995; Pennington & Ozonoff, 1996). Executive function deficits have been found in a variety of other conditions as well, including AD/HD, obsessive-compulsive disorder, schizophrenia, and various dementias (Ozonoff, 1997), but the impairment in autism does appear to be more severe, of a different type, and of different onset than the executive deficits perceived in other disorders (Pennington & Ozonoff, 1996).

Understanding of Mental States

One of the most active areas of investigation in recent psychological research has pertained to the ability of children with autism to understand mental states. As explained by Astington (1994), people typically explain and predict their own and others' behavior by imputing mental states, that is, beliefs, desires, intentions, and emotions. Children's development in this area has been described as the development of a "theory of mind." A type of task developed by Wimmer and Perner (1983) has been used widely in research in this area. In this task, a "false belief" story is acted out for the child, using toys and dolls. For example, in the story two girls are playing, and one of them, Sally, puts her marble into her picnic basket. Then Sally leaves to go for a walk. The other girl, Anne, takes the marble out of the picnic basket and puts it into a box. Sally comes back into the room and wants to play with her marble. After seeing this scenario enacted, the child is asked to predict where Sally will look for her marble. A typical 3-year-old will say that Sally will look for her marble in the box. The 3-year-old seems unable to impute a false belief to Sally, which would run contrary to the child's own knowledge that the marble is now in the box. By age 4, however, the typical child can solve this problem quite successfully. A growing number of studies have demonstrated that children with autism have difficulty with this false belief task at mental ages well above 4 years (see Happé & Frith, 1995, for a review), as well as difficulty on other tasks requiring them to respond on the basis of mental state representations (e.g., Phillips, Baron-Cohen, & Rutter, 1995). Leslie (1988) proposed that the "mind-blindness" of children with autism on tasks such as these is predictable from their earlier difficulties in understanding and engaging in symbolic play. In Leslie's view, children with autism do not develop the "metarepresentations" that permit them to pretend that an object is something other than what it is or to play with imaginary objects, pets, or people. These metarepresentations are considered essential in the development of a theory of mind. Looking at even earlier precursors, Baron-Cohen (1989) found that children with autism were impaired in their use and understanding of pointing for the purpose of sharing attention (an intention to influence another's mental state), but were not impaired in the use of pointing to get a desired object (an intention to influence another's behavior). The inability to understand mental states apparently is not universal among individuals with autism; in a number of studies, small proportions of higher-functioning children as well as older individuals with autism have passed the theory of mind tests. It may be that these individuals have developed competence in theory of mind, or alternatively, they may use some other strategies to solve the experimental tasks (Bailey, Phillips, & Rutter, 1996; Happé & Frith, 1995).

SENSORIMOTOR CHARACTERISTICS

There is a relative dearth of empirical information on the development of sensorimotor behaviors in children with autism, compared to the information available on cognitive, social, and communicative development. Yet disruptions in areas such as sensoriperceptual responses, arousal modulation, movement patterns, and object manipulations are widely reported in retrospective accounts of the early development of children with autism as well as in older children with autism (e.g., Gillberg et al., 1990; Ornitz et al., 1977). O'Neill and Jones (1997) reviewed firsthand accounts and psychological research on sensoriperceptual abnormalities in autism. Three major conclusions emerged from the clinical research they reviewed. First, unusual sensory responses are present in the majority of children with autism. Second, these unusual sensory responses may be linked to other aspects of behavior that are criterial in the diagnosis of autism, such as repetitive behaviors and social aloofness. Third, abnormal responses are apparent very early in the child's development. A recent study confirmed the early manifestation of some of these unusual behaviors. Baranek (1999) used home videotapes to compare sensorimotor behavior of three groups of infants: a typically developing group, a group with developmental delay, and a group with autism. The videotapes were made when the children were between 9 and 12 months of age, prior to the time when diagnoses of autism had been made. Symptoms that were seen at a high rate among the infants with autism compared to the other two groups included poor nonsocial visual orientation and attention, prompted or delayed responses to the child's own name, excessive mouthing of objects, and social touch aversions.

Stone (1997) listed symptoms related to "restricted and repetitive interests and behaviors" that have been found in various studies to differentiate between autism and developmental delay in children under 36 months. Most of these suggest differences in sensorimotor development and functioning:

- motor stereotypies/unusual postures
- inappropriate use of objects/unusual play
- attachment to unusual objects
- unusual visual interests
- inconsistent response to sounds/seems deaf
- insensitivity to pain, cold, or heat
- hypersensitivity to taste

SOCIAL CHARACTERISTICS

Given the centrality of social interaction difficulties to the diagnosis of PDD, understanding the social characteristics of these children is essential. Research in this area is illuminating in demonstrating that children with PDD are not devoid of social abilities or motivation; however, there are a number of qualitative differences in the social development and functioning of these children compared to children who are developing typically or children with other developmental disorders.

Development in Infancy

Recently researchers in the area of autism have devoted considerable attention to a hypothesis, initially suggested by Kanner (1943), that the syndrome of autism represents a biologically based disturbance of social/affective development. Our knowledge of development during infancy among children with autism and other PDD syndromes has been limited because these syndromes are usually not diagnosed until children are 2 years or older. In a recent review of research on the early development of children with autism, Stone (1997) listed the following behaviors in the social domain as differentiating autism from other developmental delay in children under 3 years of age:

- poor imitation
- abnormal eye contact

- poor relating or interactions
- underresponsiveness/ignores others
- little interest in social games
- preference for being alone
- little interest in being held
- little smiling/bland facial expression

Lord (1995) noted the convergence of findings from several studies, including: her own follow-up study of 2-year-olds referred for possible autism; a study of birthday videotapes of 1-year-olds later diagnosed as autistic (Osterling & Dawson, 1994); and a retrospective study of children with autism during their first 2 years of life (Dahlgren & Gillberg, 1989). Two characteristics that consistently distinguished children with autism both from children without disabilities and from children with other disabilities were a lack of initiative in directing the visual attention of others (e.g., by pointing or showing objects) and an abnormal response to voice (e.g., failing to orient to own name).

Attachment

The attachment paradigm in psychological research involves observing children's reactions to separation from, and reunions with, caregivers, compared to their reactions to strangers. Sigman and Mundy (1989) used this paradigm to study children with autism. Like children developing typically and children with mental retardation, the children with autism directed social behaviors for significantly longer periods to caregivers than to strangers. Thus, the study did show evidence of attachment behavior among children with autism, refuting earlier notions that autism was caused by a failure of attachment between children and their caregivers. This finding has been replicated by several other research teams as well (e.g., Rogers, Ozonoff, & Maslin-Cole, 1993). Sigman and Mundy (1989) observed, however, that the quality of attachment may not be the same for children with autism; for example, these children used less positive affect in expressing attachment than did children in the other two groups.

Joint Attention

In the typical sequence of development, at approximately 6 to 9 months of age, infants develop the ability to expand face-to-face interactions to include objects and events external to the dyad (Trevarthan, 1979). This type of behavior is commonly referred to as *joint attention*. Joint attention behaviors include such acts as pointing and alternating gaze between the interactive partner and an object/event, for the purpose of sharing one's interest or experience. Joint attention behaviors in children with autism have been the subject of considerable research, and various studies have consistently found joint attention to be an area of specific deficit for these children. These difficulties are so specific to the disorder that 80 to 90 percent of young children with autism can be discriminated from children with other types of developmental disabilities such as mental retardation based on their difficulties in initiating and responding to joint attention bids (see Mundy, 1995, for a review). Difficulties in this area stand in contrast to generally better skills in nonverbal requesting skills and social interactions that do not involve outside objects or events (Landry & Loveland, 1989; McEvoy, Rogers, & Pennington, 1993; Wetherby, Yonclas, & Bryan, 1989).

Eye Contact

A lack of eye contact is frequently noted clinically among children with PDD. Interestingly, several studies have found that children with autism do not differ from other children at similar developmental levels in terms of the frequency or duration of gaze (e.g., Dawson, Hill, Spencer, Galpert, & Watson, 1990; Mirenda, Donnellan, & Yoder, 1983). There do appear to be numerous qualitative differences in gaze, however. For instance, children with autism are less likely to combine eye contact with a smile (Dawson et al., 1990). As already discussed, they do not use gaze effectively to initiate or regulate joint attention.

Eye contact, which is often quite intensive in nature, has been reported in children with Rett's disorder (Trevanthan & Naidu, 1988). Another report by Cohen and his colleagues suggested variations among subgroups of children with PDD (Cohen et al., 1989). In examining boys in three age groups between the ages of 2 and 17 years, they found that males with autism and fragile X syndrome actively avoided eye contact, whereas males with autism who did not have fragile X syndrome were insensitive to antecedent social cues that could lead to mutual gaze but did not actively avoid eye contact. Once again, we are reminded to consider both the quantity and quality of responses in our clinical observations.

Imitation

Imitation can be considered in the cognitive domain, but it is important to consider the social significance of imitation as well. Mutual imitation between caregivers and infants seems to be important in sustaining early interactions (Stern, 1985). Several studies of preschoolers with autism have found delays in the development of imitation compared to object permanence skills, and have shown a correlation between imitation skills and aspects of social behavior such as social responsiveness (Curcio, 1978; Dawson & Adams, 1984). In addition, these same studies indicate that imitation skills correlate with language skills. The object permanence skills of preschool children with autism do not correlate with measures of language or social responsiveness.

These findings lend credence to consideration of imitation as a social cognitive behavior.

Social Responsiveness

The view of the child with autism as devoid of social responsiveness is too bleak and oversimplified. Research has shown that even children who are at low developmental levels initiate, and respond to, social overtures from adults through means such as eye contact, physical approaches, and nonverbal communication (Mundy, Sigman, Ungerer, & Sherman, 1986; Sigman, Mundy, Sherman, & Ungerer, 1986). Moreover, children with autism at both lower and higher developmental levels have been found to increase social behavior when adults actively solicit interaction. We would suggest that the problems in social responsiveness seen among children with PDD may be based in a lack of social understanding as much as a lack of social interest (see also Baron-Cohen, 1988).

Among older or more able children with autism, impairment in peer interaction is often even more apparent than impairment in interactions with adults (Howlin, 1986). This may be due to the fact that adults adapt their approaches and responses to the child's level and idiosyncrasies more effectively than do peers.

Affect

Clinical descriptions and controlled research have revealed quantitative and qualitative differences in the display of affect by children with autism compared to children with mental retardation at comparable developmental levels. Snow, Hertzig, and Shapiro (1987) found that preschoolers with autism displayed fewer intervals of affect and less positive affect compared to children with mental retardation. When the children with autism did show affect, it was less likely to be directed to the social partner and more likely to occur during solitary play or to appear random and unrelated to anything in the context. Kasari, Sigman, Mundy, and Yirmiya (1990) found that children with autism displayed positive affect as frequently as did children with mental retardation or children developing typically, but they were less likely than the other two groups to pair their positive affect with bids for joint attention. In addition, the children with autism showed more ambiguous displays, in which they appeared to simultaneously display positive and negative affects.

COMMUNICATION CHARACTERISTICS

Describing the communication characteristics of children with PDD must include a spectrum of individuals ranging from those who are nonverbal to those who demonstrate vocabulary and syntactic skills within the normal range for their age. This variability in developmental level of communication skills (as well as variability in cognitive developmental level) must be considered when interpreting research in this area.

Pragmatics

The term **pragmatics** refers to the interpretation and use of language in varying social, physical, psychological, and linguistic contexts. When we examine the patterns of language and communication development among children with PDD, pragmatic difficulties emerge as the best common denominator, although the types and degree of pragmatic deficits differ widely. As is true with the other areas covered in this chapter, most of the available research pertains to children with autism.

Even prior to the time when the term *pragmatics* came into common use in describing and analyzing language behavior, pragmatic deficits were described among children with autism. In his initial descriptions of children with autism, Kanner (1943) talked about a failure to use language for the purpose of communication. Cunningham (1968) said that the child with autism "shows a lack of empathy or ability to apprehend his hearer's state of mind and therefore falls back on non-communicative or demanding speech" (p. 243).

Rydell and Prizant (1995) reported that echolalia is a characteristic of at least 85 percent of verbal children with autism. Immediate echolalia is the repetition of a word or phrase just spoken by another person, whereas delayed echolalia involves the used of a phrase spoken by another person after some elapsed time. Some researchers have characterized echolalia as "meaningless" (Fay, 1969) or "nonfunctional" (Laski, Charlop, & Schreibman, 1988), whereas others have argued that echoed words and phrases are often used with some comprehension and for functional communicative purposes (Prizant & Rydell, 1984).

There is an obvious overlap between the social and communicative characteristics of children with autism. We already noted that children with autism generally have much better skills in nonverbal requesting than in establishing joint attention. In children developing typically, these two functions emerge in preverbal children at roughly the same time (Bates, 1979), so the difficulty of children with autism in establishing joint attention is not explicable solely on the basis of a generalized delay in the development of language and communication skills, but rather suggests that specific skills are more impaired than others.

Children with autism are more delayed in the development of pragmatic skills than in other aspects of language (e.g., syntax, semantics, or phonology). For example, Watson, Martin, and Schaffer (1986) found that in a sample of 17 school-age children with autism, only the 3 highest-functioning children, all of whom produced mean lengths of utterances (MLU) above

4.0, expressed a range of communicative functions comparable to those reported by Dale (1981) among typically developing children at the one-word stage of development. Ball (1978) reported that children with autism were delayed in the development of communicative functions compared to both typically developing children and children with specific language impairments.

Wetherby and Prutting (1984) investigated specific communicative functions in a small group of elementary school-aged children with autism functioning at about a 1- to 2-year-old level in their language skills. Although the overall numbers of communicative acts were similar for the children with autism and a group of language-matched, typically developing children, the children with autism requested objects and actions more and protested more than the typically developing children. On the other hand, the children with autism in their sample did not verbally request information, acknowledge others, show off, or comment. Findings by Watson et al. (1986) were only partially convergent. A number of the school-age children with autism in their sample did comment on objects or activities in the immediate environment, but efforts to get the attention of another person were very rare.

Children with autism functioning at higher language levels still exhibit numerous pragmatic difficulties. For example, they have difficulties with maintaining a conversation and monitoring their listener's needs by adjusting the information given based on whether the listener has prior knowledge of the topic (Baltaxe, 1977; Tager-Flusberg, 1981). Geller (1991), however, emphasized that the verbal school-aged children with autism in her study showed emerging abilities in adapting to the listener's perspective.

Semantics

In a comprehensive review of the existing literature on language development among children with autism, Tager-Flusberg (1981) concluded that children with autism seemed to follow a normal, albeit delayed, course of development in the areas of syntax and phonology but exhibited deviations in their development of pragmatic and semantic skills. Although pragmatic skills have been an area of considerable research since the publication of Tager-Flusberg's review, the areas of syntactic, phonological, and semantic development have been investigated much less extensively among children with autism and other types of PDD.

Tager-Flusberg did conduct some subsequent research on semantic development of children with autism (e.g., 1985a, 1985b). Based on this research, she concluded that although children with autism who function at low cognitive levels may acquire few words and use them only in limited contexts, higher-functioning children with autism do not seem to have any difficulty with organizing the conceptual knowledge of concrete objects into categories, in representing word meanings (at least for nouns), or in their productive naming abilities. In these areas, the performance of children with autism is similar to that of matched groups of children developing typically and children with mild or moderate mental retardation.

Tager-Flusberg and colleagues (Tager-Flusberg, 1989; Tager-Flusberg et al., 1990) also reported results from a longitudinal study of language development in young children with autism compared to children with Down syndrome matched for age and initial language level. The children with autism were found to use the same distribution of word classes (e.g., nouns, verbs, adjectives) as the children with Down syndrome, but they used a smaller number of different words within each category.

In their investigation, Watson et al. (1986) found that children with autism developed semantic relational categories (e.g., actor, action, object, possessor) in roughly the same developmental sequence as reported by earlier researchers of development in typically developing children. However, typically developing children were reported to exhibit the use of a range of semantic categories at MLUs of 2.5, which were only observed in the children with autism who had MLUs above 4.0. Thus, semantic development appeared to be more delayed than syntactic development. It is not clear whether this pattern is attributable to autism or to the concomitant mental retardation of the children with autism in this study.

Children with autism have often been described as being very literal. Twachtman (1995) gives an example of a 7-year-old who was asked to write a story about how to make a friend. The boy wrote, "Atoms, cells, eyes, nose, mouth, arms, legs. P.S. Then say hello." When questioned about his story, the child replied, "That's what a friend is made of." As illustrated by this example, children with autism have difficulty in understanding implied meanings and making social interpretations rather than literal interpretations.

Syntax

The level of syntactic development among young children with pervasive developmental disorders varies considerably from child to child. As discussed in the section on diagnosis, a marked delay in syntactic development is an exclusionary characteristic for a diagnosis of Asperger's disorder according to the *DSM-IV* (APA, 1994). Among children diagnosed with autism, it is common to find those who are nonverbal or using primarily single-word utterances as well as those who can produce relatively sophisticated sentence structures. In several reviews of the literature, however, investigators have concluded that problems with syntax are not a distinguishing characteristic of the autistic syndrome (Paul, 1987; Swisher & Demetras, 1985; Tager-Flusberg, 1981, 1985c). This conclusion has been drawn from analyses of cross-sectional language samples taken at a single point in time (Cantwell, Baker, & Rutter, 1978; Pierce & Bartolucci, 1977), which demonstrated that the syntax of children with autism was rule governed, varied in complexity depending on the developmental level of the child, and did not contain structures that were unusual compared to those of mental age-matched children developing typically or children with mental retardation. In a longitudinal study, Tager-Flusberg and her colleagues (Tager-Flusberg et al., 1990) found that children with autism developed syntactic structures in the same order as children with Down syndrome, although the children with autism did use a narrower range and more limited variety of syntactic structures than the other group.

Evidence regarding the acquisition of grammatical morphemes (e.g., plural /s/, past tense /ed/) is more contradictory, and across all studies the data are still very limited. Two studies (Bartolucci, Pierce, & Streiner, 1980; Howlin, 1984) reported significant differences in the acquisition of grammatical morphemes in children with autism compared to other groups of children. Tager-Flusberg (1989) also reported some evidence for subtle differences in acquisition of grammatical morphemes from her longitudinal study. Semantic and pragmatic explanations have been offered for these differences (see Tager-Flusberg, 1989).

Phonology

The area of phonology includes the acquisition of phonemes and the phonological rules governing accurate articulation (segmentals), but also prosodic rules governing intonation and stress (suprasegmentals). With respect to the segmental aspects, no striking characteristics distinguish children with autism from other children matched for developmental level (for reviews, see Paul, 1987; Tager-Flusberg, 1981). On the other hand, clinical reports and research have consistently reported differences in prosodic elements of speech production for children with autism and Asperger's disorder (see Baltaxe & Simmons, 1985; Tager-Flusberg, 1989; Wing, 1981). These authors indicated that the prosody of children with autism and Asperger's disorder has often been described as atonal or monotonic, nor is it well modulated with respect to rhythm, loudness and pitch. Baltaxe and her colleagues (Baltaxe, 1984; Baltaxe & Guthrie, 1987; Baltaxe & Simmons, 1985) have been the primary researchers examining specific parameters of prosodic development, such as the use of contrastive stress and primary sentence stress, among children with autism. Depending upon the parameter being considered, these researchers have found both similarities and differences in the use of prosody by children with autism compared to children with specific language impairments (SLI) and children developing typically. For example, the patterns of use of contrastive stress were found to be similar among all three groups, although the children with autism sometimes applied contrastive stress inappropriately to function words, a type of error not observed in the other two groups. Overall, the children with autism and the children with SLI performed more poorly than the children developing typically, even though the groups were matched for language level.

Literacy

There is limited information regarding the development of literacy skills among children with PDD. Minshew et al. (1994) found that high-functioning individuals with autism performed as well as, or better than, normal controls matched on age and IQ on tests of single-word oral reading, nonword reading, and spelling. These measures all require phonological decoding skills and thus indicate preserved or even advanced knowledge of grapheme-phoneme correspondence rules in autism. In contrast, subjects with autism in this study performed less well than controls on two measures of reading comprehension.

An early interest in letters, numbers, product logos, and similar configurations is frequently noted in clinical settings for some, but not all, children with PDD. A subgroup of these children exhibit **hyperlexia**, which has been defined as the early development of decoding skills without the benefit of reading instruction. Further, children with hyperlexia exhibit marked intellectual or language impairments and delayed reading comprehension skills, which are more commensurate with the level of intellectual and language skills than the decoding skills (Goldberg, 1987). Hyperlexia has been reported in children with a range of disabilities, including mental retardation, Down syndrome, apraxia of speech, language delay or disorder, and subtypes of PDD (see Aram & Healy, 1988, for a review), but it probably co-occurs most frequently with a diagnosis of one of the subtypes of PDD (see Whitehouse and Harris, 1984). Burd, Fisher, Knowlton, and Kerbeshian (1987) investigated the prevalence of hyperlexia among all school children with PDD in the state of North Dakota and found a prevalence rate of 6.8 percent (4 children out of 59 diagnosed with PDD). Whitehouse and Harris's (1984) investigation suggested a higher incidence, however, at least among children with autism. Records of 155 children diagnosed with infantile autism at one facility were reviewed, and, from different types of documentation in the charts, 52 cases (33.5%) were identified as hyperlexic.

As indicated by Goldberg (1987), the way hyperlexic children learn to read is uncertain. Initially, it is likely the children use visual codes and visual memory; however, many of these children go on to discover the connection between graphemes and phonemes without instruction.

The pattern exhibited by high-functioning individuals with autism, as reported by Minshew et al. (1994), and, in extreme form, by individuals with hyperlexia is quite different from that typically exhibited by individuals with reading disabilities (Pennington, 1991; Vellutino, 1979). In two studies directly comparing the reading profiles of individuals with autism versus dyslexia, the subjects with dyslexia demonstrated deficits on phonological processing measures, but strengths in comprehension and interpretation, whereas subjects with autism displayed the opposite pattern (Frith & Snowling, 1983; Rumsey & Hamburger, 1990). Thus, the profile of reading strengths and weaknesses seen in autism is not simply a reflection of general learning disability, but takes on a highly characteristic pattern.

PROGNOSIS

Follow-up studies of individuals with PDD generally demonstrate gradual improvement in social, communication, and behavioral realms, but also clear continuity of disability across the lifespan. Autism is considered a lifelong disorder with only very rare (and controversial) cases of "recovery" having been reported (Gajzago & Prior, 1974; Perry, Cohen, & DeCarlo, 1995). Gillberg (C. Gillberg, 1991) outlined four categories of outcome: individuals who deteriorate in adolescence; those who remain very handicapped; those who make substantial, but restricted progress; and those who do very well, eventually leading productive, self-supporting lives.

In virtually all individuals with autism or other PDDs, even those with the fewest and mildest symptoms, there are persistent, residual deficits apparent in adulthood (Rumsey, Rapoport, & Sceery, 1985). The most common residual deficits fall in the social realm; individuals may have little social interest, may have great difficulty making friends despite some social interest, or may demonstrate highly stereotyped social interactions (e.g., engaging in invariant scripts when meeting new people; see Rumsey et al., 1985). Thought processes continue to be concrete, literal, and perseverative on certain topics or themes (Rumsey et al., 1985). In the communication domain, the most persistent difficulties fall in the realm of pragmatics (Dewey & Everard, 1974; Ritvo, Ritvo, Freeman, & Mason-Brothers, 1994). Even individuals with the best outcomes continue to have difficulty with turn taking and reciprocity in conversations and demonstrate oddities in nonverbal communication, such as poor coordination of eye contact with speech or unusual volume or intonation when speaking. Not withstanding these residual difficulties, it is important to also emphasize that the prognosis for some individuals with autism is actually quite good, with a small proportion going on to attend college, gain employment, live independently, date, and even marry (C. Gillberg, 1991; Ritvo et al., 1994; Szatmari, Bartolucci, Bremner, Bond, & Rich, 1989).

A number of factors have been identified as predictive of a more successful outcome for individuals with autism. Several studies have converged in suggesting that the attainment of meaningful communication abilities and intellectual functioning in the nonretarded range by age 5 is most predictive of good outcomes (DeMyer et al., 1973; Gillberg & Steffenburg, 1987; Lotter, 1974; Venter, Lord, & Schopler, 1992). Conversely, a pattern in which there is a period of normal development followed by a regression in social and language functions has been associated with a poorer prognosis (Kurita, 1985). It must be remembered, however, that these patterns describe average trends or central tendencies, and, in any individual case, it is difficult to determine prognosis. Another factor that has recently been associated with better outcomes is very early intervention for the child with autism (Dawson & Osterling, 1997).

INTERVENTION ISSUES

A large number of intervention approaches have been proposed for children with pervasive developmental disorders. Treatments include educational and behavioral approaches, medications prescribed to reduce activity level, anxiety and/or agitation, sensory integration therapy, auditory integration training, special diets and dietary supplements, facilitated communication, and many others. Some approaches, especially behavioral/educational approaches, have been evaluated over a period of time, with accumulated support for their effectiveness. These approaches generally focus on improving adaptive skills, reducing behavior problems, and using strengths of the individual to maximize his/her functioning and quality of life. Research on other interventions, such as facilitated communication, has yielded little support for effectiveness (Jacobson, Mulick, & Swartz, 1995; Shane, 1994). Still other proposed approaches have not been tested in a scientific manner and instead gain popularity based on anecdotal accounts of sometimes dramatic results. As Happé (1995) notes, "Throughout the history of autism, there have been claims for miraculous cures, which raise the hopes of parents, but which fade under scrutiny and are soon forgotten" (p. 110). Professionals working with children with PDD should be aware of this history. While remaining open to the possibility of new insights and information that will improve intervention effectiveness for children with PDD, the professional must also objectively evaluate treatment efficacy. A resource that describes various treatments is provided by Gerlach (1996).

Early Intervention Programs

The goals of improving communication skills must be integrated with the educational program for a child with PDD. In the past three decades, major advances have been made in the education and treatment of individuals with autism and their families. We will illustrate the range of programs by describing three models.

In 1966, a treatment program known as TEACCH (**T**reatment and **E**ducation of **A**utistic and related **C**ommunication-handicapped **Ch**ildren) was established at the University of North Carolina at Chapel Hill (Schopler & Reichler, 1971). A cornerstone of this treatment model is parent-professional collaboration (Schopler, 1987). Thus, the model has been dubbed the "parents-as-cotherapists" model (Schopler, Mesibov, Shigley, & Bashford, 1984). Parents are given support, guidance, and supervision by a professional psychoeducational therapist, who helps them develop strategies and programs to teach their child in the home setting. Another guiding element of the

TEACCH program is structured teaching. This educational approach involves structuring and physically organizing the environment and learning materials to make them more readily understandable, predictable, and clear to the child with autism. Because individuals with autism have difficulty with abstract and language-based tasks and instructional techniques but have relatively spared visual-spatial capacities, the TEACCH program uses visual strengths to remediate other cognitive weaknesses (Schopler, Mesibov, & Hearsey, 1995). For instance, there is a use of visual schedules and other visual sequences to help the child predict what will happen next or what she or he should do next. In teaching the child to take turns, visual cues may be used to signal the child as to whose turn it is. Teaching the child new skills is balanced with making adaptations in the environment that help her or him compensate for weakness and function independently. Specifically in the area of communication, the program emphasizes the development of functional communication skills for each child, utilizing augmentative communication strategies for children who have limited verbal abilities. Several studies have demonstrated the effectiveness of the structured teaching philosophy (Marcus, Lansing, Andrews, & Schopler, 1978; Schopler, Brehm, Kinsbourne, & Reichler, 1971; Short, 1984)). The application of this model to preschool-aged children has occurred both in working with parents to develop home programs and in the development of classrooms utilizing structured teaching approaches (see Lord & Schopler, 1994).

Ozonoff and Cathcart (1998) investigated the effectiveness of this model when used to develop home programs for children with autism aged 2 to 6 years. All children were concurrently enrolled in day treatment programs, most of which relied on discrete trial training techniques (to be described subsequently). A treatment group of 11 children received approximately 4 months of home programming in addition to their day treatment programs, whereas a control group received no additional intervention. Parents of children in the treatment group met weekly with clinic staff to evaluate and revise the home program, which was individualized for each child and family but included the core elements of the TEACCH program. The parents were asked to spend 30 minutes per day implementing the home program activities developed in collaboration with the professionals. Children in the treatment group made significant gains compared to the control group in the areas of imitation, fine motor, gross motor, and nonverbal conceptual skills, as well as in total score on the pre-post measure, the Psychoeducational Profile–Revised (Schopler, Reichler, Bashford, Lansing, & Marcus, 1990). In 4 months, the treatment group showed an average of 9.3 months of developmental gain.

Another structured treatment model was developed in the 1960s by Lovaas and his collaborators. This model derived from the tradition of applied behavior analysis, in which operant conditioning principles are used to modify behavior. The approach is known more generally as "discrete trial training" or "applied behavior analysis." A hierarchical program has been outlined (see Lovaas, 1981, for a complete description of this approach and its methods), in which the treatment begins with teaching the child to sit quietly and attend to the trainer, and eventually progresses to following directions, imitation, and simple cognitive concepts. At all levels, the tasks are broken down into small steps, and the child is prompted to respond appropriately to the trainer and/or materials, with clearly specified cues and prompts at each step. Relevant to communication intervention, the emphasis in this program is on developing attention to verbal language, verbal imitation, and then unprompted verbal responses. Augmentative communication approaches are not typically included in discrete-trial training programs that closely follow Lovaas's (1981) program. In all phases of treatment, appropriate responses are reinforced, and inappropriate behaviors are followed by negative or aversive consequences, such as ignoring, time-out, overcorrection, and/or stern reprimands. The prototypical treatment program is very intensive, involving 40 or more hours of one-on-one structured training per week, which is generally provided by multiple therapists trained in the method. Major emphasis is placed on teaching parents to apply the same teaching strategies used by the therapists and require the same level of response from their child as is expected in the formal intervention. In contrast to the TEACCH approach, traditional discrete trial training programs do not focus on adaptations in the environment but instead focus on having the child learn to respond appropriately to the environment. Several follow-up studies have suggested that this type of intervention is very successful, both in reducing the abnormal behaviors of young children with autism and increasing age-appropriate cognitive, social, and other developmental skills (Birnbrauer & Leach, 1993; Harris, Handleman, Gordon, Kristoff, & Fuentes, 1991; Lovaas, 1987; McEachin, Smith, & Lovaas, 1993; Perry et al., 1995). A recent study (Sheinkopf & Siegel, 1998) supports the benefits of this type of home program but failed to find a correlation between number of hours of formal discrete-trial training (ranging from 12 to 43 hours per week) and IQ gains. The study suggests that 40 hours per week may be more formal intervention than is needed to realize the therapeutic benefits of this type of program.

A third treatment model for children with autism was developed by Rogers and her colleagues at the University of Colorado (Rogers, 1991). The theoretical view underlying this model is that the fundamental deficit in autism is social and the child with autism, due to an inborn deficit, has missed out on fundamental interactive exchanges necessary for normal development, including imitation, affect perception, joint attention, and play. To remediate these deficits, this intervention approach places a premium on developing interpersonal relationships. Therapists attempt to "turn on" the social relatedness capacity of the child through shared, highly pleasurable, emotionally charged interactions. Therapists take a very active role in entering the child's world and attempting to find anything that is of interest and pleasure to the child that can be performed with two people (and thus, by definition, is social in nature). Activities may be physical, such as bouncing on a bed, being swung through the air, or tickled—anything that brings a smile to the child's face and requires two participants. As the game becomes ritualized, predictable, and enjoyable to the child, he or she is encouraged to use verbal and nonverbal signals to maintain the interaction. Over time, as the child becomes increasingly aware of and interested in the therapist and others around her, these methods are used to develop a communication system, play schemas, imitative capacities, and interpersonal skills (Rogers, 1991). Like the other two treatment models, this approach emphasizes parent involvement and one-to-one teaching sessions. It also stresses multimodal, interdisciplinary treatment. It has been shown to be highly effective in increasing social, cognitive, and language skills in preschool children with autism (Rogers, Herbison, Lewis, Pantone, & Reis, 1986; Rogers & Lewis, 1989).

Regardless of the model of treatment used, a growing body of literature points to the critical importance of the timing of the intervention. Dawson and Osterling (1997) reviewed research indicating intensive treatment before age 5 can have a significant positive impact on the development of children with autism. Common elements of successful early intervention programs for children with autism were identified; they are outlined in Table 4-2.

As illustrated by the previous discussion, there has been a great deal of progress in the development of effective early intervention models for young children with autism, but much further investigation in this area is warranted.

Table 4-2. Common Elements of Effective Early Intervention Programs for Children with Autism

1. Curriculum content addressing the child's ability to:
   - Attend to important elements of the environment essential for learning
   - Imitate others
   - Comprehend and use language
   - Play appropriately with toys
   - Socially interact with others

2. Highly supportive teaching environments and generalization strategies

3. Predictability and routine

4. Functional approach to problem behaviors

5. Planned transition from preschool classroom

6. Family involvement

7. Intensive programming
   - 15–40 hours per week
   - Average of 27 hours per week

Adapted from Guralnick, M.J. (Ed.). (1997). *The effectiveness of early intervention* (pp. 307–326). Baltimore: Paul H. Brookes.

Dawson and Osterling (1997) identify some of the limitations of the available research on all models of early intervention with children with autism: lack of control groups in most studies, no true experimental designs involving random assignment of children to treatment and control groups, and no direct comparisons of different treatment models. Dawson and Osterling (1997) suggested several important directions for second-generation research on early intervention in autism, including the need to determine which types of intervention work best for different children (e.g., verbal versus nonverbal) and how much intervention is needed to produce optimum results. In addition, the ability to draw conclusions from research on early intervention would be aided by standardizing measures of child characteristics at entry into the intervention as well as outcome measures, such as descriptions of post-preschool placements and support services.

Guidelines and Resources for Speech, Language, and Communication Intervention

In this section, we focus on the literature offering information on communication assessment and intervention that is specific to children with autism and other PDDs. As pointed out in the discussion of development, these children share much in common with other children, both those developing typically and those with other diagnoses affecting language. Therefore, it is important for speech-language pathologists and others working with the child to be well-grounded in a knowledge of typical development and general principles of language assessment and intervention. In addressing the communication needs of these children, however, it is often their differences from other children that create the greatest challenges for their families, teachers, and other professionals who seek to help them achieve their maximum potential in developing effective communication skills.

Communication Assessment. The purpose of this section is to address issues in communication assessment which are especially pertinent to young children with autism and other pervasive developmental disorders. The chapters focusing on assessment in the *Handbook of Early Language Impairments in Children: Assessment and Intervention* (Watson, Crais, & Layton, 2000) contain information that is as important for working with children with PDD and their families as it is for children with language impairments due to other disorders. We will not attempt to replicate that information here.

Standardized measures. As with other children, standardized assessments with young children with autism have benefits and limitations. In some cases the administration of a standardized measure may be necessary to establish eligibility for services. In addition, standardized assessments perhaps offer advantages of being what they are—standardized. Thus the measure will be administered in roughly the same way under the same conditions each time, and may in that respect offer a more consistent measure of progress than nonstandardized assessments. On the other hand, standardized assessments are also limited in that they are standardized and for that reason may not tap into many emerging skills that are apparent only under certain conditions, which may be idiosyncratic to the child or to the routines between a child and her or his partner. This is a consideration for any young child but may be a more serious limitation in assessment of children with PDD, who are characterized by idiosyncratic patterns of communication. Another limitation of most standardized assessments for young children is that they do little to describe and measure a child's pragmatic skills. Yet it is in the area of pragmatics that children with PDD are most at variance in their pattern of development from other children. One measure that does look at the interactional and pragmatic abilities of children in the developmental age range of birth to 2 years is the Communication and Symbolic Behavior Scales (CSBS) (Wetherby & Prizant, 1993). This assessment instrument uses a variety of communication "temptations," which provide good contexts for examining the communicative intentionality of young children and their ability to establish joint focus, as well as the means by which they communicate and the phonetic repertoire exhibited. In addition, the CSBS includes combinatorial and symbolic play probes and book sharing as mechanisms for profiling the child's skills across related domains.

For profiling a young child's skills across additional communication-related domains, the MacArthur Communicative Development Inventories (MCDI), (Fenson et al., 1993) can be useful. This set of two instruments (Words and Gestures, Words and Sentences) covers the age range from 8 to 30 months. The Words and Gestures form (8-16 months) covers both comprehension and production of early words, as well as gestures, games and routines, actions on objects, pretend play, and imitation of others. The Words and Sentences form (16-30 months) covers word production and several grammatical areas (word endings, plurals, verb forms, complexity of sentences). An advantage of this instrument is that it is based on parent report, and thus provides information on communication skills a young child may have but not exhibit in a controlled testing environment.

Another instrument developed for children between the ages of 3 and 8 years is the Test of Pragmatic Skills (Shulman, 1986). This test sets up several play situations with children, and uses these to examine the functions of communication and children's ability to use their communication skills when the routine expectations of a given situation are violated. The standardization sample for this instrument was limited to middle-class white children in the United States, so its applicability to assessment of children from other sociocultural backgrounds is questionable.

Nonstandardized assessment. Two general strategies for nonstandardized assessment will be discussed: the collection of communication samples through observation in a natural setting, and interviews with parents, teachers, and others who are familiar with the child's communicative interactions. It is important to examine the way the child with PDD communicates in her or his everyday environment. We have seen some children with PDD who look more capable in their everyday environments than in standardized assessment activities, and some children who looked much less capable in their everyday environments than we would have expected based on their performance on a standardized test. Watson, Lord, Schaffer, and Schopler (1989) offered guidelines for collecting a communication sample by making notes about a child's spontaneous communication during "online" observation of the child in a classroom or at home. These procedures include recording all forms of communication judged to be intentional, not just vocal and/or verbal behavior. The behaviors are then analyzed according to the purposes or functions of communication, the form(s) of communication, the vocabulary used, the semantic categories represented by the vocabulary, and the contexts in which communication was observed. For children functioning at slightly higher levels, Twachtman (1995) described a similar procedure for collecting a sample, but offers some suggestions for analyzing conversational skills exhibited by the child.

Parents, teachers, and others who have frequent opportunities to observe the child during daily routines are also critical to the assessment process. There are interview protocols suggested in the CSBS (Wetherby & Prizant, 1993), as well as in Watson et al. (1989), Layton and Watson (1995), and Quill (1995). Information from interviewing individuals who spend regular time with a child across varied situations offers the advantage of providing a more comprehensive picture of a child's communication skills and needs than is possible with a limited period of direct observation. Also, as Rydell and Prizant (1995) pointed out, this information is invaluable in interpreting idiosyncratic behavior and speech used by the child. Direct observation may provide more detail than an interview along with both quantifiable as well as qualitative information. Thus the two methods of assessment are complementary and neither is a substitute for the other.

For children with hyperlexia or a demonstrated interest in print, an assessment of literacy skills is appropriate. These skills can be used to good advantage in language and social interventions. One standardized test appropriate for young children is the Test of Early Reading Abilities–2nd edition (TERA-2), (Reid, Hresko, & Hammill, 1989), which examines the child's ability to recognize logos as well as letters, numbers, and words. Children with autism and other PDDs may have reading abilities that are not exhibited under conventional testing conditions, so observation, informal probes, and interviewing are also appropriate in the assessment of literacy skills. It is of interest to know whether the child is memorizing words visually or has strategies for decoding unfamiliar words; can associate individual words with meaningful stimuli; understands sentence length material in print (e.g., can follow simple printed directions); and has the ability to comprehend printed discourse. Children with autism may be much more knowledgeable about the forms of written language than about its various functions; thus, the assessment should address the knowledge of written language functions as well. Assessment should evaluate the child for evidence of understanding that reading and writing can serve varied purposes, including entertainment, information, instruction, memory aids, social interaction, and so forth.

Communication Intervention. Data on the efficacy of interventions to improve communication skills are limited. This is a concern for professionals in the area of autism, whether at the level of an individual child or at the level of larger subgroups of children with autism. Accountability is an ethical mandate.

With respect to strategies, there is discussion among professionals and parents concerned with children with pervasive developmental disorders as well as other disabilities regarding whether a structured, teacher/parent/clinician-directed approach or a facilitative, naturalistic, child-centered approach is optimal in promoting language and communication skills. There is evidence for the efficacy of both types of approaches, and insufficient research comparing different approaches and examining the interaction of child characteristics with teaching strategies. We will review some of the available literature next.

With respect to clinician-structured approaches, the Lovaas program described earlier in this section is an example of a program that is highly structured and directive, in addition to being very intensive. Communication skills are addressed along with other skill areas. Although the outcome data are not specific to communication skills, improved communication skills would seem to be an essential component of the improved intelligence test scores and the successful regular education classroom placements for many of the children included in the evaluation research on this program (Lovaas, 1987). It is not possible to know which aspects of the Lovaas program account for its apparent effectiveness: selection criteria for children enrolled in the program, structure of the program, specific skills taught, intensity, involvement of children in preschool programs for typically developing children, or any of a number of other possible variables.

There have been numerous investigations of clinician-directed interventions to teach specific language/communication skills to children with autism which have demonstrated such structured approaches can result in an increased use of the targeted skill (see Carr, 1985, for a review). Concerns about such approaches include whether they result in the child becoming prompt dependent, whether skills generalize to new contexts, and whether the skills taught are pivotal skills that result in improvements in other related, untrained skills. Recent research has increasingly focused on these issues (Koegel & Koegel, 1995).

Results of investigations by the Koegels and their colleagues indicate that an approach which is further on the continuum toward the "child-centered" end may be more effective in improving language skills and reducing behavior problems than a highly adult-directed approach (Koegel, Koegel, & Surratt, 1992; Koegel, O'Dell, & Koegel, 1987). The approach used was called the "natural language-teaching paradigm (NLP)," which incorporated components of incidental teaching and a facilitative style which was very responsive to the child's interests and behavior. Results indicated that this approach was superior to an "analog" training program, which incorporated discrete trial training. The NLP was also associated with many fewer disruptive behaviors during intervention sessions than were evident in sessions using the analog approach.

Early intervention for children with no or minimal verbal skills. Layton and Watson (1995) addressed communication intervention with this population. For very young children and/or children whose social communication skills are less than those of a typically-developing 2-year-old, much of the initial intervention will likely be directed at improving social awareness and interaction more than directly working on verbal language skills. Klinger and Dawson (1992) provide a rationale based on research for a child-centered program developed to improve social awareness, imitation, and eye contact.

Children with autism who are using little or no language often communicate their wants to adults by moving the other person's hand toward an object the child wants to have or wants the other person to act on (e.g., pushing the adult's hand toward a bubble bottle to get the adult to blow bubbles). An early strategy for moving the child toward a more symbolic form of communication is to implement an object exchange system. The goal is to have the child give the adult an object related to her or his desire in order to get the desired object or action. For instance, the child might learn to hand the adult a bubble wand to get the adult to blow bubbles, give a cup to get juice, and give a knife to get peanut butter. The representation of the child's wish by the object is still very concrete, but the act of giving the object to communicate a want is a less direct means for achieving a communicative end than manipulating the adult's hand. Objects can also be used to improve the child's comprehension of language at early developmental levels. For example, if it is time to go to the table to eat, the parent or teacher might give the child a plate while saying, "Time to eat." A set of associated objects might be identified for various routine activities in the child's day, and then used in conjunction with consistent verbal cues when giving the child directions about those activities.

Although we are aware of no formal efforts to evaluate an object exchange system, there are some evaluation data for a similar, but symbolically higher-level, picture exchange system. Bondy and Frost (1995) have formalized steps for teaching young children with autism to use the Picture Exchange Communication System (PECS) and have reported on the results of implementing this approach with 66 preschool children with autism. All of the children were able to learn to use PECS at some level, and 73 percent of the children went on to develop verbal skills. There was no comparison group included in the study, but Bondy and Frost pointed out that this percentage is higher than figures cited in the literature, which suggest that only around 50 percent of children with autism develop useful verbal skills. The results of this study are another indication that early and appropriate intervention may positively alter the developmental trajectory of children with autism.

Sign language is another system of communication which has been used with children with autism. Evidence indicates that for children with limited verbal imitation skills, teaching sign language or using a "total communication" approach (sign and speech) is more effective than teaching speech alone (Layton, 1988).

An additional augmentative communication option for children with autism is programmable devices which can incorporate voice output. These include personal computers as well as dedicated communication devices such as the Hawk™, Touchtalker™, and McCaw™. Again, there is little literature published on the use of programmable devices with children with autism. Our experience is that these devices often hold intrinsic interest for the children, perhaps because of their cause-and-effect relations (e.g., push the panel, and the device "speaks"). Children with autism must still learn the communicative potential of the device, however, and not just its potential as a cause-and-effect toy. Thus the challenges involved in using programmable devices with children with autism at young developmental ages are similar to the challenges of using any other communicative system.

Intervention for verbal children. For children who are beginning to use meaningful verbal language, there have been some data published regarding the efficacy of both highly structured, clinician-directed approaches and more naturalistic approaches. The work of the Koegels and their colleagues evaluating the NLP with children with autism was described earlier (see also Koegel, 1995).

Scherer and Olswang (1989) reported on the use of a structured discourse approach to teach two-word phrases, including action-object, adjective-object, and possessor-object semantic relations. In this training program, the clinician presented stimuli using real toys in a discrete trial format and asked the child a consistent stimulus question for each two-word relation (e.g., "What's he doing?"). If the child responded with the targeted phrase, she or he was given the toys to play with briefly as a reinforcer. If the child responded with only one of the targeted words, the clinician modeled the targeted phrase and cued the child to imitate. Once the child imitated the two-word phrase, the toys were offered as a reinforcer. The authors found that this strategy was not only successful in teaching the targeted set of two-word phrases, it also generalized in that the children produced similar two-word phrases in response to a new set of stimuli that had not been specifically taught.

Rydell and Prizant (1995) discussed recommended strategies for intervention with echolalic children to encourage more spontaneous, generative use of language. Given that echolalia increases with greater demands for comprehension and production, Rydell and Prizant emphasize the importance of keeping language input and demands well within the child's level of comprehension. Less echolalia is used in situations in which the interactive partners use a more facilitative style, as discussed above.

Twachtman (1995) discussed approaches for young children with autism who are "higher functioning," emphasizing the importance of concrete environmental supports and predictable routines and sequences even for these more capable children. She also described strategies for "indexing" the environment verbally for children to increase the child's understanding of the social world and appropriate responses to varying situations. A specific strategy that accomplishes the purpose of indexing the environment was described by Gray (1995), who developed written "social stories" to promote appropriate social behavior among children with autism. Stories specific to a particular child are written to give her or him explanations of a social situation that are tailor-made to her or his level of comprehension. Most stories include both descriptive statements and directive statements. The descriptive statements help the child understand the situation and provide words for the situation that she or he may not be able to generate alone. The directive statements tell the child things that she or he can do in a situation that will be more socially appropriate than the current responses. For children who can read or are interested in having other people read to them, this approach can provide a script to use in difficult social situations and may be effective in helping them develop some ability to self-regulate. Taking an alternative approach, Charlop and Milstein (1989) used video modeling to provide scripts for children with autism to help them improve their conversational speech.

Recently the importance of teaching "self-learning" language strategies has been emphasized by Koegel (1995). These strategies involve learning to ask questions in increasingly natural contexts, so that the child has a way of having others supply verbal information and models even in situations in which there is no interventionist present. Koegel discussed strategies for teaching the following question types: What's that? Where is it? Where + *noun*? Whose is it? Whose + *noun*? What happened?

For children with hyperlexia, the visual strengths apparent in the child's ability to decode written language can be used to enhance communication development. Written cues can be used to prompt the child to take an appropriate verbal turn in the interaction. This is often less confusing for the child than a verbal prompt such as "You say, . . ." We have used reading skills in young children with autism for a number of different intervention goals (Watson & Ward, 1994). For example, for one child who had very limited verbal communication, printed cards were used to prompt basic requests for objects and actions. Another child was developing language and communication skills at a good rate but had numerous phonological processes persisting in his speech which often made him unintelligible (e.g., an unusual backing process in which /g/ was substituted for voiced /th/). His motivation to read proved to be the key to addressing his phonological problems. Yet another child was working on learning to ask questions. Verbal cues by the clinician such as, "You ask, 'Who took the ball?'" consistently led him to try to answer the question even though he did not know the answer. However, the printed cue, "Who took the _____?" was effective in cueing him to ask the question instead of trying to answer it.

CASE STUDY: ERIC

Eric is an 8-year-old boy whose mother is a native of Taiwan and whose father is a native of the United States. English is the only language regularly spoken in the home. Eric's mother is fluent in English, but her speech reflects some errors in syntax and vocabulary related to learning English as a second language. Eric has a 10-year-old brother who was diagnosed with autism at the age of 3. Eric was diagnosed with a language delay at the age of 3 years, with skills estimated at the 1- to-1½-year-old level. After this evaluation, Eric began receiving services in a preschool classroom for children with special needs. When Eric was 3½ years old, his family moved to North Carolina, at which time he was enrolled in a language preschool operated by the Division of Speech and Hearing Sciences at the University of North Carolina at Chapel Hill. Local school district personnel scheduled him for a full evaluation in order to determine his eligibility for other services. The school system evaluation team diagnosed Eric as having autism, a diagnosis later confirmed by TEACCH division staff. This was a very difficult diagnosis for Eric's parents to hear, because his development was much different, and closer to typical, than that of his brother. They had expected him to catch up with his age peers in his language skills with intervention and did not suspect that he was also autistic. The parents' expectations for Eric's success undoubtedly were based in part on their observation of his above average performance in some areas. Evaluation information confirmed that Eric was exceptionally intelligent in some ways. For example, at age 3;8, he was tested on the Leiter International Performance Scale (Leiter, 1979) and attained a nonverbal mental age of 5½ years. He showed hyperlexic abilities in being able to read a number of single words. However, his skills in verbal language, imitation, and imaginative play were well below the expected level for his chronological age.

The stress on Eric's family increased following his diagnosis of autism. Eric's mother shared the fact that in her culture, a common belief is that if parents have a child with a disability, it is a punishment for something they have done wrong. Thus, learning that she and her husband had two children with serious disabilities was especially hard for her. Eric's parents made the decision not to have a third child as they had planned, due not only to the financial and energy resources required to meet the needs of Eric and his brother, but also to their fears of having a third child with autism. In addition, Eric's father took a higher-paying job that required him to be gone for long hours every day. The job helped the family meet its financial needs but resulted in Eric's mother having very little daily support in the care of the two boys.

Eric continued in the language preschool placement three mornings a week for 1½ years. In this setting Eric received intensive group and individual language therapy in a small group of six children, with a 2:1 child-to-clinician ratio. For the other two mornings of the school week, Eric was enrolled in a regular preschool in the community. A special education teacher spent 1 hour per week with him in this setting to help promote social adaptation and interactions with the teachers and other children.

Eric's mother educated herself about language, communication, and social development, and strategies for helping children with autism. She observed Eric's therapy in the language preschool regularly, and she found multiple opportunities each day to teach verbal concepts and the use of emerging language and social skills that were being targeted in his language therapy program. She attended parent group meetings offered through Division TEACCH, and also participated in a series of individual parent/child sessions with the TEACCH staff to help her develop home-teaching strategies and activities for Eric. About a year after Eric's diagnosis, she was able to obtain funding through an area mental health program to provide some extra support to the family. Although this support was targeted to the needs of the older son, who has more severe autism, Eric unquestionably benefited from this support as well, because his mother had more time and energy to interact with him as well as to advocate for the services he needed.

When Eric first entered the language preschool, he had a number of verbal skills. He could identify many objects and could label all letters of the alphabet as well as colors, numbers, and shapes. However, Eric infrequently initiated verbal interactions in the classroom. Some of the spontaneous language heard at that point included the following: "Purple, green, yellow, pink, orange, green (labeling colors of markers on the table)," "Mine (claiming ownership)," "Cheese (requesting)," "Upside-down (commenting)." As is characteristic of children with autism, most of Eric's spontaneous utterances were used to request things or activities he wanted. An individual strength for Eric, and probably the reason why autism was not diagnosed earlier, was his attention to verbal directions and requests and his consistent attempts to comply with these. Initially, Eric often arrived at the preschool with a spoon in his hand and would resist giving it up. He did not initiate play or verbal interactions with the other children. However, he found the smallest child in the classroom very amusing and would laugh at him, say his name over and over, and imitate his behaviors, such as falling down and running away from the group. Eric's interest in this child was so intense during the first several months he was enrolled in the language preschool that it was difficult for him to focus his attention on group activities. Although it interfered with his learning in some ways, one benefit of this intense interest was that Eric's commenting and use of action words first increased in relation to describing the activities of this peer.

Eric was retested using the Clinical Evaluation of Language Fundamentals-Preschool (CELF-P), (Wiig, Secord & Semel, 1992), when he was 4;11. He had a standard score of 85 on this test, with receptive and expressive scores being *very similar to each other. The corresponding age equivalent score was 3;5. In the classroom at that point in time, Eric was demonstrating excellent progress in social interactions with peers and was observed to ask to play with his peers, to initiate trading toys, to verbally protest a peer's action ("Andy, I told you to stop!"), and to assign roles to peers and himself for pretend play (e.g., scenarios about school or taking a trip).*

Just prior to his 5th birthday, Eric transferred to a full-time placement in a Headstart classroom, where he continued to receive 2 hours per week of special services (speech-language therapy and special education). The teachers reported that he did well in that setting, with the biggest problem being his obsession with a particular classmate. Subsequently, Eric has continued in regular education classrooms for his kindergarten, first-, and second-grade years, with support services provided by a special education resource teacher and speech-language pathologist. Eric's mother reported that during his kindergarten year, he began to sometimes correct her errors in speaking English, an indication of his progress in developing greater competency with the structural aspects of language. Each year in the regular classroom, however, the demands on Eric to process more abstract, complex verbal information increase, creating greater challenges to the educational team in making adaptations and providing support services that enable him to remain successful in the regular classroom. Eric's mother continues to be a very active advocate for him, but as both her sons have gotten older and are spending full days in their school programs, she has also begun to share what she has learned by serving as a parent mentor to other families of newly diagnosed children with autism. She reports deriving a great deal of satisfaction from this new role.

SUMMARY

Children with pervasive developmental disorders have characteristic impairments in social interaction, communication, and range of behaviors and interests. Although there is no single known etiologic factor common to all individuals with PDD, the evidence that these disorders are biologically based is irrefutable. There is a large literature describing the developmental characteristics of children with autism, but much more limited information on children with other PDDs. The need for continued research on treatment efficacy is apparent; however, available studies on children with autism support the use of early, intensive intervention using predictable routines, visual and other environmental supports, and activities designed to maximize the child's engagement in social interactions.

References

American Psychiatric Association. (1980). *Diagnostic and statistical manual of mental disorders* (3rd ed.). Washington, D.C.: Author.

American Psychiatric Association. (1994). *Diagnostic and statistical manual of mental disorders* (4th ed.). Washington, D.C.: Author.

Aram, D. M., & Healy, J. M. (1988). Hyperlexia: A review of extraordinary word recognition. In L. K. Obler & D. Fein (Eds.), *The exceptional brain* (pp. 70–102). New York: Guilford.

Asperger, H. (1944). "Autistic psychopathy" in childhood. *Archiv fur Psychiatrie und Nervenkrankheiten, 117,* 76–136.

Astington, J. W. (1994). Children's developing notions of others' minds. In J. F. Duchan, L. E. Hewitt, & R. M. Sonnenmeier (Eds.), *Pragmatics: From theory to practice* (pp. 72–87). Englewood Cliffs, N.J.: Prentice-Hall.

Bailey, A., Bolton, P., Butler, L., LeCouteur, A., Murphy, M., Scott, S., Webb, T., & Rutter, M. (1993). Prevalence of the fragile X anomaly amongst autistic twins and singletons. *Journal of Child Psychology and Psychiatry, 34,* 673–688.

Bailey, A. J., LeCouteur, A., Gottesman, I., Bolton, P., Simonoff, E., Yuzda, E., & Rutter, M. (1995). Autism as a strongly genetic disorder: Evidence from a British twin study. *Psychological Medicine, 25,* 63–77.

Bailey, A., Phillips, W., & Rutter, M. (1996). Autism: Towards an integration of clinical, genetic, neuropsychological, and neurobiological perspectives. *Journal of Child Psychology and Psychiatry, 37,* 89–126.

Ball, J. (1978). *A pragmatic analysis of autistic children's language with respect to aphasic and normal language development.* Unpublished honors thesis, Melbourne University, Melbourne, Australia.

Baltaxe, C. A. M. (1977). Pragmatic deficits of autistic adolescents. *Journal of Pediatric Psychology, 2,* 176–180.

Baltaxe, C. A. M. (1984). The use of contrastive stress in normal, aphasic, and autistic children. *Journal of Speech and Hearing Research, 27,* 97–105.

Baltaxe, C. A. M., & Guthrie, D. (1987). The use of primary sentence stress by normal, aphasic, and autistic children. *Journal of Autism and Developmental Disorders, 17,* 255–271.

Baltaxe, C. A. M., & Simmons, J. Q. (1985). Prosodic development in normal and autistic children. In E. Schopler & G. Mesibov (Eds.), *Communication problems in autism* (pp. 95–125). New York: Plenum.

Baranek, G. (1996). Autism during infancy: A retrospective video analysis of sensory-motor and social behaviors at 9–12 months of age. *Journal of Autism and Developmental Disorders, 29,* 213–224.

Baron-Cohen, S. (1988). Social and pragmatic deficits in autism: Cognitive or affective? *Journal of Autism and Developmental Disorders, 18,* 379–402.

Baron-Cohen, S. (1989). Perceptual role-taking and protodeclarative pointing in autism. *British Journal of Developmental Psychology, 7,* 113–127.

Bartolucci, G., Pierce, S. J., & Streiner, D. (1980). Cross-sectional studies of grammatical morphemes in autistic and mentally retarded children. *Journal of Autism and Developmental Disorders, 10,* 39–50.

Bates, E. (1979). *The emergence of symbols: Cognition and communication in infancy.* New York: Academic.

Bauman, M., & Kemper, T. L. (1985). Histoanatomic observations of the brain in early infantile autism. *Neurology, 35,* 866–874.

Bauman, M., & Kemper, T. L. (1988). Limbic and cerebellar abnormalities: Consistent findings in infantile autism. *Journal of Neuropathology and Experimental Neurology, 47,* 369.

Bettelheim, B. (1967). *The empty fortress.* New York: Free Press.

Birnbrauer, J. S., & Leach, D. J. (1993). The Murdoch early intervention program after 2 years. *Behavior Change, 10,* 63–74.

Bolton, P., MacDonald, H., Pickles, A., Rios, P., Goode, S., Crowson, M., Bailey, A., & Rutter, M. (1994). A case control family history study of autism. *Journal of Child Psychology and Psychiatry, 35,* 877–899.

Bondy, A. S., & Frost, L. A. (1995). Educational approaches in preschool. In E. Schopler & G. Mesibov (Eds.), *Learning and cognition in autism* (pp. 311–333). New York: Plenum.

Buchsbaum, M. S., Siegel, B. V., Wu, J. C., Hazlett, E., Sicotte, N., Haier, R., Tanguay, P., Asarnow, R., Cadorette, T., Donoghue, D., Lagunas-Solar, M., Lott, I., Paek, J., & Sabalesky, D. (1992). Attention performance in autism and regional brain metabolic rate assessed by positron emission tomography. *Journal of Autism and Developmental Disorders, 22,* 115–125.

Burd, L., Fisher, W., Knowlton, D., & Kerbeshian, J. (1987). Hyperlexia: A marker for improvement in children with pervasive developmental disorder? *Journal of the American Academy of Child and Adolescent Psychiatry, 26,* 407–412.

Cantwell, D., Baker, L., & Rutter, M. (1978). A comparative study of infantile autism and specific developmental receptive language disorder: IV. Analysis of syntax and language function. *Journal of Child Psychology and Psychiatry, 19,* 351–362.

Carr, E. G. (1985). Behavioral approaches to language and communication. In E. Schopler & G. B. Mesibov (Eds.), *Communication problems in autism* (pp. 37–57). New York: Plenum.

Casey, B. J., Gordon, C. T., Mannheim, G. B., & Rumsey, J. M. (1993). Dysfunctional attention in autistic savants. *Journal of Clinical and Experimental Neuropsychology, 15,* 933–946.

Charlop, M. H., & Milstein, J. P. (1989). Teaching autistic children conversational speech using video modeling. *Journal of Applied Behavior Analysis, 22,* 275–285.

Chess, S., Korn, S. J., & Fernandez, P. B. (1971). *Psychiatric disorders of children with congenital rubella.* New York: Brunner-Mazel.

Cohen, I. L., Vietze, P. M., Subhalter, V., Jenkins, E. C., & Brown, W. T. (1989). Parent-child dyadic gaze patterns in fragile X males and in non–fragile X males with autistic disorder. *Journal of Child Psychology and Psychiatry, 30,* 845–856.

Coleman, M. (1987). The search for neurological subgroups in autism. In E. Schopler & G. B. Mesibov (Eds.), *Neurobiological issues in autism* (pp. 163–178). New York: Plenum.

Cook, E. H., Courchesne, R., Cox, N. J., Lord, C., Gonen, D., Guter, S. J., Lincoln, A., Nix, K., Haas, R., Leventhal, B. L., & Courchesne, E. (1998). Linkage disequilibrium mapping with 15q11–13 markers in autistic disorder. *American Journal of Human Genetics, 62,* 1077–1083.

Courchesne, E., Lincoln, A. J., Kilman, B. A., & Galambos, R. (1985). Event-related brain potential correlates of the processing of novel visual and auditory information in autism. *Journal of Autism and Developmental Disorders, 15,* 55–75.

Courchesne, E., Press, G. A., & Yeung-Courchesne, R. (1993). Parietal lobe abnormalities detected with MR in patients with infantile autism. *American Journal of Roentgenology, 160,* 387–393.

Courchesne, E., Townsend, J., Akshoomoff, N. A., Saitoh, O., Yeung-Courchesne, R., Lincoln, A. J., James, H. E., Haas, R. H., Schreibman, L., & Lau, L. (1994). Impairment in shifting attention in autistic and cerebellar patients. *Behavioral Neuroscience, 108,* 848–865.

Courchesne, E., Yeung-Courchesne, R., Press, G. A., Hesselink, J. R., & Jernigan, T. L. (1988). Hypoplasia of cerebellar vermal lobules VI and VII in autism. *New England Journal of Medicine, 318,* 1349–1354.

Cunningham, M. A. (1968). A comparison of the language of psychotic and non-psychotic children who are mentally retarded. *Journal of Child Psychology and Psychiatry, 9,* 229–244.

Curcio, F. (1978). Sensorimotor functioning and communication in mute autistic children. *Journal of Autism and Childhood Schizophrenia, 8,* 282–292.

Dahlgren, S. O., & Gillberg, C. (1989). Symptoms in the first two years of life: A preliminary population study of infantile autism. *European Archives of Psychiatric and Neurological Science, 283,* 169–174.

Dale, P. S. (1981). Is early pragmatic development measurable? *Journal of Child Language, 7,* 1–12.

Dawson, G., & Adams, A. (1984). Imitation and social responsiveness in autistic children. *Journal of Abnormal Child Psychology, 12,* 209–226.

Dawson, G., Finley, C., Phillips, S., & Galpert, L. (1986). Hemispheric specialization and the language abilities of autistic children. *Child Development, 57,* 1440–1453.

Dawson, G., Hill, D., Spencer, A., Galpert, L., & Watson, L. (1990). Affective exchanges between autistic children and their mothers. *Journal of Abnormal Child Psychology, 18,* 335–345.

Dawson, G., & Osterling, J. (1997). Early intervention in autism. In M. J. Guralnick (Ed.), *The effectiveness of early intervention* (pp. 307–326). Baltimore: Brookes.

DeLong, G. R., Bean, S. C., & Brown, F. R. (1981). Acquired reversible autistic syndrome in acute encephalopathic illness in children. *Archives of Neurology, 38,* 191–194.

DeLong, R. (1994). Children with autistic spectrum disorder and a family history of affective disorder. *Developmental Medicine and Child Neurology, 36,* 674–688.

DeMyer, M. K., Barton, S., Alpern, G. D., Kimberlin, C., Allen, J., Yang, E., & Steele, R. (1974). The measured intelligence of autistic children. *Journal of Autism and Childhood Schizophrenia, 4*, 42–60.

DeMyer, M. K., Barton, S., DeMyer, W. E., Norton, J. A., Allen, J., & Steele, R. (1973). Prognosis in autism: A follow-up study. *Journal of Autism and Childhood Schizophrenia, 3*, 199–246.

Dewey, P., & Everard, P. (1974). The near-normal autistic adolescent. *Journal of Autism and Childhood Schizophrenia, 4*, 348–356.

Douglas, V. I., & Peters, K. G. (1979). Toward a clearer definition of the attentional deficit of hyperactive children. In G.A. Hale & M. Lewis (Eds.), *Attention and cognitive development* (pp. 173–247). New York: Plenum.

Elliott, C. D. (1990). *The Differential Abilities Scales.* San Antonio: Psychological Corporation.

Fay, W. (1969). On the basis of autistic echolalia. *Journal of Communication Disorders, 2*, 38–47.

Fenson, L., Dale, P., Reznick, S., Thal, D., Bates, E., Hartung, J., Pethick, S., & Reilly, J. (1993). *MacArthur Communicative Development Inventories.* San Diego: Singular.

Filipek, P. A., Richelme, C., Kennedy, D. N., Rademacher, J., Pitcher, D. A., Zidel, S., & Caviness, V. S. (1992). Morphometric analysis of the brain in developmental language disorders and autism. *Annals of Neurology, 32*, 475.

Fombonne, E., Bolton, P., Prior, J., Jordan, H., & Rutter, M. (1997). A family study of autism: Cognitive patterns and levels in parents and siblings. *Journal of Child Psychology and Psychiatry, 38*, 667–683.

Freeman, B. J., Rahbar, B., Ritvo, E. R., Bice, T. L., Yokota, A., & Ritvo, R. (1991). The stability of cognitive and behavioral parameters in autism: A twelve-year prospective study. *Journal of the American Academy of Child and Adolescent Psychiatry, 30*, 479–482.

Freeman, B. J., Ritvo, E. R., Needleman, R., & Yokota, A. (1985). The stability of cognitive and linguistic parameters in autism: A five-year prospective study. *Journal of the American Academy of Child Psychiatry, 24*, 459–464.

Frith, U., & Snowling, M. (1983). Reading for meaning and reading for sound in autistic and dyslexic children. *British Journal of Developmental Psychology, 1*, 329–342.

Gajzago, C., & Prior, M. (1974). Two cases of "recovery" in Kanner syndrome. *Archives of General Psychiatry, 31*, 264–268.

Garretson, H. B., Fein, D., & Waterhouse, L. (1990). Sustained attention in children with autism. *Journal of Autism and Developmental Disorders, 20*, 101–114.

Geller, E. (1991). The interplay between linguistic and social-cognitive knowledge in perspective-taking by autistic children. *Journal of Childhood Communication Disorders, 14*, 23–44.

George, M. S., Costa, D. C., Kouris, K., Ring, H. A., & Ell, P. J. (1992). Cerebral blood flow abnormalities in adults with infantile autism. *Journal of Nervous and Mental Disease, 180*, 413–417.

Gerlach, E. K. (1996). *Autism treatment guide* (rev. ed.). Eugene, Ore.: Four Leaf Press.

Gillberg, C. (1986). Onset at age 14 of a typical autistic syndrome: A case report of a previously normal girl with herpes encephalitis. *Journal of Autism and Developmental Disorders, 16,* 369–375.

Gillberg, C. (1991). Outcome in autism and autistic-like conditions. *Journal of the American Academy of Child and Adolescent Psychiatry, 30,* 375–382.

Gillberg, C., Ehlers, S., Schaumann, H., Jakobsson, G., Dahlgren, S., Lindblom, R., Bagenholm, A., Tjuus, T., & Blidner, E. (1990). Autism under 3 years of age: A clinical study of 28 cases referred for autistic symptoms in infancy. *Journal of Child Psychology and Psychiatry and Allied Disciplines, 31,* 921–931.

Gillberg, C., & Gillberg, I. C. (1983). Infantile autism: A total population study of reduced optimality in the pre-, peri-, and neonatal period. *Journal of Autism and Developmental Disorders, 13,* 153–166.

Gillberg, C., & Steffenburg, S. (1987). Outcome and prognostic factors in infantile autism and similar conditions: A population-based study of 46 cases followed through puberty. *Journal of Autism and Developmental Disorders, 17,* 273–287.

Gillberg, I. C. (1991). Autistic syndrome with onset at age 31 years: Herpes encephalitis as a possible model for childhood autism. *Developmental Medicine and Child Neurology, 33,* 920–924.

Gillberg, I. C., Gillberg, C., & Ahlsen, G. (1994). Autistic behavior and attention deficits in tuberous sclerosis: A population based study. *Developmental Medicine and Child Neurology, 36,* 50–56.

Goldberg, T. E. (1987). On hermetic reading abilities. *Journal of Autism and Developmental Disorders, 17,* 29–44.

Goodman, R. (1990). Are perinatal complications causes or consequences of autism? *Journal of Child Psychology and Psychiatry, 31,* 809–812.

Grandin, T. (1995). How people with autism think. In E. Schopler and G. B. Mesibov (Eds.), *Learning and cognition in autism* (pp. 137–156). New York: Plenum.

Gray, C. (1995). Teaching children with autism to "read" social situations. In K. A. Quill (Ed.), *Teaching children with autism: Strategies to enhance communication and socialization* (pp. 219–241). Albany, NY: Delmar.

Groden, G., & Mann, L. (1988). Intellectual functioning and assessment. In G. Groden & M. G. Baron (Eds.), *Autism: Strategies for change* (pp. 75–97). New York: Gardner.

Happé, F. (1995). *Autism: An introduction to psychological theory.* Cambridge, Mass.: Harvard University Press.

Happé, F., & Frith, U. (1995). Theory of mind in autism. In E. Schopler & G. B. Mesibov (Eds.), *Learning and cognition in autism* (pp. 177–197). New York: Plenum.

Harris, S. L., Handleman, J. S., Gordon, R., Kristoff, B., & Fuentes, F. (1991). Changes in cognitive and language functioning of preschool children with autism. *Journal of Autism and Developmental Disorders, 21,* 281–290.

Holm, V. A. (1985). Rett's syndrome: A progressive developmental disability in girls. *Developmental and Behavioral Pediatrics, 6,* 32–36.

Hoon, A. H., & Reiss, A. L. (1992). The mesial temporal lobe and autism: Case report and review. *Developmental Medicine and Child Neurology, 34,* 278–279.

Horwitz, B., Rumsey, J. M., Grady, C. L., & Rapoport, S. I. (1988). The cerebral metabolic landscape in autism: Intercorrelations of regional glucose utilization. *Archives of Neurology, 45,* 749–755.

Howlin, P. (1984). The acquisition of grammatical morphemes in autistic children: A critique and replication of the findings of Bartolucci, Pierce and Streiner, 1980. *Journal of Autism and Developmental Disorders, 14,* 127–136.

Howlin, P. (1986). An overview of social behavior in autism. In E. Schopler & G. Mesibov (Eds.), *Social behavior in autism* (pp. 63–70). New York: Plenum.

Hunt, A., & Shepherd, C. (1993). A prevalence study of autism in tuberous sclerosis. *Journal of Autism and Developmental Disorders, 23,* 323–339.

Hutt, S. J., Hutt, C., Lee, D., & Ounsted, C. (1964). Arousal and childhood autism. *Nature, 204,* 908–909.

Jacobson, J. W., Mulick, J. A., & Swartz, A. A. (1995). A history of facilitated communication: Science, pseudoscience, and antiscience. *American Psychologist, 50,* 750–765.

Johnson-Martin, N. M. (1988). Assessment of low-functioning children. In E. Schopler & G. B. Mesibov (Eds.), *Diagnosis and assessment in autism* (pp. 303–319). New York: Plenum.

Kanner, L. (1943). Autistic disturbances of affective content. *Nervous Child, 2,* 217–250.

Kasari, C., Sigman, M., Mundy, P., & Yirmiya, N. (1990). Affective sharing in the context of joint attention interactions of normal, autistic, and mentally retarded children. *Journal of Autism and Developmental Disorders, 20,* 87–100.

Klin, A. (1994). Asperger syndrome. *Child and Adolescent Psychiatric Clinics of North America, 3,* 131–148.

Klinger, L. G., & Dawson, G. (1992). Facilitating early social and communicative development in children with autism. In S. F. Warren & J. Reichle (Eds.), *Causes and effects in communication and language intervention* (pp. 157–186). Baltimore: Brookes.

Klinger, L. G., & Dawson, G. (1995). A fresh look at categorization abilities in persons with autism. In E. Schopler & G. B. Mesibov (Eds.), *Learning and cognition in autism* (pp. 119–136). New York: Plenum.

Koegel, L. K. (1995). Communication and language intervention. In R. L. Koegel & L. K. Koegel (Eds.), *Teaching children with autism* (pp. 17–32). Baltimore: Brookes.

Koegel, R. L., & Koegel, L. K. (1995). *Teaching children with autism.* Baltimore: Brookes.

Koegel, R. L., Koegel, L. K., & Surratt, A. V. (1992). Language intervention and disruptive behavior in preschool children with autism. *Journal of Autism and Developmental Disorders, 22,* 141–153.

Koegel, R. L., O'Dell, M. C., & Koegel, L. K. (1987). A natural language paradigm for teaching nonverbal autistic children. *Journal of Autism and Developmental Disorders, 17,* 187–199.

Kurita, H. (1985). Infantile autism with speech loss before the age of thirty months. *Journal of the American Academy of Child Psychiatry, 24,* 191–196.

Landry, S., & Loveland, K. (1989). The effect of social context on the functional communication skills of autistic children. *Journal of Autism and Developmental Disorders, 19,* 282–287.

Laski, K., Charlop, M., & Schreibman, L. (1988). Training parents to use the natural language paradigm to increase their autistic children's speech. *Journal of Applied Behavior Analysis, 21,* 391–400.

Layton, T. L. (1988). Language training with autistic children using four different modes of presentation. *Journal of Communication Disorders, 21,* 333–350.

Layton, T. L., & Watson, L. R. (1995). Enhancing communication in nonverbal children with autism. In K. A. Quill (Ed.), *Teaching children with autism: Strategies to enhance communication and socialization* (pp. 73–103). Albany: Delmar.

Leiter, R. G. (1979). *Leiter International Performance Scale* (rev. ed.). Wood Dale, Ill.: Stoelting.

Leslie, A. M. (1988). Some implication of pretence for mechanisms underlying the child's theory of mind. In J. W. Astington, P. L. Harris, & D. R. Olson (Eds.), *Developing theories of mind* (pp. 19–46). New York: Cambridge University Press.

Lincoln, A. J., Allen, M. H., & Kilman, A. (1995). The assessment and interpretation of intellectual abilities in people with autism. In E. Schopler & G. B. Mesibov (Eds.), *Learning and cognition in autism* (pp. 89–117). New York: Plenum Press.

Lord, C. (1995). Follow-up of two-year-olds referred for possible autism. *Journal of Child Psychology and Psychiatry, 36,* 1365–1382.

Lord, C., Rutter, M., & DiLavore, P. C. (1998). *Autism Diagnostic Observation Schedule–Generic.* Unpublished manuscript, University of Chicago.

Lord, C., Rutter, M. L., Goode, S., Heemsbergen, J., Jordan , H., Mawhood, L., & Schopler, E. (1989). Autism Diagnostic Observation Schedule: A standardized observation of communicative and social behavior. *Journal of Autism and Developmental Disorders, 19*(2), 185–212.

Lord, C., Rutter, M., & LeCouteur, A. (1994). Autism Diagnostic Interview—Revised: A revised version of a diagnostic interview for caregivers of individuals with possible pervasive developmental disorders. *Journal of Autism and Developmental Disorders, 24,* 659–685.

Lord, C., & Schopler, E. (1985). Differences in sex ratios in autism as a function of measured intelligence. *Journal of Autism and Developmental Disorders, 15,* 185–193.

Lord, C., & Schopler, E. (1988). Intellectual and developmental assessment of autistic children from preschool to school age: Clinical implications of two follow-up studies. In E. Schopler & G. B. Mesibov (Eds.), *Diagnosis and assessment in autism* (pp. 167–181). New York: Plenum.

Lord, C., & Schopler, E. (1989). The role of age at assessment, developmental level, and test in the stability of intelligence scores in young autistic children. *Journal of Autism and Developmental Disorders, 19,* 483–499.

Lord, C. & Schopler, E. (1994). TEACCH services for preschool children. In S. Harris & J. Handleman (Eds.), *Preschool education programs for children with autism* (pp. 87–106). Austin, Tex.: Pro-Ed.

Lotter, V. (1974). Factors related to outcome in autistic children. *Journal of Autism and Childhood Schizophrenia, 4,* 263–277.

Lovaas, O. I. (1981). *Teaching developmentally disabled children: The ME book.* Austin, Tex.: Pro-Ed.

Lovaas, O. I. (1987). Behavioral treatment and normal educational and intellectual functioning in young autistic children. *Journal of Consulting and Clinical Psychology, 55,* 3–9.

Lovaas, O. I., Koegel, R. L., & Schreibman, L. (1979). Stimulus overselectivity in autism: A review of research. *Psychological Bulletin, 86,* 1236–1254.

Marcus, L. M., Lansing, M., Andrews, C. E., & Schopler, E. (1978). Improvement of teaching effectiveness in parents of autistic children. *Journal of the American Academy of Child Psychiatry, 17,* 625–639.

McEachin, J. J., Smith, T., & Lovaas, O. I. (1993). Long-term outcome for children with autism who received early intensive behavioral treatment. *American Journal on Mental Retardation, 97,* 359–372.

McEvoy, R., Rogers, S., & Pennington, R. (1993). Executive function and social communication deficits in young, autistic children. *Journal of Child Psychology and Psychiatry, 34,* 563–578.

Minshew, N. J., Goldstein, G., & Siegel, D. J. (1997). Neuropsychologic functioning in autism: Profile of a complex information processing disorder. *Journal of the International Neuropsychological Society, 3,* 303–316.

Minshew, N. J., Goldstein, G., Taylor, H. G., & Siegel, D. J. (1994). Academic achievement in high-functioning autistic individuals. *Journal of Clinical and Experimental Neuropsychology, 16,* 261–270.

Mirenda, P. L., Donnellan, A., & Yoder, D. (1983). Gaze behavior: A new look at an old problem. *Journal of Autism and Developmental Disabilities, 13,* 397–409.

Mullen, E. (1989). *Infant Mullen Scales of Early Learning.* Cranston, RI: TOTAL Child.

Mullen, E. (1992). *Mullen Scales of Early Learning.* Cranston, RI: TOTAL Child.

Mundy, P. (1995) Joint attention and social-emotional approach behavior in children with autism. *Development and Psychopathology, 7,* 63–82.

Mundy, P., Sigman, M., Ungerer, J. A., & Sherman, T. (1986). Defining the social deficits in autism: The contribution of non-verbal communication measures. *Journal of Child Psychology and Psychiatry, 27,* 657–669.

National Society for Autistic Children. (1978). NSAC definition of the syndrome of autism. *Journal of Autism and Developmental Disorders, 8,* 162–167.

O'Neill, M., & Jones, R. S. P. (1997). Sensory-perceptual abnormalities in autism: A case for more research? *Journal of Autism and Developmental Disorders, 27,* 283–293.

Ornitz, E. M., Guthrie, D., & Farley, A. H. (1977). The early development of autistic children. *Journal of Autism and Childhood Schizophrenia, 7,* 207–229.

Ornitz, E. M., & Ritvo, E. R. (1968). Perceptual inconstancy in early infantile autism. *Archives of General Psychiatry, 18,* 76–98.

Osterling, J., & Dawson, G. (1994). Early recognition of children with autism: A study of first birthday home videotapes. *Journal of Autism and Developmental Disorders, 24,* 247–259.

Ozonoff, S. (1995). Executive functions in autism. In E. Schopler & G. B. Mesibov (Eds.), *Learning and cognition in autism* (pp. 199–219). New York: Plenum.

Ozonoff, S. (1997). Components of executive function in autism and other disorders. In J. Russell (Ed.), *Autism as an executive disorder* (pp. 179–211). New York: Oxford University Press.

Ozonoff, S., & Cathcart, K. (1998). Effectiveness of a home program intervention for young children with autism. *Journal of Autism and Developmental Disorders, 28,* 25–32.

Ozonoff, S., & Strayer, D. L. (1997). Inhibitory function in nonretarded children with autism. *Journal of Autism and Developmental Disorders, 27,* 59–77.

Paul, R. (1987). Communication. In D. J. Cohen & A. M. Donnellan (Eds.), *Handbook of autism and pervasive developmental disorders* (pp. 61–84). New York: Wiley.

Pennington, B. F. (1991). Genetics of learning disabilities. *Seminars in Neurology, 11,* 28–34.

Pennington, B. F., & Ozonoff, S. (1996). Executive functions and developmental psychopathologies. *Journal of Child Psychology and Psychiatry Annual Research Review, 37,* 51–87.

Perry, R., Cohen, I., & DeCarlo, R. (1995). Deterioration, autism, and recovery in two siblings. *Journal of the American Academy of Child and Adolescent Psychiatry, 34,* 232–237.

Phillips, W. L., Baron-Cohen, S., & Rutter, M. (1995). To what extent do children with autism understand desire? *Development and Psychopathology, 7,* 151–169.

Pierce, S. J., & Bartolucci, G. (1977). A syntactic investigation of verbal autistic, mentally retarded and normal children. *Journal of Autism and Childhood Schizophrenia, 7,* 121–134.

Piven, J., Arndt, S., Bailey, J., & Andreasen, N. (1996). Regional brain enlargement in autism: A magnetic resonance imaging study. *Journal of the American Academy of Child and Adolescent Psychiatry, 35,* 530–536.

Piven, J., Palmer, P., Jacobi, D., Childress, D., & Arndt, S. (1997). Broader autism phenotype: Evidence from a family history study of multiple incidence families. *American Journal of Psychiatry, 154,* 185–190.

Prizant, B. M. & Rydell, P. J. (1984). An analysis of the functions of delayed echolalia in autistic children. *Journal of Speech and Hearing Research, 27,* 183–192.

Quill, K. A. (1995). Enhancing children's social-communicative interaction. In K. A. Quill (Ed.), *Teaching children with autism: Strategies to enhance communication and socialization* (pp. 163–189). Albany: Delmar.

Reed, T., & Peterson, C. C. (1990). A comparative study of autistic subjects' performance at two levels of visual and cognitive perspective taking. *Journal of Autism and Developmental Disorders, 20,* 555–567.

Reid, D. K., Hresko, W. P., & Hammill, D. D. (1989). *Test of Early Reading Ability–Second Edition.* Austin, Tex.: Pro-Ed.

Rimland, B. (1964). *Infantile autism: The syndrome and its implications for a neural theory of behavior.* New York: Appleton-Century-Crofts.

Ritvo, E. R., Freeman, B. J., Pingree, C., Mason-Brothers, A., Jorde, L., Jenson, W. R., McMahon, W. M., Petersen, P. B., Mo, A., & Ritvo, A. (1989). The UCLA–University of Utah epidemiologic survey of autism: Prevalence. *American Journal of Psychiatry, 146,* 194–199.

Ritvo, E. R., Freeman, B. J., Scheibel, A. B., Duong, T., Robinson, H., Guthrie, D., & Ritvo, A. (1986). Lower purkinje cell counts in the cerebella of four autistic subjects: Initial findings of the UCLA-NSAC autopsy research report. *American Journal of Psychiatry, 143,* 862–866.

Ritvo, E. R., Ritvo, R., Freeman, B. J., & Mason-Brothers, A. (1994). Clinical characteristics of mild autism in adults. *Comprehensive Psychiatry, 35,* 149–156.

Rogers, S., Ozonoff, S., & Maslin-Cole, C. (1993). Developmental aspects of attachment behavior in young children with pervasive development disorders. *Journal of the American Academy of Child and Adolescent Psychiatry, 32,* 1274–1282.

Rogers, S. J. (1991). A psychotherapeutic approach for young children with pervasive developmental disorders. *Comprehensive Mental Health Care, 1,* 91–108.

Rogers, S. J., Herbison, J. M., Lewis, H. C., Pantone, J., & Reis, K. (1986). An approach for enhancing the symbolic, communicative, and interpersonal functioning of young children with autism or severe emotional handicaps. *Journal of the Division for Early Childhood, 10,* 135–145.

Rogers, S. J., & Lewis, H. (1989). An effective day treatment model for young children with pervasive developmental disorders. *Journal of the American Academy of Child and Adolescent Psychiatry, 28,* 207–214.

Rumsey, J. M., Duara, R., Grady, C., Rapoport, J. L., Margolin, R. A., Rapoport, S. I., & Cutler, N. R. (1985). Brain metabolism in autism: Resting cerebral glucose utilization rates as measured with positron emission tomography. *Archives of General Psychiatry, 42,* 448–455.

Rumsey, J. M., & Hamburger, S. D. (1988). Neuropsychological findings in high-functioning men with infantile autism, residual state. *Journal of Clinical and Experimental Neuropsychology, 10,* 201–221.

Rumsey, J. M., & Hamburger, S. D. (1990). Neuropsychological divergence of high level autism and severe dyslexia. *Journal of Autism and Developmental Disorders, 20,* 155–168.

Rumsey, J. M., Rapoport, J. L., & Sceery, W. R. (1985). Autistic children as adults: Psychiatric, social, and behavioral outcomes. *Journal of the American Academy of Child Psychiatry, 24,* 465–473.

Rutter, M. (1978). Diagnosis and definition. In M. Rutter & E. Schopler (Eds.), *Autism: A reappraisal of concepts and treatment* (pp. 1–25). New York: Plenum.

Rutter, M., Bailey, A., Bolton, P., & LeCouteur, A. (1994). Autism and known medical conditions: Myth and substance. *Journal of Child Psychology and Psychiatry, 35,* 311–322.

Rutter, M., MacDonald, H., LeCouteur, A., Harrington, R., Bolton, P., & Bailey, A. (1990). Genetic factors in child psychiatric disorders: Empirical findings. *Journal of Child Psychology and Psychiatry, 31,* 39–83.

Rutter, M. & Schopler, E. (1987). Autism and pervasive developmental disorders: Concepts and diagnostic issues. *Journal of Autism and Developmental Disorders, 17,* 159–186.

Rydell, P. J., & Prizant, B. (1995). Assessment and intervention strategies for children who use echolalia. In K. A. Quill (Ed.), *Teaching children with autism: Strategies to enhance communication and socialization* (pp. 105–132). Albany: Delmar.

Scherer, N. J. & Olswang, L. B. (1989). Using structured discourse as a language intervention technique with autistic children. *Journal of Speech and Hearing Disorders, 54,* 383–394.

Schopler, E. (1987). Specific and nonspecific factors in the effectiveness of a treatment system. *American Psychologist, 43,* 376–383.

Schopler, E., Brehm, S. S., Kinsbourne, M., & Reichler, R. J. (1971). Effect of treatment structure on development in autistic children. *Archives of General Psychiatry, 24,* 416–421.

Schopler, E., Mesibov, G. B., & Hearsey, K. (1995). Structured teaching in the TEACCH system. In E. Schopler & G. B. Mesibov (Eds.), *Learning and cognition in autism* (pp. 243–268). New York: Plenum.

Schopler, E., Mesibov, G. B., Shigley, R. H., & Bashford, A. (1984). Helping autistic children through their parents: The TEACCH model. In E. Schopler & G. B. Mesibov (Eds.), *The effects of autism on the family* (pp. 65–81). New York: Plenum.

Schopler, E., & Reichler, R. J. (1971). Parents as co-therapists in the treatment of psychotic children. *Journal of Autism and Childhood Schizophrenia, 1,* 87–102.

Schopler, E., Reichler, R. J., Bashford, A., Lansing, M. D., & Marcus, L. M. (1990). *Psychoeducational Profile–Revised.* Austin, Tex.: Pro-Ed.

Schopler, E., Reichler, R. J., & Renner, B. R. (1986). *The Childhood Autism Rating Scale (CARS)*. Los Angeles: Western Psychological Services.

Schroer, R. J., Phelan, M. C., Michaelis, R. C., Crawford, E. C., Skinner, S. A., Cuccaro, M., Simensen, R. J., Bishop, J., Skinner, C., Fender, D., & Stevenson, R. E. (1998). Autism and maternally derived aberrations of chromosome 15q. *American Journal of Medical Genetics, 76*, 327–336.

Shane, H. C. (Ed.). (1994). *Facilitated communication: The clinical and social phenomenon.* San Diego: Singular.

Sheinkopf, S. J. & Siegel, B. (1998). Home-based behavioral treatment of young children with autism. *Journal of Autism and Developmental Disorders, 28*, 15–23.

Sherman, M., Nass, R., & Shapiro, T. (1984). Regional cerebral blood flow in autism. *Journal of Autism and Developmental Disorders, 14*, 439–446.

Short, A. B. (1984). Short-term treatment outcome using parents as co-therapists for their own autistic children. *Journal of Child Psychology and Psychiatry, 25*, 443–458.

Shulman, B. B. (1986). *Test of Pragmatic Skills: Revised edition.* Tucson: Communication Skill Builders.

Siegel, D. J., Minshew, N. J., & Goldstein, G. (1996). Wechsler IQ profiles in diagnosis of high-functioning autism. *Journal of Autism and Developmental Disorders, 26*, 389–406.

Sigman, M. & Mundy, P. (1989). Social attachments in autistic children. *Journal of the American Academy of Child and Adolescent Psychiatry, 28*, 74–81.

Sigman, M., Mundy, P., Sherman, T., & Ungerer, J. (1986). Social interactions of autistic, mentally retarded and normal children and their caregivers. *Journal of Child Psychology and Psychiatry, 27*, 647–656.

Smalley, S. L., Asarnow, R. F., & Spence, M. A. (1988). Autism and genetics: A decade of research. *Archives of General Psychiatry, 45*, 953–961.

Snow, M., Hertzig, M., & Shapiro, T. (1987). Expressions of emotion in young autistic children. *Journal of the American Academy of Child and Adolescent Psychiatry, 26*, 836–838.

Sparrow, S. (1997). Developmentally based assessments. In D. J. Cohen & F. R. Volkmar (Eds.), *Handbook of autism and pervasive developmental disorders* (2nd ed., pp. 411–447). New York: Wiley.

Stern, D. N. (1985). *The interpersonal world of the infant.* New York: Basic Books.

Stone, W. L. (1997). Autism in infancy and early childhood. In D. J. Cohen & F. R. Volkmar (Eds.), *Handbook of autism and pervasive developmental disorders* (2nd ed., pp. 266–282). New York: Wiley.

Swanson, J. M., Posner, M., Potkin, S., Bonforte, S., Youpa, D., Fiore, C., Cantwell, D., & Crinella, F. (1991). Activating tasks for the study of visual-spatial attention in ADHD children: A cognitive anatomic approach. *Journal of Child Neurology, 6* (Suppl.) S119–S127.

Swisher, L., & Demetras, M. J. (1985). The expressive language characteristics of autistic children compared with mentally retarded or specific language-impaired children. In E. Schopler & G. Mesibov (Eds.), *Communication problems in autism* (pp. 147–162). New York: Plenum.

Szatmari, P., Bartolucci, G., Bremner, R., Bond, S., & Rich, S. (1989). A follow-up study of high-functioning autistic children. *Journal of Autism and Developmental Disorders, 19,* 213–225.

Szatmari, P., Bremner, R., & Nagy, J. (1989). Asperger's syndrome: A review of clinical features. *Canadian Journal of Psychiatry, 34,* 554–560.

Tager-Flusberg, H. (1981). On the nature of linguistic functioning in early infantile autism. *Journal of Autism and Developmental Disorders, 11,* 45–54.

Tager-Flusberg, H. (1985a). Basic level and superordinate level categorization in autistic, mentally retarded and normal children. *Journal of Experimental Child Psychology, 40,* 450–469.

Tager-Flusberg, H. (1985b). The conceptual basis for referential word meaning in children with autism. *Child Development, 56,* 1167–1178.

Tager-Flusberg, H. (1985c). Psycholinguistic approaches to language and communication in autism. In E. Schopler & G. Mesibov (Eds.), *Communication problems in autism* (pp. 69–87). New York: Plenum.

Tager-Flusberg, H. (1989). A psycholinguistic perspective on language development. In G. Dawson (Ed.), *Autism: Nature, diagnosis and treatment* (pp. 92–115). New York: Guilford.

Tager-Flusberg, H. Calkins, S., Nolin, R., Baumberger, T., Anderson, M., & Chadwick-Dias, A. (1990). A longitudinal study of language acquisition in autistic and Down syndrome children. *Journal of Autism and Developmental Disorders, 20,* 1–21.

Trevanthan, E., & Naidu, S. (1988). The clinical recognition and differential diagnosis of Rett syndrome. *Journal of Child Neurology, 3* (Suppl.), S6–S16.

Trevarthan, C. (1979). Communication and cooperation in early infancy: A description of primary intersubjectivity. In M. Bullowa (Ed.), *Before speech* (pp. 321–347). New York: Cambridge University Press.

Tsai, L. Y. (1987). Pre-, peri-, and neonatal factors in autism. In E. Schopler & G. B. Mesibov (Eds.), *Neurobiological issues in autism* (pp. 180–189). New York: Plenum.

Twachtman, D. (1995). Methods to enhance communication in verbal children. In K. A. Quill, (Ed.), *Teaching children with autism: Strategies to enhance communication and socialization* (pp. 133–162). Albany: Delmar.

Van Acker, R. (1991). Rett syndrome: A review of current knowledge. *Journal of Autism and Developmental Disorders, 21,* 381–406.

Vellutino, F. (1979). *Dyslexia: Theory and research.* Cambridge, Mass.: MIT Press.

Venter, A., Lord, C., & Schopler, E. (1992). A follow-up study of high-functioning autistic children. *Journal of Child Psychology and Psychiatry, 33,* 489–507.

Volkmar, F. R. (1992). Childhood disintegrative disorder: Issues for DSM-IV. *Journal of Autism and Developmental Disorders, 22,* 625–642.

Volkmar, F. R., & Cohen, D. J. (1989). Disintegrative disorder or "late onset" autism. *Journal of Child Psychology and Psychiatry, 30,* 717–724.

Volkmar, F. R., Klin, A., Siegel, B., Szatmari, P., Lord, C., Campbell, M., Freeman, B. J., Cicchetti, D. V., Rutter, M., Kline, W., Buitelaar, J., Hattab, Y., Fombonne, E., Feuntes, J., Werry, J., Stone, W., Kerbeshian, J., Hoshino, Y., Bregman, J., Loveland, K., Szymanski, L., & Towbin, K. (1994). Field trial for autistic disorder in DSM-IV. *American Journal of Psychiatry, 151,* 1361–1367.

Volkmar, F. R., & Rutter, M. (1995). Childhood disintegrative disorder: Results of the DSM-IV autism field trial. *Journal of the American Academy of Child and Adolescent Psychiatry, 34,* 1092–1095.

Wainwright-Sharp, J. A., & Bryson, S. E. (1993). Visual orienting deficits in high-functioning people with autism. *Journal of Autism and Developmental Disorders, 23,* 1–13.

Warren, R. P. (1998). An immunologic theory for the development of some cases of autism. *CNS Spectrum, 3,* 71–79.

Watson, L. R., Lord, C., Schaffer, B., & Schopler, E. (1989). *Teaching spontaneous communication to autistic and developmentally handicapped children.* Austin, Tex.: Pro-Ed.

Watson, L. R., Martin, J., & Schaffer, B. (1986). Form, content, and function of the spontaneous communication of autistic children. *Australian Journal of Human Communication Disorders, 17,* 91–102.

Watson, L. R., & Marcus, L. M. (1988). Diagnosis and assessment of preschool children. In E. Schopler & G. B. Mesibov (Eds.), *Diagnosis and assessment in autism* (pp. 271–301). New York: Plenum.

Watson, L. R., Crais, E. R., & Layton, T. L. (eds.) (in press). *Handbook of early language impairments: Assessment and intervention.* Albany, NY: Delmar.

Watson, L. R., & Ward, L. (1994). *Clinical implications of hyperlexia in children with autism.* Paper presented at the annual convention of the North Carolina Speech, Hearing and Language Association, Asheville.

Wechsler, D. (1974). *Manual for the Wechsler Intelligence Scale for Children–Revised.* New York: Psychological Corporation.

Wechsler, D. (1981). *Manual for the Wechsler Adult Intelligence Scale–Revised.* New York: Psychological Corporation.

Weidmer-Mikhail, E., Sheldon, S., & Ghaziuddin, M. (1998). Chromosomes in autism and related pervasive developmental disorders: A cytogenetic study. *Journal of Intellectual Disability Research, 42,* 8–12.

Wetherby, A. M., & Prizant, B. M. (1993). *Communication and Symbolic Behavior Scales.* Chicago: Riverside.

Wetherby, A. M., & Prutting, C. (1984). Profiles of communicative and cognitive-social abilities in autistic children. *Journal of Speech and Hearing Research, 27,* 364–377.

Wetherby, A., Yonclas, D., & Bryan, A. (1989). Communicative profiles of handicapped preschool children: Implication for early identification. *Journal of Speech and Hearing Disorders, 54,* 148–158.

White, C. P., & Rosenbloom, L. (1992). Temporal lobe structures and autism. *Developmental Medicine and Child Neurology, 34,* 556–559.

Whitehouse, D., & Harris, J. C. (1984). Hyperlexia in infantile autism. *Journal of Autism and Developmental Disorders, 14,* 281–289.

Wiig, E. H., Secord, W., & Semel, E. (1992). *Clinical Evaluation of Language Fundamentals–Preschool.* San Antonio: Psychological Corp.

Wimmer, H. & Perner, J. (1983). Beliefs about beliefs: Representation and the constraining function of wrong beliefs in young children's understanding of deception. *Cognition, 13,* 103–128.

Wing, L. (1981). Asperger's syndrome: A clinical account. *Psychological Medicine, 11,* 115–129.

Wing, L. (1988). The continuum of autistic characteristics. In E. Schopler & G. B. Mesibov (Eds.), *Diagnosis and assessment in autism* (pp. 91–110). New York: Plenum.

World Health Organization. (1977). *Manual of the international classification of diseases* (9th rev.). Geneva, Switzerland: Author.

World Health Organization. (1992). *Manual of the international classification of diseases: Diagnostic criteria for research* (10th rev., draft). Geneva, Switzerland: Author.

Zilbovicius, M., Garreau, B., Samson, Y., Remy, P., Barthelemy, C., Syrota, A., & Lelord, G. (1995). Delayed maturation of the frontal cortex in childhood autism. *American Journal of Psychiatry, 152,* 248–252.

Zilbovicius, M., Garreau, B., Tzourio, N., Mazoyer, B., Bruck, B., Martinot, J. L., Raynaud, C., Samson, Y., Syrota, A., & Lelord, G. (1992). Regional cerebral blood flow in childhood autism: A SPECT study. *American Journal of Psychiatry, 149,* 924–930.

Fragile X Syndrome in Young Children

Gail A. Spiridigliozzi, Ph.D.
Assistant Clinical Professor
Duke University Medical Center
Durham, North Carolina

Ave M. Lachiewicz, M.D.
Assistant Clinical Professor
Duke University Medical Center
Durham, North Carolina

Penny Mirrett, Ph.D., CCC-SLP
Project Director
Frank Porter Graham Child Development Center
University of North Carolina, Chapel Hill
and
Allyn McConkie-Rosell, Ph.D., CGC
Clinical Associate
Duke University Medical Center
Durham, North Carolina

Key Terms

CGG repeat	mosaic
FMR1 gene	premutation
full mutation	transmitting male

Overview

Fragile X syndrome is the leading known X-linked cause of mental retardation. It also causes specific learning disabilities and can be associated with a diagnosis of autism in some individuals. Unlike conditions such as Down syndrome, which typically affect only one family member, fragile X syndrome has implications for the entire family. It is not uncommon for siblings, cousins, and other relatives of a person with fragile X also to be affected. In addition, some relatives who do not have fragile X may nevertheless be carriers of the gene and have a high risk for having affected children. It is now estimated that 1 out of 4,000 males carries the full mutation, but as many as 1 out of 250 women and 1 out of 700 males may carry the gene for this condition (Turner, Webb, Wake, & Robinson, 1996). Fragile X syndrome has been reported throughout the world and is believed to be present in all ethnic groups. Still, the condition is underdiagnosed, and many affected individuals have yet to come to the attention of medical professionals.

This chapter is designed to provide an overview of children with fragile X syndrome and issues important to their assessment and treatment. Boys are often distinguished from girls with the condition because males tend to be more severely affected. Not all children with fragile X syndrome will show all of the characteristics described here. The goal of this chapter is to give clinicians a framework for better understanding children with fragile X and to help clinicians develop appropriate treatment plans.

ETIOLOGY AND CHARACTERISTICS OF FRAGILE X SYNDROME

The clinical and developmental manifestations of fragile X syndrome have been linked to a specific gene on the X chromosome. In 1991, this gene was isolated and named the FMR1 gene (Fragile X Mental Retardation–1). Our understanding of this gene and its mechanism of inheritance has increased dramatically in recent years. Fragile X syndrome was found to be caused by an unstable expansion of a triplet repeat. We now understand that fragile X was only the first of many triplet repeat disorders to be described. Other conditions that were subsequently found to have the same mechanism of inheritance include Huntington's disease, myotonic muscular dystrophy, and other neurodegenerative disorders (Ashley & Warren, 1995).

All individuals carry the gene for fragile X syndrome, or FMR1. What distinguishes those families with members affected by fragile X syndrome from others is the instability of this gene. The instability results from the size of a particular DNA fragment or "switch" controlling the gene called the **CGG repeat**. CGG repeat refers to a particular sequence of amino acids, cytosine (C), guanine (G), and guanine (G). In most people, this CGG sequence is repeated about 29 times. In those individuals identified as carriers of fragile X syndrome, however, this CGG sequence is repeated anywhere from 54 to 230 times and the gene is said to be in the **premutation** stage. This stage is represented by an unstable gene in which the CGG repeat number is between 50–54 to approximately 230 without methylation. Here, the switch is enlarged but has not yet shut down the gene (i.e., the gene is not methylated). In those individuals clearly affected by fragile X syndrome, the CGG repeat size typically ranges from 230 to 4,000 repeats. Here, the gene is in the **full mutation** stage, and the switch is both expanded and methylated, or shut off. When the FMR1 gene shuts down, it no longer produces the specific protein (known as the FMR1 protein) it was intended to make. Although the exact function of the FMR1 protein is not yet understood, its presence is believed to be essential to normal brain development and function.

Some individuals with fragile X syndrome carry the gene in the premutation stage in some cell lines and the gene in the full mutation stage in other cell lines. Such an individual is referred to as a **mosaic**. Often, mosaics are less severely affected because some amount of FMR1 protein is being produced in their bodies.

The FMR1 gene can be transmitted from fathers to daughters and from mothers to sons and daughters. The gene cannot be passed from a father to his sons because the gene is located on the X chromosome, whereas fathers pass the Y chromosome to their sons. When the FMR1 gene passes from one generation to the next, the number of CGG repeats, or the size of the switch, typically increases. This switch controlling the gene remains relatively stable in size when passed from a father to his daughter and generally expands when passed from a mother to her son or daughter.

Another unique feature of families with fragile X syndrome is the presence of a **transmitting male**. These males carry the FMR1 gene in the premutation stage and do not show any obvious clinical manifestations of fragile X syndrome. They will pass the gene to all of their daughters, however, and the daughters will be carriers. The risk of having affected children will be in the next generation, when these women have children of their own. Once again, the FMR1 gene is more likely to expand when passed down from a mother to her children. Her risk of transmitting the unstable FMR1 gene is 50 percent. However, her risk of having an affected son is 25 percent (.50 chance for transmitting the unstable X and .50 chance the baby is a boy). Since girls can also be affected, the risk of having a child that would be affected with fragile X to some degree is 50 percent. It is important to remember that the clinical manifestations of fragile X syndrome are quite variable. Although it is possible to determine the risk of transmitting the unstable FMR1 to offspring, it can be difficult to predict the severity of the condition in an individual child.

The genetics of fragile X syndrome are complicated. This information is generally conveyed to families by a physician and/or a genetic counselor when a diagnosis of fragile X syndrome is made or is being considered. We recommend genetic counseling for all families who have had a member diagnosed with fragile X. This is important not only in helping families understand the inheritance pattern, but also in identifying other relatives who are at risk of having affected children or passing the gene to subsequent generations.

DIAGNOSIS

Prior to 1991, fragile X syndrome was diagnosed through a procedure called karyotyping or chromosome analysis. This involves taking blood from an individual's arm and directly visualizing the chromosomes under a microscope. The chromosome analysis that was done to diagnose fragile X syndrome involved growing the blood sample in a special folate-depleted tissue culture medium and looking for the fragile site. Under the microscope, the fragile site for which fragile X syndrome was named made the long arm of the X chromosome appear to be unraveling. This fragile site was found only in those individuals with the full mutation. It was not found in individuals carrying the premutation. Therefore, the chromosome study was not accurate in detecting carriers of fragile X syndrome. We now understand that the fragile X site corresponds to the region of the expansion of the switch known to be the cause of fragile X syndrome.

The fragile X gene (FMR1) was isolated and partially characterized in 1991 (Tarleton & Saul, 1993). The most immediate benefit of this discovery was the addition of direct DNA testing as a diagnostic option. This meant that a diagnosis of fragile X could be made with greater accuracy (particularly for females) and less cost to families. As a result, some individuals previously diagnosed with fragile X were found to be negative for the condition. Others who were negative on karyotyping have been found to carry the FMR1 gene. This is because the DNA testing is clearly the more accurate of the two methods. Individuals diagnosed with fragile X syndrome before 1991 should have the diagnosis confirmed by DNA testing, and those who were thought to be negative for fragile X prior to 1991 should also be retested with the DNA method to be certain that they are not carrying the FMR1 gene. DNA testing is performed in specialized laboratories using blood drawn from the patient. The results include information about the number of CGG repeats and whether or not the gene is methylated (i.e., turned off).

Prenatal testing for fragile X syndrome is also available, although it is not done unless a pregnant woman or her physician requests it. This can be accomplished through chorionic villi sampling (CVS) at about 10 to 11 weeks into the pregnancy or amniocentesis at about 14 to 16 weeks into the pregnancy.

PHYSICAL CHARACTERISTICS

The physical characteristics of children with fragile X syndrome differ in boys and girls. Each will be discussed briefly below.

Boys with Fragile X Syndrome

A number of physical characteristics have been described in boys with fragile X syndrome (Freund, 1994; Hagerman, 1996). Some boys display more of these features than others. Although there is a characteristic "look" to boys with fragile X, it is not as obvious as those with other genetic conditions such as Down syndrome. However, the physical features of fragile X often become more evident as a boy grows older. Young boys with fragile X are often very attractive and difficult to distinguish physically from peers. Because boys with fragile X may not look different, a referral for fragile X DNA testing and subsequent diagnosis may not be made based on physical characteristics. Other factors, such as the child's family history, abnormal behaviors, and developmental functioning must be considered when requesting a referral for fragile X DNA testing.

Some primary physical characteristics of boys with fragile X syndrome include an elongated face, large ears, and a highly arched palate. The boys tend to have low muscle tone and hyperextensible finger joints. Hand calluses are often seen in boys with fragile X due to their tendency to bite their fingers and hands. Large testicles in boys with fragile X are apparent after about age 8 years. They may also have flat feet. Although these boys are generally average in their height, they tend to have a larger-than-average head size.

Boys with fragile X syndrome tend to have frequent ear infections. Many parents report that their sons have had pressure equalizing (PE) tubes inserted one or more times. In addition, there may be an increased frequency of eye problems, such as strabismus (Hatton, Buckley, Lachiewicz, & Roberts, in press). About 10 to 20 percent of the males are also diagnosed with a seizure disorder.

Girls with Fragile X Syndrome

Girls with fragile X syndrome may have a normal appearance or have some of the same features as the boys, including a long face, prominent ears, and a highly arched palate. They also tend to have low muscle tone and hyperextensible finger joints (Davis, Hagerman, & Eilert, 1990) which contribute to their difficulty with fine motor tasks.

SENSORIMOTOR CHARACTERISTICS

Information regarding the sensorimotor characteristics of boys with fragile X syndrome is based largely on clinical experience. Some information has been gained from studies of specific behaviors that distinguish boys with fragile X from boys with developmental disabilities who are negative for this condition (Lachiewicz, Spiridigliozzi, Gullion, Ransford, & Rao, 1994). Additional studies are needed in this area to confirm the clinical impressions that have been reported.

Boys with fragile X syndrome often demonstrate problems with tactile defensiveness, a tendency to react with negative emotions or behaviors to information received through the tactile (touch) sensory system. For example, the boys may become upset when touched lightly on the shoulder or dislike activities such as playing in the sand or finger painting. Having their hair combed may be highly aversive, as well as the feel of certain fabrics on their skin. This increased sensitivity to certain kinds of touch can lead to temper tantrums or crying, which may persist even after the sensory input is withdrawn.

In addition, some boys with fragile X are overly sensitive to sights or sounds. This is called sensory defensiveness. It is not uncommon to see boys with fragile X put their hands over the ears and became upset if the noise level is high. Even when an activity is a very desirable one, the child's sensitivity to sound can interfere with the ability to participate. For example, one boy in our clinic trained extensively for the Special Olympics but could not take part in the games after hearing the opening gun shot. This noise was so unsettling to him that he was unable to regain control of his emotions and take part in the races. Similarly, bright lights can be unsettling to boys with fragile X. One adolescent male frequently wears sunglasses to the hospital clinic because he is bothered by the fluorescent lighting.

Boys with fragile X syndrome may also show signs of gravitational insecurity. This refers to poorly developed postural responses to the gravitational forces needed during movement and particularly in response to sudden or complex movement patterns (Gilfoyle, Grady, & Moore, 1981). The inability to adjust quickly and smoothly to these changes makes the child feel insecure and distressed. For instance, boys with fragile X may be fearful of being in high places, climbing on playground equipment, riding on escalators, or being placed on a physician's examining table. They prefer to have both feet on the ground at all times. Once again, the negative emotions associated with these activities may result in significant behavioral problems.

An understanding of these sensory processing issues is important as a way of interpreting many of the behaviors shown by boys with fragile X. Because they often experience incoming sensory information in such a negative way, these boys may react with disruptive behaviors that are largely outside of their control. In addition, these outbursts are likely to occur with strangers or outside the home, where the typical diversions available for children such as playground equipment, loud music, animated characters, and so forth are often movement and sensation oriented. Therefore, a preventive approach to understanding, anticipating, and modifying the child's environment will be more helpful than providing a consequence for each behavioral outburst. Some examples of preventive sensory interventions are provided in Table 5-1.

Fine and Gross Motor Characteristics

Boys with fragile X syndrome generally have poorly developed fine motor skills (Anderson, 1992). This is most obvious in their difficulty with hand-

Table 5-1. Sensory Integration Problems Frequently Seen in Boys with Fragile X Syndrome

WORRISOME BEHAVIOR	SENSORY SYSTEM THAT MAY BE AFFECTED	SUGGESTIONS FOR INTERVENTION
• Makes poor eye contact • Looks away from another person's face • Seems sensitive to bright light	VISUAL sight	• Don't demand eye contact when giving verbal instructions • Allow child to wear sunglasses • Provide natural light when possible • Provide environment with decreased visual stimulation (e.g., blank walls or simple decorations only, low light)
• Reacts negatively to loud noises • Covers ears to reduce noise • Talks self through tasks	AUDITORY hearing	• Use soft, calm voice • Provide calming background noise (e.g., classical music, sounds from nature, etc.) • Gradually introduce child to noisy environments (e.g., the cafeteria) • Consider use of ear plugs or ear muffs • Try to keep competing noise to a minimum
• Is hypersensitive to smell • Is distracted by smells • Smells objects to explore them	OLFACTORY smell	• Use natural odors and food smells (e.g., strawberry or banana) • Be aware that perfume can be distracting • Avoid strong cleaners, paints • Encourage exploring with other senses such as tactile (touch)
• Has strong negative reaction to touch, especially light touch • Becomes upset by some clothes or labels • Has difficulty tolerating tooth brushing, hair combing, hair washing, or bathing UNDERSTAND THAT THESE BEHAVIORS MAY BE A PROTECTIVE RESPONSE	TACTILE touch	• Alert child before touching • Use firm but gentle touch • Consult occupational therapist about brushing techniques to decrease negative reactions to touch • Place child first or last in school lines and assign seat in front of bus to avoid bumping into other children • Give "bear" hugs and use bean-bag chairs to create a "nest-like" space • Encourage exploration or touch at the child's pace • Use natural fibers in clothes • Wash new clothes before wearing
• Avoids many types of movement • Seeks out rocking • Avoids physical activities	VESTIBULAR involves receptors in inner ear that help regulate sense of balance,	• If movement elicits fear, encourage but do not force • Provide rocking chair • Provide playground activities that will stimulate the vestibular system (e.g., jungle gyms, spinning toys, swings)

(continues)

Table 5-1. Sensory Integration Problems Frequently Seen in Boys with Fragile X Syndrome (continued)

WORRISOME BEHAVIOR	SENSORY SYSTEM THAT MAY BE AFFECTED	SUGGESTIONS FOR INTERVENTION
	movement and posture	• Provide alternative work positions (e.g., lying on stomach, beanbag chair • Encourage athletic activities and noncompetitive sports

• Jumps in place
• Flaps hands
• Bites hands
• Excessively restless or distractible
	PROPRIOCEPTIVE sensations from the muscles, joints, and tendons that let us know how body parts (e.g., legs, arms, mouth, and tongue) are positioned	• Provide opportunities for increased stimulation to muscles by allowing child to perform "heavy work." For example:
		   Move chairs or tables
		   Break down boxes
		   Hand out heavy textbooks
		   Wash chalkboard
		   Do push-ups off wall or chair
		   Pull or push wagons, book carts, or wheelbarrow
		• Allow child to change positions when needed (e.g., changing from sitting to standing)
		• Apply deep pressure (e.g., place beanbag chair on back of child while while he is lying on stomach)
		• Allow chewing gum (two pieces)
		• Encourage oral-motor games (e.g., blowing whistles, bubbles, or using cocktail straws or long crazy straws)
		• Give thick drinks for straw drinking
		• Encourage child to eat hard or chewy foods with texture and resistance (e.g., carrots, bagels, fruit chews, licorice, pretzels, and pickles)

PRECAUTIONS:
• Try one approach several times before rejecting
• Only change one intervention at a time to see if it improves the situation
• Work closely with an occupational or physical therapist who has training in sensory integration therapy

writing and other tasks such as fastening their clothes, cutting, and eating skillfully. The boys' low cognitive ability, low muscle tone, hyperextensible finger joints, and weak motor planning skills all seem to contribute to these difficulties. In addition, the boys may have a genuine sensory aversion to holding things in their hands, such as pencils or eating utensils, which may further decrease their motivation to attempt or practice these skills.

Boys with fragile X syndrome typically demonstrate only mild gross motor delays. Their acquisition of motor milestones, such as walking, may be within the normal range. Prouty, Rogers, and Stevenson (1988) reported a mean age of 10 months for sitting alone and 20.6 months for walking unassisted in a group of 25 males with fragile X. Four of these boys were walking before 15 months of age. Other gross motor weaknesses have been described clinically, such as postural mechanism difficulties (Wilson, Stackhouse, O'Connor, Scharfenaker, & Hagerman, 1994). For example, the boys may have trouble staying seated in an upright position. They may also show signs of dyspraxia or difficulty with motor planning. Boys with fragile X syndrome often benefit from adaptive physical education services in school.

In general, girls with fragile X syndrome are likely to show more subtle sensory-processing and motor deficits. They may not display the same magnitude or frequency of negative behaviors often associated with these difficulties in boys. All children with an early diagnosis of fragile X syndrome will benefit from a comprehensive occupational therapy evaluation to determine their profile of strengths and weaknesses and need for early intervention services. This may help prevent long-term delays in these areas.

BEHAVIORAL AND SOCIAL CHARACTERISTICS

Boys with fragile X syndrome may exhibit a number of challenging behaviors. Often, it is the behavioral issues more than cognitive weaknesses that interfere with their ability to function at home or school. Therefore, it is helpful to think about these behaviors from several different perspectives and adopt a preventive approach to managing them.

Many boys with fragile X have been diagnosed with attention deficit/hyperactivity disorder. They are often extremely distractible, impulsive, and have a short attention span. Their overall level of motor activity is typically high. It is not uncommon for the parents of young boys with fragile X to report sleep problems, including difficulty falling asleep and early awakening.

Many of these boys display unusual hand movements. These include flapping their hands and/or biting them, particularly when they are excited or overstimulated. About 25 percent of the boys will have calluses on their hands or fingers from biting them repeatedly.

Boys with fragile X also tend to make poor eye contact. This may improve over time in a familiar situation, presumably as their level of anxiety decreases. Demanding that the child make good eye contact is not helpful, however, and may trigger other negative behaviors (Sudhalter, Cohen, Silverman, & Wolf-Schein, 1990).

Boys with fragile X often have trouble dealing with changes in their routine. When unexpected changes do occur and the child does not understand what will be happening next, tantrums or other behavior problems may result. Dealing with multiple transitions in a short time period can also be problematic.

Our clinical experience has been that boys with fragile X do not show a strong drive to try new things or seek out information. Many prefer to watch specific television shows or movies that capture their attention. These boys often need to be "pushed" to try things that may be uncomfortable for them initially. Although some boys may be very active, they are not particularly organized in their play or work. It is important that parents, teachers, and other professionals set some clearly defined expectations for these children, so that they will reach their maximum potential. For example, some parents insist that their boys participate in a structured physical activity, such as T-ball or horseback riding. Even though the boys may protest going to the activity, they generally do fine once they are there and grow accustomed to the routine.

Some investigators have attempted to determine those behaviors that distinguish boys with fragile X syndrome from others with pervasive developmental delays who are negative for fragile X syndrome. Lachiewicz et al. (1994) asked mothers or the female caregivers of boys with fragile X and a control group of boys without fragile X (matched on age, socioeconomic status, level of cognitive functioning, and race) to complete a variety of behavioral rating scales. The behaviors seen more often in the boys with fragile X included tactile defensiveness, the use of abnormal language, hand flapping, poor self-control, and poor eye contact.

There is also an association between fragile X syndrome and the behaviors seen in individuals with autism. Some investigators have reported that up to 16 percent of males with autism may also have fragile X syndrome (Blomquist et al., 1985). Reports on the frequency of autism in males with fragile X syndrome range from 5 to 54 percent (Hagerman, 1991). The variability in these findings is probably due, in part, to differences in the criteria used to make a diagnosis of autism. Frequently, boys with fragile X syndrome exhibit some behaviors that make a clinician consider this diagnosis, but they may not meet the full criteria for the autistic disorder, as specified in the *Diagnostic and Statistical Manual of Mental Disorders, 4th Edition (DSM-IV)* (American Psychiatric Association [APA], 1994).

In a study by Reiss and Freund (1992), boys with fragile X (ages 3 to 18 years) were compared to an IQ- and age-matched control group of boys who had developmental delays but were negative for fragile X. These investigators looked at the specific behaviors outlined in *DSM-IV* to make a diagnosis of autism. Boys with fragile X had more trouble with social play and showed more dysfunction in their verbal and nonverbal communication skills than boys with developmental delays and other diagnoses. The boys with fragile X also had more problems with repetitive motor behaviors, such as hand flapping, hand biting, and rocking. These behaviors rarely occurred in the control group. Reiss and Freund (1992) also noted that the specific behaviors from the autism spectrum manifested in boys with fragile X are not generally seen until the "preschool years."

Most boys with fragile X syndrome seem genuinely interested in making social contacts, forming attachments, and being around other children and adults, but experience significant anxiety in social situations related to their language and motor deficits (Hagerman, 1991). Reiss and Freund (1992) found that infants and toddlers with fragile X did not differ from controls in terms of attachment behaviors with caregivers. As the children with fragile X enter the preschool years, however, impairments in their social behaviors become more evident. They may appear to be shy or uncomfortable in new situations, but generally become more at ease over time and with repeated contacts. This may be evident in their increased eye contact or verbal communication. Boys with fragile X syndrome often have difficulty initiating social contacts in an appropriate way but will be responsive to the overtures of others. They are also likely to imitate the social and play behaviors displayed by peers, such as joining a game on the playground. These boys tend to have difficulty using appropriate language in social situations, such as making their needs known verbally or expressing their displeasure in words.

Girls with fragile X syndrome tend to have milder behavioral and social difficulties than the boys, although some of their issues may fall on the same continuum. For example, the girls often have attention problems that interfere with their learning and may have been diagnosed with attention deficit/hyperactivity disorder. They are less likely than the boys, however, to show excessive motor activity.

Girls with fragile X are often described as being overly shy or anxious in social situations (Freund, Reiss, & Abrams, 1993). They may want to have friends but find it difficult to talk in groups or relate to peers. These girls often appear to be socially immature. They seem to do best in small, structured activities such as church youth groups or choir.

In one study looking specifically at the behaviors of girls with fragile X, each mother was asked to complete a variety of behavioral checklists regarding her daughter (Lachiewicz, 1992; Lachiewicz & Dawson, 1994). In comparison to a control group matched for age, IQ level, and diagnosis of a chronic medical or developmental disorder, the girls with fragile X were described as having an increased incidence of poor attention, poor interactive skills, and symptoms of social withdrawal (Lachiewicz, 1992). According to Lachiewicz and Dawson (1994), the mothers of girls with fragile X also endorsed more behaviors than controls on the Anxiety factor and Hyperactivity Index of the Conners' Parent's Questionnaire (Connors, 1990). In addition, Freund et al. (1993) found that 65 percent of girls with fragile X, versus 12 percent of a control group (matched for age, IQ, and socioeconomic status), showed shyness and social avoidance to the extent that it interfered with their social relationships with peers.

COGNITIVE CHARACTERISTICS

Children with fragile X syndrome show a range of cognitive functioning. Approximately 2/3 of girls with fragile X have IQ scores in the average range (Freund, 1994). Some girls, in particular, have average or low-average IQ scores but manifest specific learning disabilities in one or more areas. Boys with fragile X syndrome are generally more severely impaired. Their level of cognitive functioning may range from borderline to moderate or severe mental retardation (Pennington, O'Connor, & Sudhulter, 1991). It is important to keep in mind that although cognition and behavior may be described separately, they constantly influence one another in day-to-day functioning and across the child's course of development. As Shopmeyer and Lowe (1992) explain, "The behaviors children exhibit based on their neurology influence cognitive characteristics" and "The ways in which children cognitively understand the world around them in turn influences their behavior" (p. 36).

Cognitive Strengths in Males

Boys with fragile X syndrome often show an uneven profile of cognitive skills that can be puzzling to families and professionals. Several studies (Dykens, Hodapp, & Leckman, 1987; Kemper, Hagerman, & Altshul-Stark, 1988) have shown that boys with fragile X do better on tasks emphasizing simultaneous-processing abilities versus sequential-processing skills, as measured on the Kaufman Assessment Battery for Children (K-ABC) (Kaufman & Kaufman, 1983). For example, these boys are likely to identify a picture of an object even when important parts of it are missing (simultaneous processing). Their performance on this particular subtest (Gestalt Closure) can be in the average range in comparison to peers.

Long-term memory appears to be a relative strength for boys with fragile X syndrome. They tend to remember factual information for a long time, particularly when it relates to an area of interest. Boys with fragile X have strong visual memory skills as well. For example, they can often recall the directions to a particular spot after only visiting it once. They can also learn to spell and read many words by memorizing their visual configuration. Systematic assessment of memory functioning in these boys may lead to a better understanding of their learning style and effective educational interventions.

Another strength for boys with fragile X syndrome appears to be their imitation skills. They are very good at imitating what they see and hear. In regard to their verbal imitation skills, boys with fragile X often repeat what they hear, especially if it is a word that sounds interesting or pleasurable to them (for example, "ridiculous"). Unfortunately, they also repeat words and phrases that are less than desirable. Therefore, it is critical that the boys be exposed to good language role models at home and school. This was illustrated to us by one boy with good verbal skills but moderate mental retardation. When he was placed in a classroom setting with nonverbal peers, his language skills quickly deteriorated.

Boys with fragile X also seem to imitate the behaviors that they see, both positive and negative. For example, one boy with fragile X was placed in a self-contained classroom with two other brothers with fragile X who were more impaired. Within weeks, the boy's caregivers began seeing many of the old "fragile X behaviors" that they had worked hard to eliminate, such as hand flapping and hand biting. Another boy with fragile X who was in a class with students who were nonambulatory requested a wheelchair for Christmas. On the other hand, many boys with fragile X are benefitting from placement in a regular classroom setting. Their parents often report a decrease in negative behaviors and an increase in positive interactions with peers. Once again, it is very important that boys with fragile X be exposed to good behavioral models in all settings to capitalize positively on their strong imitation skills.

Cognitive Weaknesses in Males

Boys with fragile X syndrome often show significant weaknesses in their abstract reasoning, problem-solving abilities, and calculation skills (Wilson et al., 1994). Most of these have been described clinically, although some formal research studies have been completed (Hodapp, Dykens, Ort, Zelinsky, & Leckman, 1991; Kemper et al., 1988).

Boys with fragile X have more trouble recalling a series of elements in the right order (sequential processing). This relative difficulty with sequencing may impact on their functioning in a number of different areas, such as applying a phonetic approach to reading, learning the steps necessary to form letters, and counting with one-to-one correspondence.

Boys with fragile X may have trouble starting and completing tasks that emphasize fine motor and motor planning skills. For example, worksheets that involve coloring, drawing, and handwriting skills will be difficult for them and not particularly meaningful. The boys will also have trouble copying material from a book or the board.

A number of studies, both retrospective and prospective, have shown that the boys' scores on intelligence tests (IQs) decline over time (Lachiewicz, Gullion, Spiridigliozzi, & Aylsworth, 1987). Although their IQs may be in the borderline to mild range of mental retardation as preschoolers, boys with fragile X are more likely to function in the mild-to-moderate range of mental retardation by late childhood. There are several factors that may influence this trajectory of cognitive development. First, there is no evidence that the boys lose skills over time. Rather, their rate of development appears to slow down. This may be due to the impact of their attentional problems on learning and/or the increased emphasis on abstract reasoning skills and speed of processing in IQ tests for older children.

Cognitive Variation in Females

Girls with fragile X syndrome are generally not as severely impaired in their cognitive abilities as the boys, although approximately one-third are mentally retarded (Reiss, Freund, Abrams, Boehm, & Kazazian, 1993). In addition, girls carrying the gene in the premutation stage will have fewer or no striking deficits in comparison to girls carrying the gene in the full mutation stage. Clinicians and researchers are now looking more closely at these two groups of females to better understand their profile of skills (e.g., Borghgraef, Umans, Steyaert, Leguius, & Fryns, 1996; Reiss et al., 1993).

Researchers have described a characteristic profile of cognitive weaknesses often seen in females with fragile X syndrome (Pennington et al., 1991). On the Wechsler Scales of Intelligence (Wechsler, 1974, 1981), their scores on the Arithmetic, Digit Span, and Block Design subtests tend to be significantly lower than their performance on the other subtests. Miezejeski et al. (1986) described a math learning disability in their sample of females with fragile X. The issue of visual-spatial deficits and difficulty with math continues to be an important area of study among girls and women with the FMR1 gene. In our clinical work, these females frequently report having trouble with math courses and math applications in their lives, such as computing fractions or balancing a checkbook. However, reading appears to be a particular area of strength.

COMMUNICATION SKILLS

The communication style and speech pattern of males with fragile X has generally been described as distinctive or characteristic. Although the factors contributing to this distinctive speech and language pattern have been described by several authors (Freund, 1994; Shopmeyer & Lowe, 1992; Wilson et al., 1994), controlled studies are just beginning to emerge in the literature. This section will focus on several areas of development that impact on the speech and language functioning of children with fragile X syndrome. It should be noted that the degree of impact on specific individuals varies substantially.

Early Markers of Speech-Language Impairment

Given that fragile X syndrome is the most common inherited cause of developmental disabilities and learning problems and the fact that measured IQs range from normal to severe mental retardation, it is not surprising that early patterns of speech and language development are also highly variable. There are, however, some key features to look for in the toddler and preschool aged child that may facilitate early diagnosis and early intervention focused on preverbal and verbal skills.

Generalized hypotonicity that also affects the oral structures is a common finding in fragile X (Abbeduto & Hagerman, 1997; Wilson et al., 1994). Oral sensory defensiveness is another early hallmark (Shopmeyer & Lowe, 1992; Wilson et al., 1994). These two factors underlie common parental reports of difficulty sucking, poor chewing with food loss (i.e., poor lip seal), and poor tolerance of different food textures. Shelhart, Casamassimo, Hagerman, and

Belanger (1986) also note excessive gagging in their patients with fragile X, which is consistent with tactile defensiveness. Shopmeyer and Lowe (1992) provide a number of clinical examples of persistent intolerance of two textures in the mouth or one texture plus a utensil in the mouth. Parents frequently report persistent finger feeding and/or regression to finger feeding when a new texture or food is introduced. Simko, Hornsteir, Soukup, and Bagamery (1989) also report mouthing of objects past a young age as a frequent finding in children with fragile X. Inadequate sensory awareness and hypotonicity in the mouth can lead to increased drooling. Parents frequently report stuffing of food into the mouth before swallowing a previous bite.

All of these behaviors and issues can become frustrating for parents and teachers. It is much more helpful for caregivers to understand that these behaviors arise from very real sensory and motor impairments. Providing motor and sensory integration interventions can eliminate or minimize the child's need for such behaviors.

The onset of functional speech and language skills is almost universally delayed in boys with fragile X syndrome. Simko et al. (1989) reported that 95 percent of children in their sample were characterized by language delay. Freund (1994) reported that boys with fragile X typically evidence skills 18 to 29 months below chronological age expectations for the onset of clearly spoken words, performance 45 to 56 months below age for phrases of two or more words, and delays of up to 60 months below age for functional sentences.

Speech Intelligibility

Although the perception of clear speech is a holistic phenomenon, there are at least four distinct factors that impact speech intelligibility: articulation, prosody, fluency, and voice. Boys with fragile X, in particular, present with difficulties in each of these areas to varying degrees.

Articulation.   Articulation may be affected in several ways. Developmental substitutions of the consonants /r/, /l/, /s/, /v/ and voiced and unvoiced /th/ have frequently been described (Paul, Cohen, Breg, Watson, & Herman, 1984; Prouty et al., 1988). It is important to note, however, that these errors are usually consistent with developmental age and do not differ significantly from the consonant errors of other children who are mentally retarded or from the speech of many normal preschoolers as they acquire the complete consonant sound repertoire of the language. Several researchers have also noted features in the speech of males with fragile X that are consistent with developmental dyspraxia—that is, impairment in the planning, sequencing, and execution of smooth, fluent speech (Madison, George, & Moeschler, 1986; Paul et al., 1984; Vilkman, Niemi, & Ikonen, 1988). Vilkman et al. (1988) noted vowel substitutions and omissions, which are not normal developmental variations. Further, in 88 percent of these errors, Vilkman et al. (1988) found the productions to be off by one feature only, which is consistent with the presence of developmental dyspraxia. Madison et al. (1986) observed the most impaired intelligibility in children with fragile X who spoke in the longest sentences. This is often seen in children with dyspraxia. Other characteristics common to verbal dyspraxia and frequently noted in the speech of boys with fragile X include: incorrect sequencing of nonreduplicated syllables (e.g., puh-tuh-kuh) and greater difficulty pronouncing multisyllable words (e.g., refrigerator, ridiculous) than one- or two-syllable words (Paul et al., 1984).

Prosody.   Prosody or prosodic features include rate, intonation, stress, junction (or pauses) and rhythm. The rapid, uneven, staccato-like aspects of connected speech often described in males with fragile X reflect prosodic problems. This pattern may be related to persistent low muscle tone (hypotonia), developmental dyspraxia, or other difficulties in language learning not yet delineated. Shopmeyer and Lowe (1992) point out that these aberrations can significantly impact intelligibility, since the rhythm and pauses in normal speech serve grammatical and semantic functions in organizing or "staging" the message for the listener.

Fluency.   Fluency is often impaired in males with fragile X, but is more consistent with the profile of "cluttering" than stuttering. Cluttering is described by Hanson, Jackson, and Hagerman (1986) as fast and fluctuating in rate with random repetitions in sounds, words, and phrases. These dysfluencies tend to increase with an increase in the boys' agitation and can be decreased with calming techniques (Shopmeyer & Lowe, 1992).

Voice.   Voice quality may also be distinctive in children with fragile X. It has been described as hoarse or harsh (Palmer, Gordon, Coston, & Stevenson, 1988; Prouty et al., 1988), although the boys seen in our clinic often speak with a high-pitched voice. Shopmeyer and Lowe (1992) report reduced or uneven loudness and a "mumbling" quality to speech in many children with fragile X. These vocal characteristics could also be related to low muscle tone.

Language Processing and Language Production Skills

Across the spectrum of severity in children with fragile X syndrome, nearly all acquire some degree of functional speech and language skills. This potential, even in children with quite low measured IQs, suggests the need for a more creative use of both formal and informal test measures to determine the aspects of language involved in reception, association, formulation, and execution that seem to interfere with their communication skills in different contexts. The child with fragile X offers the language clinician and language researcher unique and exciting opportunities to delineate the influence of behavior on communication and the influences of communication demands on behavior. Given the presence of varying, but persistent, degrees of sensory impairment in this population, these children also offer excellent models for the study of the ability of sensory integration techniques to enhance attention, learning, and language processing. No one professional can accomplish the latter alone. Rather, combined speech/language and occupational therapy becomes a critical element in "bringing body and mind together" (Wilson et al., 1994). These strategies will be further discussed under "Intervention Issues."

Listening. There is some evidence that deficient listening skills in children with fragile X may be related to at least three specific factors: (1) an increased incidence of persistent otitis media during the first 5 years of life; (2) central auditory-processing dysfunction; and (3) attentional problems.

To date, the incidence of otitis media in boys with fragile X has only been formally studied by Hagerman, Altshul-Stark, and McBogg (1987). They found that 63 percent of the 30 boys followed had six or more ear infections in their first 5 years. These researchers hypothesize that several factors may contribute to recalcitrant otitis related to impaired eustachian tube functioning—namely, the generalized hypotonia, connective tissue dysplasia (abnormal tissue development), and the typical craniofacial variations of a long, narrow face and highly arched palate.

Evidence of possible central auditory pathway dysfunction in a high percentage of males with fragile X has been described by Arinami, Sato, Nakajima, and Kondo (1988). These investigators studied auditory brain stem responses in 12 men with fragile X syndrome. They found prolonged I-IV interpeak latencies in almost 50 percent of their subjects, which indicates delayed conduction time along the auditory neural pathways. Prolonged interpeak latencies can be related to early recurrent otitis. It is difficult to speculate on any lasting functional impact on listening skills or auditory attentive behaviors without the benefit of further studies.

Attentional problems have been described repeatedly in children with fragile X syndrome. Hagerman (1991) states that "attentional deficits with or without hyperactivity are significant problems for almost all young males with fragile X and for many cognitively impaired females" (p. 290). Hagerman also emphasizes that the ongoing management for the attention deficits and accompanying behavioral issues is most effective when it is multimodal. Medication may significantly reduce hyperactivity and enhance concentration, but learning and carryover of positive behaviors appears to be dependent on a combination of medication, occupational therapy, language therapy, and appropriate modifications in the home and school settings.

Receptive and Expressive Language. Several researchers have described the general learning style as well as the language learning style in boys with fragile X as being stronger for simultaneous tasks versus sequential tasks. That is, information is more successfully learned and remembered if processed as a whole rather than in sequential parts. Although this learning style may be more exaggerated in the children with fragile X, it is also fairly common among other children with specific language impairment. Wetherby (1992) describes this type of child as a "gestalt learner" and contrasts this style with the "analytic learner." For several decades, researchers in the area of child language development have used a variety of descriptors to explain observed dichotomies in the language learning strategies of both typical and atypical children. Wetherby (1992) combines this information in a useful way to describe a continuum of style and strategies among language learners. On one end of the continuum is the gestalt language learner, and on the other end is the analytic language learner. Children with fragile X syndrome and others with significant language impairments tend to be on the extreme end of the gestalt learning style.

According to Wetherby (1992), the gestalt child learns the tune before the words. He or she produces whole phrases or sentences rather than single words without evidence of using the words referentially (e.g., uses word chunks like, "Umunuhh boh bubbows," for, "I want to blow bubbles"). The analytic child produces one-word utterances of one to two syllables in length, closely approximates the adult target, and uses them referentially and differentially. Table 5-2 contains a list of speech and language behaviors typical of a child with a gestalt learning style.

Perseverative speech is common in boys with fragile X syndrome. In fact, Wolf-Schein et al. (1987) found repetition of words or phrases and fixation on specific topics to be some of the language characteristics that differentiated boys with fragile X from matched control subjects with Down syndrome. The use of redundant "familiar" phrases is not surprising, if the child's learn-

---

Table 5-2.   Gestalt Learner's Language Behaviors

- Impulsive cognitive style/demanding temperament; acts and talks before thinking
- Expressive language more advanced than symbolic play
- Higher proportion of communication to regulate others' behavior
- Frequent formulaic chunks (i.e., knows the tune, but not the exact words) and utterances
- Language production better than language comprehension, "poor listener"
- Continued repetition of given information
- Intonation-oriented; suprasegmental orientation
- High use of imitation as a language strategy
- Strengths in episodic memory; memory for personal events stored by spatial and temporal aspects of events
- High proportion of pronouns to nouns
- Inflections and function words in early multi-word stage
- Context bound use of names
- Less variety within lexical categories

Reprinted by permission from Wetherby, A.M. (1992). *Communication and language interventions for preschool children.* (pp. 20–21). Chicago, Ill.: Applied Symbolix.

ing style also appears to be gestalt in nature—for example, involving strengths in imitation and difficulty with specific word retrieval. Sudhalter, Scarborough, and Cohen (1991) and Sudhalter, Maranion, and Brooks (1992) sought to investigate syntactic versus semantic competence in relation to the use of perseverative utterances. Sudhalter et al. (1991) found that syntax was not significantly below age expectations in the boys they tested with fragile X. However, most studies have reported that syntax is delayed but typically consistent with the individual's cognitive development. Their progress in syntax tends to follow a normal developmental trajectory, just at a slower rate (Abbeduto & Hagerman, 1997; Palmer, et al., 1988).

In a follow-up study of semantic competence in males with fragile X, Sudhalter et al. (1992) analyzed responses to a sentence completion task. The 99 sentences were administered to 11 males with fragile X matched for developmental age with 11 typically developing 4-year-olds. The males with fragile X made significantly more semantic errors and had particular difficulty with sentences that could be correctly completed with a wider choice of words. These results suggest that the expressive semantic system is a particular area of deficit for males with fragile X and may explain, at least in part, their perseverative expressive language patterns and heightened level of anxiety when specific responses to questions are requested of them outside of a familiar context.

Clinicians and researchers working with boys with fragile X often observe a relative strength in single word vocabulary knowledge and use. Kemper and colleagues (1988) found that boys with fragile X demonstrated a relative strength identifying pictures of common objects, as measured specifically on the Peabody Picture Vocabulary Test–Revised (Dunn & Dunn, 1981). Shopmeyer and Lowe (1992) hypothesize that humorous and high-interest words (e.g., "Scoo-bee-doo," and "big Mac") are among the most easily acquired for these children. This predisposition would also be consistent with the gestalt learning style and suggests the need to include novel pictures and humorous situations to teach vocabulary and concepts to students with fragile X.

For all of the reasons discussed here, boys with fragile X syndrome have particular difficulty formulating verbal responses upon demand. They have trouble answering direct questions and expressing all that they know verbally about a subject. It is not uncommon for a boy with fragile X to say little in class about a lesson yet talk about the material in detail at home. Although the presence of good language role models is important, these children are easily overwhelmed by too much verbal input or noise. For example, if an immediate response is not provided, it is important to wait quietly, with a patient, expectant affect, rather than to repeat a direction over. Similarly, it would be better to "show and tell" the child what result is expected (i.e., "the goal" or "the finish line"), rather than issuing a series of directions.

Little information is available regarding the speech and language characteristics of girls with fragile X syndrome. Hagerman, Jackson, and Amiri (1992) reported that 13 girls in their sample of 32 females with fragile X syndrome were receiving speech and language therapy. Our experience has been that there is a very wide range of skills, but that overall the weaknesses in preschool girls are relatively mild and may not qualify them for intervention services. They need to be closely monitored, however, particularly for language processing deficits that may become more apparent over time.

INTERVENTION ISSUES

Most parents and professionals involved with children with fragile X recognize the benefits of early diagnosis and early intervention. Confirming that a child has fragile X syndrome can provide parents, teachers, and other professionals with a framework for better understanding his or her profile of strengths and weaknesses. In addition, the diagnosis of a genetic condition can be helpful in securing intervention services through the public school system. This is particularly true for girls with fragile X, who often show only subtle deficits in their early years and who may not otherwise be identified. Even though a learning disability profile may not be apparent at a young age, an educational label of "Other Health Impaired" (or similar category, depending upon the state) can help secure intervention services before significant delays develop.

A multidisciplinary team approach to treatment is also important, given the complex nature of fragile X syndrome. Generally, assessment and treatment by a team that includes the following professionals is recommended for young children with fragile X syndrome.

Speech-Language Pathologist

The speech-language pathologist, along with the child's pediatrician, may be the most likely professional to identify a child who may have fragile X as a toddler or preschooler. This is because significant delays in the onset of expressive speech and early oral-motor/feeding problems are common in these children. Although delayed speech and oral-motor difficulties are common to a variety of etiologies, fragile X should be considered and should trigger probes for other features such as sensory defensiveness, the typical craniofacial attributes, and/or a family history of learning problems or mental retardation. Once the diagnosis is confirmed by DNA testing, the speech-language pathologist should become an ongoing consultant for the family and teachers and vice-versa. The speech-language pathologist must identify the child's strengths and weaknesses in oral-motor, sensory, speech production, listening, receptive language, expressive language, and social interactions. The parents and teachers, in collaboration with the team, must identify the child's preferences and needs, so that specific goals focused on topics of interest to each child can be developed.

In addition, ample clinical evidence and some research data now exist to support the importance of collaboration between occupational therapy and speech-language therapy for children with fragile X (Scharfenaker, Hickman, & Braden, 1991; Shopmeyer & Lowe, 1992; Wilson et al., 1994). The techniques comprising sensory integration treatment, developed by Ayres (1979), have been particularly helpful. Shopmeyer and Lowe (1992) provide a useful discussion for clinicians of various models for combined speech-language and occupational therapy treatment, including consultative, observational, side-by-side, supportive, and transdisciplinary. All of these models may prove to be useful with the same child in different situations or at different points in their developmental course.

Occupational Therapist

Children with fragile X syndrome have a number of weaknesses that can be addressed by an occupational therapist. Their fine motor deficits, low muscle tone, and motor-planning problems are among those that are within the realm of occupational therapy. Although some goals may focus on strengthening the child's abilities in these areas, an occupational therapist can also help identify ways of compensating for these relative weaknesses. For example, developing keyboarding skills and adaptations for the use of a computer could be one alternative to handling the handwriting demands of lengthy assignments.

Many occupational therapists are beginning to develop expertise in the area of sensory integration theory and treatment (Shopmeyer & Lowe, 1992). Since children with fragile X often have difficulty processing sensory information in an appropriate way, sensory integration therapy is strongly recommended. Sensory integration treatment goals often address the tactile and sensory defensiveness displayed by children with fragile X as well as the attentional issues and negative behaviors that may result from a dysfunctional sensory system. For example, in the case of one young boy with fragile X syndrome who was having frequent behavioral outbursts in his preschool classroom, a close look at a videotaped segment of his school day showed that the classroom was very noisy and unstructured. When changes were made in the classroom structure, routine, and physical environment, his outbursts diminished in frequency and intensity.

Developmental Pediatrician

In spite of the numerous developmental and educational issues facing children with fragile X syndrome, it is important to keep in mind that fragile X is a medical condition. Ongoing input and monitoring from a medical professional, such as a developmental pediatrician, are critical for each child's treatment program. Although children with fragile X are generally healthy, issues such as repeated ear infections, pronated feet, eye problems, and the possibility of seizures need to be followed. The use of medication is often an important part of the child's treatment. Many children with fragile X benefit from stimulant medication, for instance, to address their attentional problems and hyperactivity. Medication may also be useful in decreasing the anxiety experienced by many of the children. We believe that many children with fragile X do best with medication in combination with behavior management strategies and extensive special education and related services.

Child Psychologist, Educational Specialist, and Classroom Teacher

These individuals are instrumental in determining the cognitive and academic profile of children with fragile X syndrome and addressing behavior management issues. In addition, input from these professionals in conjunction with the speech-language pathologist and occupational therapist is often helpful in developing an appropriate educational program for children with fragile X syndrome. This can be challenging given the children's multiple needs and uneven profile of skills. Some children with fragile X also benefit from individual counseling and/or social skills instruction.

Genetic Counselor

Our understanding of the genetics of fragile X syndrome has increased dramatically in recent years and continues to be the focus of considerable research efforts. It is essential that this information be conveyed to families in a way that is accurate, understandable, and useful in their particular situation. Therefore, periodic contact with a genetic counselor is critical. Since this information is very complicated, it is unlikely that any family will be able to fully comprehend and understand its implications for specific family members based on one contact with a geneticist or genetic counselor. These professionals can also help parents convey information about fragile X syndrome to other relatives who are at risk for the condition.

Family Support Person

An integral member of the Fragile X Clinic at Duke University Medical Center is the mother of a boy with fragile X syndrome. Her perspective on the many issues facing families with fragile X syndrome has been invaluable. In addition to providing families with information about fragile X syndrome and available resources for their children, she has founded a non-profit organization and sponsors social events so that families may network with one another. This has permitted parents to share their experiences and benefit from each other's knowledge. Because many mothers of our patients have also experienced learning challenges, such networking is often more difficult for families with fragile X syndrome.

Parents of Children with Fragile X Syndrome

Each child's parents should also be an integral part of the multidisciplinary treatment team. They are truly the resident "experts" on their child's strengths and weaknesses and on what has proven useful in the past. In addition, parents often find themselves in the position of "linking" the professionals involved with their children and even providing them with information about fragile X syndrome.

DEVELOPING AN APPROPRIATE EDUCATIONAL PROGRAM

As is true for any child with special needs, considering individual strengths and weaknesses, as well as the family's preferences and capabilities, is the best starting point for developing an appropriate educational program. There is no set educational plan, classroom, or program that is optimal for all children with fragile X syndrome. Some children have been highly successful in a total inclusion program, where they spend all, or the majority, of their day in a mainstream classroom with appropriate support. Given the children's strong imitation skills, they are often able to "rise to the occasion" and benefit a great deal from the incidental learning that occurs from interacting with typically developing peers.

There are several resources that may be helpful in implementing an inclusive program. For example, one mother of a son with fragile X prepared detailed presentations for school personnel regarding the condition and how it manifests in her child (Weber, 1994). There is also an excellent book written for children that describes a boy with fragile X syndrome and his behavior in understandable terms (O'Connor, 1995).

Other children with fragile X syndrome, particularly boys, are being educated in programs that include separate classrooms for students with special needs. This may provide the benefit of a smaller group setting and more individualized attention. On the other hand, the role models and expectations for such children may be less than optimal. Some of these classrooms are also very busy and can be overstimulating.

Another key issue is the flexibility of the child's primary teachers and related professionals. Children with fragile X syndrome often require extra planning, "brainstorming," and problem solving throughout the school year. A particular approach may be successful for a while and then need to be modified. Rigidly adhering to one strategy or approach, though successful for other students, may be problematic for children with fragile X.

PROGNOSIS

Since there is no cure for fragile X syndrome at this time, management of the condition is a long-term issue. Prospective longitudinal studies examining the developmental profile of children with fragile X syndrome are now being conducted (Bailey, Hatton, & Skinner, 1998). Although many adult males have been diagnosed and described in the literature, the services provided throughout their lifetime have probably not been as extensive as the services children are currently receiving. Therefore, it is difficult to say if their level of functioning is representative of their potential. In addition, the wide range of functioning observed in children is also seen in adults. For example, some are employed in the mainstream with support while others find it difficult to function in a sheltered workshop environment. Some individuals are institutionalized.

We have observed that the individuals' level of behavioral control appears to be more predictive of their functioning as adults than their cognitive abilities per se. As with children, behavioral issues may be related to the frustration resulting from language and sensory integration issues and low tolerance for stress. In many cases these problems are not solved by medication management alone, but require the same multidisciplinary approach that we advocate for young children.

It is also important to remember that many of the issues described in children with fragile X persist into adolescence and adulthood. For instance, many adult males with fragile X continue to have problems with sensory defensiveness. This means that the level of stimulation in their home and/or work environment may impact on their behavior, and must be considered. Our hope is that a greater understanding of fragile X syndrome will lead to more targeted interventions and a better prognosis over time.

CASE STUDY: RYAN

Ryan is a 5½-year-old boy who was seen at the Duke University Medical Center Fragile X Clinic. He was recently diagnosed with fragile X syndrome at a nearby medical center. Ryan and his family were referred to the clinic for follow-up and additional treatment recommendations.

According to his parents, Ryan was born at full-term, weighing 7 pounds, 2 ounces. Reportedly, he sat alone at 8 months, crawled at 10 months, and started walking at 14–15 months of age. Ryan said his first word at 1 year and began to speak in phrases at about 3 years. He is not yet fully toilet trained and still has accidents. Ryan has been healthy, other than having about three ear infections per year for the first 3 years of his life.

Ryan was initially seen for a speech and language evaluation at a local clinic at 4;1. At that time, he earned a receptive language score of 24–27 months and an expressive language score of 20–22 months on the Receptive-Expressive Emergent Language Scale, 2nd edition (REEL-2), (Bzoch & League, 1991). Shortly after this evaluation, Ryan was seen by a local pediatric neurologist. He had an abnormal EEG at 4;3. The neurologist started Ryan on Depakote (i.e., compound for use in seizures) and shortly after this his speech improved significantly. Due to these findings and his severe expressive and receptive language delays, Ryan was given a tentative diagnosis of Landau-Kleffner syndrome. Ryan's parents were relieved to have a diagnosis of some kind and began researching this condition. They also made contact with a parent information and support group.

At 4½ years of age, Ryan completed a multidisciplinary assessment at the state-supported developmental evaluation center. The evaluation summary indicated that Ryan's cognitive skills were at the 23-month level and his nonverbal, preacademic skills were at the 21-month level. His gross motor skills were at the 17-month level, and his fine motor skills were at the 19-month level. Ryan was reported to be extremely active and had difficulty attending to tasks. He was also described as being a "self-directed child." Ryan was referred for preschool services, including speech and language therapy. A referral to the statewide autism diagnostic and treatment program was also recommended. A progress note after 15 sessions of speech and language therapy indicated that: "Significant progress has been made in the area of attentional skills through use of sensory integration techniques (barriers to prevent view of external visual stimuli, brushing, and joint compression techniques). Ryan has made slow, steady progress in his language development. Language development has been facilitated through use of sign language, some communication boards, and scripting techniques."

At about 5 years of age, Ryan was tested for fragile X syndrome by his neurologist. DNA testing revealed that he had more than 200 CGG repeats, which is consistent with the full mutation. His infant brother was subsequently tested, and the results were normal.

Ryan began attending a preschool program for children with special needs at age 4;10 (through his public school system). He also received speech and language therapy through the public school. Ryan's current educational label is "preschool developmentally delayed." Although Ryan is now 5 years old, he will remain in the preschool program another year. He is scheduled to receive speech and language therapy for two 30-minute sessions each week. He is also scheduled to receive consultation from an occupational therapist twice each month. Ryan will be mainstreamed with the kindergarten classes for assemblies and field trips.

As part of Ryan's visit to the Fragile X Clinic, we recommended that he receive more intensive occupational therapy services through the school system, with a focus on sensory integration issues and oral-motor development. Ryan's speech and language therapist should also work on oral-motor development as part of his treatment plan. In addition, Ryan should be provided with more opportunities for mainstreaming (with appropriate support). It is very important that he be exposed to good language role models. The developmental pediatrician also recommended that Ryan's parents consider a trial of low-dose stimulant medication to help with hyperactivity and attentional problems. Finally, we strongly urged the parents to pursue more genetic counseling services and testing of extended family members, particularly those who have mental retardation.

SUMMARY

Fragile X syndrome is the leading known X-linked cause of mental retardation and is also associated with specific learning disabilities and autism. This condition can affect males and females, although males are generally more severely affected. Boys with fragile X may exhibit some or all of the characteristic physical features, behaviors, speech, language, motor, and sensory integration problems seen in this condition. Girls with fragile X tend to show milder variants of these features. The genetics of fragile X syndrome are complex; however, it is important for parents and professionals to understand this information and the implications for immediate and extended family members.

Children with fragile X syndrome have a variety of strengths and needs, which are best addressed by a multidisciplinary team approach. Some of their characteristics distinguish them from peers with mental retardation who are negative for fragile X syndrome. Early diagnosis and early intervention are critical to unlocking each child's developmental and academic potential. By helping family members and professionals understand the strongest and most vulnerable areas in each child's profile, learning challenges can be minimized and even overcome for some children. Additional research is needed to better describe the unique aspects of motor, sensory, and speech and language functioning in children with fragile X syndrome, and those of effective treatment strategies.

APPENDIX 5

Resources

National Fragile X Foundation
P.O. Box 190488
San Francisco, CA 94119-0488
1-800-688-8765
e-mail: NATLFX@sprintmail.com
website: www.FragileX.org

FRAXA Research Foundation
45 Pleasant Street
Newburyport, MA 01950
1-978-462-1866
e-mail: info@fraxa.org
Web site: www.fraxa.org

References

Abbeduto, L., & Hagerman, R. J. (1997). Language and communication in fragile X syndrome. *Mental Retardation and Developmental Disabilities, 3,* 313–322.

American Psychiatric Association. (1994). *Diagnostic and statistical manual of mental disorders*. (Fourth Edition). Washington, D.C..: Author.

Anderson, S. (1992). Motor and sensory characteristics of fragile X. In B. B. Shopmeyer & F. Lowe (Eds.), *The fragile X child* (pp. 59–70). San Diego: Singular.

Arinami, T., Sato, M., Nakajima, S., & Kondo, I. (1988). Auditory brain-stem responses in the fragile X syndrome. *American Journal of Human Genetics, 43*, 46–51.

Ashley, C. T., Jr., & Warren, S. T. (1995). Trinucleotide repeat expansion and human disease. *Annual Review of Genetics, 29*, 703–728.

Ayres, A. J. (1979). *Sensory integration and the child*. Los Angeles: Western Psychological Services.

Bailey, D. B., Hatton, D. D., & Skinner, M. (1998). Early developmental trajectories of males with fragile X syndrome. *American Journal of Mental Retardation, 103*, 29–39.

Blomquist, M. K., Bohman, M., Edvinston, S., Gillberg, C., Gustavson, K. H., Holmgren, G., & Wanstrom, J. (1985). Frequency of the fragile X syndrome in infantile autism: A Swedish multicenter study. *Clinical Genetics, 27*, 113–117.

Borghgraef, M., Umans, S., Steyaert, J., Legius, E., & Fryns, J. P. (1996). New findings in the behavioral profile of young Fragile X females. *American Journal of Medical Genetics, 64*, 346–349.

Bzoch, K. R., & League, R. (1991). *Receptive-Expressive-Emergent Language Scale–2*. Austin, Tex.: Pro-Ed.

Connors, C. K. (1990). *Conner's Rating Scales manual*. North Tonawanda, N.Y.: Multi-Health Systems.

Davis, J. R., Hagerman, R. J., & Eilert, R. E. (1990). The orthopaedist and fragile X syndrome. *Journal of Bone and Joint Surgery, 72*, 889–896.

Dunn, L. M. & Dunn, L. M. (1981). *The Peabody Picture Vocabulary Test-Revised manual*. Circle Pines, Minn.: American Guidance Service.

Dykens, E. M., Hodapp, R. M., & Leckman, J. F. (1987). Strengths and weakness in the intellectual functioning of males with fragile X syndrome. *American Journal of Mental Deficiency, 92*, 234–236.

Freund, L. (1994). Diagnosis and developmental issues for young children with fragile X syndrome. *Infants and Young Children, 6*, 34–45.

Freund, L., Reiss, A., & Abrams, M. (1993). Psychiatric disorders associated with fragile X in the young female. *Pediatrics, 92*, 321–329.

Gilfoyle, E. M., Grady, A. D. & Moore, J. C. (1981). *Children adapt*. Throrfare, N.J.: Slack.

Hagerman, R. J. (1991). Medical follow-up and pharmacotherapy. In R. J. Hagerman & A. Silverman (Eds.), *Fragile X syndrome: Diagnosis, treatment, and research*. Baltimore: Johns Hopkins University Press.

Hagerman, R. J. (1996). Physical and behavioral phenotype. In R. J. Hagerman & A. Silverman (Eds.), *Fragile X syndrome: Diagnosis, treatment, and research* (Ed. 2, pp. 3-87). Baltimore: Johns Hopkins University Press.

Hagerman, R. J., Altshul-Stark, D., & McBogg, P. (1987). Recurrent otitis media in boys with the fragile X syndrome. *American Journal of Disabilities of Childhood, 141,* 184–187.

Hagerman, R. J., Jackson, C., & Amiri, K. (1992). Girls with fragile X syndrome: Physical and neurocognitive status and outcome. *Pediatrics, 89,* 395–400.

Hanson, D. M., Jackson, A. W., & Hagerman, R. J. (1986). Speech disturbances (cluttering) in mildly impaired males with the Martin-Bell fragile X syndrome. *American Journal of Medical Genetics, 23,* 195–206.

Hatton, D. D., Buckley, E. G., Lachiewicz, A. M., & Roberts, J. E. (in press). Ocular status of boys with fragile X syndrome: A prospective study. *Journal of the American Association for Pediatric Ophthalmology and Strabismus.*

Hodapp, R. M, Dykens, E. E., Ort, S. I., Zelinsky, D. G., & Leckman, J. F. (1991).Changing patterns of intellectual strengths and weakness in males with fragile X syndrome. *Journal of Autism and Developmental Disorders, 21,* 503–516.

Kaufman, A. S., & Kaufman, N. L. (1983). *Kaufman Assessment Battery for Children,* Interpretive Manual. Circle Pines, Minn.: American Guidance Service.

Kemper, M. B., Hagerman, R. J., & Altshul-Stark, D. (1988). Cognitive profiles of boys with the fragile X syndrome. *American Journal of Medical Genetics, 30,* 191–200.

Lachiewicz, A. M. (1992). Abnormal behaviors of young girls with fragile X syndrome. *American Journal of Medical Genetics, 43,* 72–77.

Lachiewicz, A. M., & Dawson, D. V. (1994). Behavior problems of young girls with fragile X syndrome: Factor scores on the Conners' Parent's Questionnaire. *American Journal of Medical Genetics, 51,* 364–369.

Lachiewicz, A. M., Gullion, C. M., Spiridigliozzi, G. A., & Aylsworth, A. S. (1987). Declining IQ scores of young males with fragile X syndrome. *American Journal of Mental Retardation, 92,* 272–278.

Lachiewicz, A. M., Spiridigliozzi, G. A., Gullion, C. M., Ransford, S. N., & Rao, K. (1994). Aberrant behaviors of young boys with fragile X syndrome. *American Journal on Mental Retardation, 98,* 567–579.

Madison, L. S., George, C., & Moeschler, J. B. (1986). Cognitive functioning in the fragile X syndrome: A study of intellectual, memory, and communication skills. *Journal of Mental Deficiency Research, 30,* 129–148.

Miezejeski, C. M., Jenkins, E. C., Hill, A. L., Wisniewski, K., French, J. H., & Brown, W. T. (1986). A profile of cognitive deficit in females from fragile X families. *Neuropsychologica, 24*(3), 405–409.

O'Connor, R. (1995). *Boys with fragile X syndrome.* Child Development Unit. The Children's Hospital, Denver.

Palmer, K. K., Gordon, J. S., Coston, G. N., & Stevenson, R. E. (1988). Fragile X syndrome IV, speech and language characteristics. *Proceedings, Greenwood Genetic Center, 7,* 93–97

Paul, R., Cohen, D. J., Breg, W. R., Watson, M. & Herman, S. (1984). Fragile X syndrome: Its relation to speech and language disorders. *Journal of Speech and Hearing Disorders, 49*, 328–332.

Pennington, B. F., O'Connor, R. A., & Sudhalter, V. (1991). Toward a neuropsychology of fragile X syndrome. In R.J. Hagerman & A. C. Silverman (Eds.), *Fragile X Syndrome: Diagnosis, treatment, and research* (pp. 173–201). Baltimore: The Johns Hopkins University Press.

Prouty, L. A., Rogers, R. C., & Stevenson, R. E. (1988). Fragile X syndrome: Growth, development, and intellectual function. *American Journal of Medical Genetics, 30*, 123–142.

Reiss, A. L., & Freund, L. (1992). Behavioral phenotype of fragile X syndrome: DSM-III-R autistic behavior in male children. *American Journal of Medical Genetics, 43*, 35–46.

Reiss, A. L., Freund, L., Abrams, M. T., Boehm, C., & Kazazian, H. (1993). Neurobehavioral effects of the fragile X presentation in adult women: A controlled study. *American Journal of Human Genetics, 52*, 884–894.

Scharfenaker, S., Hickman, L., & Braden, M. (1991). An integrated approach to intervention. In R.J. Hagerman & A. Silverman (Eds.), *Fragile X syndrome: Diagnosis, treatment and research* (pp. 327–372). Baltimore: Johns Hopkins University Press.

Shelhart, W. C., Casamassimo, P. S., Hagerman, R. J., & Belanger, G. K. (1986). Oral findings in fragile X syndrome. *American Journal of Medical Genetics, 23*, 179–187.

Shopmeyer, B. B. & Lowe, F. (1992). *The fragile X child.* San Diego: Singular.

Simko, A., Hornsteir, L., Soukup, S., & Bagamery, N. (1989). Fragile X syndrome: Recognition in young children. *Pediatrics, 84*, 547–552.

Spiridigliozzi, G. A., Lachiewicz, A. M., MacMurdo, C. S., Vizoso, A. D., O'Donnell, C. M., McConkie-Rosell, A., & Burgess, D. J. (1994). *Educating boys with fragile X syndrome: A guide for parents and professionals.* Durham, N.C.: Duke University Medical Center.

Sudhalter, V., Cohen, I. L., Silverman, W., & Wolf-Schein, E. (1990). Conversational analyses of males with fragile X, Down syndrome, and autism: Comparisons of the emergence of deviant language. *American Journal on Mental Retardation, 94*, 431–441.

Sudhalter, V., Maranion, M., & Brooks, P. (1992). Expressive semantic deficit in the productive language of males with fragile X syndrome. *American Journal of Medical Genetics, 43*, 65–71.

Sudhalter, V., Scarborough, H. S., & Cohen, I. L. (1991). Syntactic delay and pragmatic deviance in the language of fragile X males. *American Journal of Medical Genetics, 38*, 493–497.

Tarleton, J. C., & Saul, R. A. (1993). Molecular genetic advances in fragile X syndrome. *Journal of Pediatrics, 122*(2), 169–185.

Turner, G., Webb, T., Wake, S., & Robinson, H. (1996). The prevalence of the fragile X syndrome. *American Journal of Medical Genetics, 64*, 196–197.

Vikman, E., Niemi, J., & Ikoneu, V. (1988). Fragile X speech phonology in Finnish. *Brain and Language, 34*, 203–221.

Weber, J. D. (1994). *Transitioning "special" children into elementary school.* Boulder, Colo.: Books Beyond Borders.

Wechsler, D. (1974). *Wechsler Intelligence Scale for Children–Revised manual.* New York: Psychological Corporation.

Wechsler, D. (1981). *Wechsler Adult Intelligence Scale–Revised manual.* New York: Psychological Corporation.

Wetherby, A. (1992). Individual validations in learning style. In A. Wetherby (Ed.), *Communication and language intervention for preschool children* (pp. 19–26). Chicago: Applied Symbolix.

Wilson, P., Stackhouse, T., O'Conner, R. Scharfenaker, S., & Hagerman, R (1994). *Issues and strategies for educating children with fragile X syndrome.* Dillon, Colo.: Spectra.

Wolf-Schein, E. G., Sudhalter, V., Cohen, I. L., Fisch, G. S., Hanson, D., Pfadt, A. G., Hagerman, R. J., Jenkins, E. C., & Brown, W. T. (1987). Speech and language and the fragile X syndrome: Initial findings. *Asha, 29*, 35–38.

Young Children with Down Syndrome

Thomas L. Layton, Ph.D., CCC-SLP
Professor, Communication Sciences and Disorders
North Carolina Central University
Durham

Key Terms

hypotonia
lexical acquisition
oral-motor
speech intelligibility

symbolic play
syntax
thematic and semantic relations

Overview

The first known description of a child with Down syndrome was reported by Esquirol in 1838, followed soon after by Seguin's (1846) description of a child manifesting a condition he called "furfuraceous (scaly) idiocy." Then, in 1866, Duncan described a girl who presented "a small round head, Chinese looking eyes, projecting a large tongue who only knew a few words." During that same year, an English physician, Down (1866), published a paper describing a group of patients he called "mongoloids" because, like Duncan, he thought they resembled the peoples of east Asia, for whom the general racial term *mongoloid* was then accepted among anthropologists (along with *caucasoid* and *negroid*). The term was used for these patients until 1967, when a study group at a medical conference in Edinburgh concluded that the term was, essentially, racist, and suggested as an alternative the expression "Down's Syndrome"—to characterize the syndrome rather than the person exhibiting it, and to acknowledge Down's work. This form prevailed until, recently, the possessive marker was removed from "Down's" (to eliminate the grammatical implication that Down himself was such a patient) and the capital letter in "syndrome" was replaced by lower case—producing its current form, Down syndrome. Readers will often find the other forms in older textbooks and journal articles, but the current term, Down syndrome (DS), is clearly to be preferred and will be used in this chapter.

The purpose of this chapter is to provide an overview of the diagnosis and behaviors of children with DS. Besides etiological considerations, speech, language, communication and cognitive-social skills will be addressed. Intervention issues will complete the chapter.

ETIOLOGY AND CHARACTERISTICS OF DOWN SYNDROME

In 1959, Lejeune, Turpin, and Gautier reported that Down syndrome was the result of a chromosomal abnormality, resulting in an extra 21st chromosome. They also found that individuals with DS could be divided into three karyotypes based on genetic makeup: the most common type was trisomy 21 (accounting for 70 percent of the population), followed by translocation (15 percent), and then mosaicism (10 percent).

In the general population, individuals typically have 23 pairs of chromosomes in each cell, whereas most individuals with Down syndrome (trisomy 21) have an extra, or third, 21st chromosome, yielding a total of 47 chromosomes (Polani, 1976). The translocation group, on the other hand, occurs as a result of a rearrangement in the 21st chromosome material (Rondal, 1988). In this instance, an extra 21st chromosome occurs and attaches to the other pair. Since the translocation group is inherited, the risk of recurrence for this type of DS is quite high (Polani, 1976). The third type of DS, mosaicism, occurs when the abnormal separation of the 21st chromosome occurs sometime after conception, or when the cell division has already begun. In these individuals, some cells contain 46 chromosomes while others contain 47. The risk of recurrence for this type of DS is no different from that of the general population (Blackman, 1983).

Individuals with mosaic DS have been reported to have the highest intelligence and the best nonverbal cognitive abilities among the three etiologies of DS. Individuals with trisomy 21 are considered the next highest, followed by individuals with translocation (see Gibson, 1981, for a review). These reports are, however, far from conclusive (Johnson & Abelson, 1969) and have caused a good deal of controversy in the literature.

A search through the literature has failed to identify any studies investigating the relationship between the three karyotypes and possible language differences. Most of the descriptions of speech, language, and cognitive abilities have involved only children with trisomy 21. It is important to point out that all children with DS present a wide variety of abilities and constitute a heterogeneous group. Therefore, any planned assessment or intervention strategy should be geared toward the child as an individual, and not as a member of a group with general cognitive and language deficits.

PARENTAL PERCEPTIONS OF EARLY INTERACTIONS WITH PROFESSIONALS

The first contact that parents of children with special needs have with a professional is likely to have an impact on all subsequent interactions (Cunningham & Sloper, 1977; McWilliam, Winton, & Crais, 1996). Even when parents forget the specifics of what they had been told, they tend to remember the attitude of the person who informed them (D'Arcy, 1968; Konstantareas, 1989). Parents are, therefore, more likely to follow through on recommendations given by professionals who demonstrate an interest in their concerns, trust the parents' ability to do what is best for their child, and maintain a sense that the parents' concerns are primary at the time (Cadman, Shurvell, Davies, & Bradfield, 1984; Korsch & Negrete, 1972).

There has been a general consensus that parental satisfaction with the initial contact is related to how the parents are told about their child's condition (Cunningham, Morgan, & McGucken, 1984; Doherty & Baird, 1986; Pueschel & Murphy, 1976; Quine & Pahl, 1986). Most parents are satisfied when they are informed as soon as possible of their child's special needs, with their spouse or a close friend present; in an honest, direct manner; with simple language; empathetically; and with overt concern and interest in the parents' questions (Doherty & Baird, 1986). However, the kind of information parents usually receive has focused on the child's needs or what the professional *perceives* are the family needs at the time (Martin, George, O'Neal, & Daly, 1987). Too frequently, this information involves specific facts about the child's condition, such as causes of Down syndrome, effects on physical condition, genetic counseling, and common characteristics (Cunningham & Sloper, 1977; Gayton & Walker, 1974). However, studies have indicated that what many parents want is information about expectations for the future, effects on the family, a list of additional services available in the community, educational opportunities and options, home activities, access to other parents with similar children, and strategies for coping (Hadadian & Merbler, 1995; Martin et al., 1987; Power, 1989). The overwhelming amount of technical information provided initially to parents can explain why many parents are dissatisfied with the initial interaction with professionals and why many professionals often regard parents as denying the diagnosis or being unable to process the information (Cunningham & Sloper, 1977). The technical information may be necessary but inadequate by itself (Konstantareas, 1989; Martin et al., 1987).

In one study regarding discretionary treatment of children with DS, Springer and Steele (1980) found that physicians often made decisions on what to tell parents based on social criteria (i.e., the threat to family stability posed by the presence of the infant and the expected quality of life and social value the infant might experience). Springer and Steele also found that many parents did not follow the advice given by the physician because it was deemed too pessimistic. In fact, parents preferred that the professionals err slightly on the side of overoptimism than pessimism. Wolraich and Siperstein (1983) found when it came to making decisions regarding their child's future, most parents responded to their own personal feelings and to the input obtained from other parents, and not to the advice of the professionals. Therefore, professionals need to be careful in making assumptions about what individual families want and/or need from them and instead should let families play a part in determining the type and amount of information to be shared in the early stages.

DEVELOPMENTAL CHARACTERISTICS OF CHILDREN WITH DOWN SYNDROME

Down syndrome occurs in about 1 in every 800 births, making it the most common organic form of mental retardation. Most individuals with DS have some degree of mental retardation, which ranges from mild to profound, but with most persons with DS functioning in the moderate range (Gibson, 1981). The developmental delays in individuals with DS are generally moderate during the early years of life but become more severe in later life. Gibson (1981) has identified three mental age (MA) growth periods, with the first two periods being followed by temporary plateaus, and the third, by a gradual decline. The first plateau is reached between 4 and 6 years of age and occurs with an MA of about 18 months. The second plateau is reached around 8 to 11 years of age, with an MA of about 30 months. The third plateau is reached between 12 and 17 years of age and corresponds to an MA of approximately 48 months. Gibson reports that the majority of individuals with DS obtain an MA of 48 months, but the third plateau is not always reached. These three plateaus are important benchmarks when considering the levels and stages of language acquisition obtained by children with DS. Furthermore, the effects of early intervention (which has recently been encouraged) on the development of children with Down syndrome may indicate that Gibson's three stages occur earlier than previously thought and may even need to be reconfigured.

Some 50 years ago, the life-span expectancy for individuals with DS was around 12 years, or during Gibson's third plateau. More recently, with trends promoting deinstitutionalization and with medical progress, life expectancy has reached 50 years or more and is expected to increase (Baird & Sadovnick, 1988; Strauss & Eyman, 1996). Because individuals with DS are living longer than in previous years, it is important that they learn the necessary social and cognitive skills that will allow them to live as independently as possible and to be productive members of society. Early education, such as full inclusion during the preschool years and elementary grades, can help to establish these skills. Unfortunately, too many programs continue to isolate children with

DS from the mainstream of society, which impacts directly on their ability to function independently as adults.

Growth Patterns

Cronk and Annerén (1992) reported the growth patterns among children with DS differ at various ages and stages. Beginning during the second or third trimester of fetal life, the length and weight of the fetus are only slightly less than normal. During infancy, however, deficits in length, weight, and head circumference become marked, being smaller, by as much as 25 percent, than the normal growth rates. By age 3 years, children with DS are, on average, smaller than 90 percent of typically developing children. During adolescence, youngsters with DS typically present smaller pubescent growth spurts and present height that is two standard deviations below the mean. Weight gain during adolescence, however, is often excessive and frequently results in individuals becoming overweight; this only compounds serious health problems such as congenital heart disease, which occurs in 44 percent of children with DS (Pueschel, 1991), and hypotonia (loss of muscle tone) (Griffiths, 1976).

Hearing Pathology

Anatomical differences of the ear are present in children with DS. One of the most common findings is a small pinna (external ear), which may be lower and more oblique than in typically developing children (Dahle & Baldwin, 1992), as well as smaller and shorter external ear canals (Strome, 1981). Other anatomical differences include an overlapping helix (rim-like periphery of the pinnae), a prominent antihelix (semicircular ridge, just anterior to the helix), projecting pinnae, and absent or malformed ear lobes (Dahle & Baldwin, 1992).

It has been reported that over 75 percent of children with DS present with frequent hearing losses due to otitis media or fluid buildup in the middle ear space (Cooley & Graham, 1991). Schwartz and Schwartz (1978) have reported that 67 percent of their sample of children with DS (mean age of 3 years) demonstrated otoscopic pathologic ear conditions, and Balkany, Downs, Jafek, and Krajicek (1978) reported 78 percent of their 107 children with DS (mean age of 12 years) had a hearing loss. Since it has been documented that a mild conductive hearing loss can affect language and cognitive development (Telle, 1984), Strome (1981) recommends early detection and aggressive management to reduce middle ear pathology. Otologic management for children with DS can be problematic as otoscopic viewing and the surgical placement of tubes may be made difficult by the small ear canals that characterize these children (Balkany, Mischke, Downs, & Jafek, 1979; Strome, 1981). Consequently, it is important to find experienced specialists when seeking medical services for children with DS.

In addition to middle ear pathologies, inner ear pathologies are also common in children with DS. Igrashi, Takahashi, Alford, and Johnson (1977) reported that individuals with DS frequently have alterations in the development of the inner ear, which may include both the cochlear and vestibular portions. Sensorineural hearing losses have been reported as being more prevalent in children with DS than in age-matched peers (Dahle & Baldwin, 1992; Dahle & McCollister, 1986; Whiteman, Simpson, & Compton, 1986).

Dahle and Baldwin (1992) recommend regular and systematic hearing evaluations for all children with DS. They suggest that infants with DS should receive an audiologic evaluation within a few months of birth and be checked every 6-12 months thereafter. If a conductive hearing loss is detected, Dahle and Baldwin recommend monitoring the middle ear function as dictated by the treatment regimen.

SOCIAL AND COMMUNICATION ISSUES

Several social, interactive, and communicative issues have been reported among children with DS and will now be discussed.

Play Behavior

Play behavior, especially symbolic play, is considered by Westby (1980) to be one of the most significant cognitive developments in early childhood and the precursor of representational thought and language (Piaget, 1957; Unger, Zelazo, Kearsley, & O'Leary, 1981). Westby (1980) further suggests that symbolic play can be a means of assessing a child's representational ability. Fein (1981) concluded that children with imaginary play skills use much more sophisticated language than do children who play at less developed or more concrete levels of play.

Several investigations have focused on the play of children with DS. The overwhelming conclusion is that their play follows a similar sequence to and is as well organized and as consistent across different domains as that of cognitively matched, typically developing children (Beeghly, Weiss-Perry, & Cicchetti, 1990; Cicchetti & Stroufe, 1976; Krakow & Kopp, 1983; Mans, Cicchetti, & Stroufe, 1978; Motti, Cicchetti, & Stroufe, 1983). Motti et al. (1983), for instance, examined the symbolic play of a group of children with DS and found that, when adjusted for mental age, the play of the group with DS proceeded through the same sequence and at approximately the same time schedule as that of typically developing peers. Beeghly et al. (1990) described symbolic play from mother-child play sessions involving children with DS and cognitively matched, typically developing children. The symbolic play in the children with DS emerged in a delayed manner but did progress through the typical stages of decentration, decontextualization, and integration in both object and social play. In a third study, Chuang and Layton (1992) assessed the play behaviors of two groups of Chinese toddlers, one with DS and the other typically developing and matched by chronological age, gender, birth order, and mother's education. They used Westby's (1980) Symbolic Play Scale to assess play behaviors. The children with DS were found overall to be functioning at approximately the same stage on Westby's scale as were the typically developing children, but the former group exhibited quantitatively more presymbolic behaviors during their early stages and fewer play behaviors at the higher levels of the scale. These results suggest that the children with DS had acquired the same level of play skills as the age-related peers but used less sophisticated play behaviors during their daily routines.

Voice Quality

Researchers have recognized the unusual voice quality of children with Down syndrome for over 50 years. A distinctively rough, breathy, low-pitched voice is a well-recognized feature that distinguishes children with Down syndrome from other children (Blanchard, 1964; Montague & Hollien, 1973). Two areas of investigation related to vocal quality differences have been pursued. The first area of investigation involves a range of physiological factors that have been proposed as underlying the cause of the atypical voice quality. Benda (1960), for instance, attributes deviant voice quality to the short, broad neck and high larynx of children with DS, whereas Engler (1949) and Strazzula (1953) suggest the deviations of the facial bones, such as the small, blunt styloid processes, as possible contributors. Other anatomical differences, such as a high palate, short buccal cavity, obstructed nasal passage, and large tongue relative to the small oral cavity are possible causes of the unusual voice (Lind, Uvorenski, Rosberg, & Partanen, 1970; Novak, 1972; Pentz, 1987). Muscle hypotonia, thickened and fibrotic laryngeal mucosa, and pharyngeal mucosa that shows signs of atrophy and dryness are further factors (Lind et al., 1970; Novak, 1972; Pentz, 1987). No one physiological factor, as of yet, clearly stands out as the cause of the vocal deviation in children with Down syndrome.

A second area of investigation has focused on measuring the acoustic quality of the speech signal. Pitch, or fundamental frequency (F_0), has been investigated thoroughly, yet the results have been inconclusive. Weinburg and Zlatin (1970), for example, found that half of the children with DS had significantly higher F_0 than did matched controls, despite a perceived lower pitch judged by a panel of experts. In contrast, Hollien and Copeland (1965) and Lind et al. (1970) found lower F_0 in their subject children with DS, while Montague, Brown, and Hollien (1974) and Michel and Carney (1964) reported findings of essentially no differences in F_0. In a recent study, Hays, Layton, and Hooper (1991) attempted to control for several of the design problems of the earlier investigations and found that children with DS, when compared to age-matched controls, produced essentially the same F_0, but that unlike the controls, the children with DS produced many of their vowels with an open, relaxed vocal tract (like low-back vowels).

Apparently, the unusual voice qualities among children with DS are not related to differences in fundamental frequency, but they could be due to differences in resonating cavities or formant frequencies. Formants reflect the shape and size of the vocal tract (Baken, 1987). In one investigation, Pentz (1987) reported on the formants of 14 children with DS, matched with a set of same-age and -gender peers, using a narrowband, real-time spectrograph and found: (1) no differences occurred in the first formant on sustained vowels /a, i, u/ between the groups, but a lower second formant existed for the children with DS; (2) productions of different vowels by the children with DS tended to have greater variability in formant amplitudes than in the control group; and (3) the children with DS showed significantly reduced formant amplitudes compared to age- and gender-matched controls.

Pentz reasoned that these differences could be due to the children with DS having an overall reduction in muscle tone, which could permit excessive air to escape. The excessive escaping air, along with increased noise, could account for the perceived hoarse and breathy voice quality commonly associated with these children. Furthermore, children with DS frequently present poor speech intelligibility (Dodd, 1975, 1976; Dodd & Leahy, 1989), with imprecision of articulators and an anatomically variant resonating cavity (Novak, 1972). Together, these characteristics could alter the formant acoustic signals, as noted by Pentz (1987), and could account for the atypical voice quality among these children.

Phonology and Speech Intelligibility

As noted earlier, problems with **speech intelligibility** are common among children with DS (Dodd, 1976; Dodd & Leahy, 1989). Ingram (1976) reported on the phonological processes and articulation disorders among children with DS, in general, and other children with mental retardation. For the other children with mental retardation, phonological errors appeared to be similar to those of younger, typically developing children, whereas for the children with DS, both similarities and differences occurred in their substitution patterns. The differences consisted of unique phonological substitutions, higher instances of omissions, and poorer speech intelligibility.

In a related study, Bodine (1974) reported on the first naturalistic investigations of speech acquisition in two boys with Down syndrome, ages 5 years, 9 months (5; 9), and 6; 2. Both boys were recorded in their home while wearing a wireless microphone. For one of the boys, 2 hours of taping occurred, and for the other, 4 hours were recorded. Bodine completed both narrow and wide phonetic transcriptions of the two samples. The speech for both boys was characterized as presenting several omissions and substitutions. Specifically, frequent initial consonant deletions included /b, d, g, m, n, w, y/, whereas glottal stops were frequently used as substitutions. Also, fricatives were either distorted or substituted by earlier phonological forms, and final voiced stops and voiced fricatives were deleted. Both boys were reported to use a relatively restricted range of vowels, with low vowels frequently being produced, supporting the work of Hays et al. (1991) and Pentz (1987). Thus, the poor vowel productions, frequent substitutions, and omissions made intelligibility a major problem. For one of the boys, only 33 percent of utterances were intelligible; the other boy produced 75 percent intelligible utterances. Dodd (1976) reported that children with DS produced more than twice as many articulation errors and twice as many error inconsistencies as did mental age (MA)-matched children with other types of mental retardation.

Dodd and Leahy (1989), in a more recent study, suggest that poorer speech intelligibility among children with Down syndrome may be a specific or unique occurrence. That is, they report that children with DS have greater problems with intelligibility and different phonological errors than do children with mental retardation associated with other etiologies (Dodd, 1975, 1976; Rosin, Swift, Bless, & Vetter, 1988; Stoel-Gammon, 1981). Furthermore, the speech productions for these children are inconsistent, such that the same individual may produce a single word three or four different ways during a single conversation (Dodd & Leahy, 1989). This inconsistency, along with poor intelligibility, is not present among other children with mental retardation (Dodd & Leahy, 1989), and it seems to remain a persistent problem even after intense therapy (Dodd & Iacano, 1989; Horstmeier, 1987).

Despite the many organic factors that could contribute to the poor speech intelligibility of children with DS, none has completely accounted for the fact that these children imitate words better than they produce them spontaneously (Miller, 1988). Certainly, organic factors cannot account for the inconsistent speech productions, nor for the improved speech skills during imitation. Consequently, Dodd, McCormack, and Woodyatt (1994) believe that a central specific deficit in speech-motor control exists among these children and accounts for the unique speech behavior. Furthermore, their overall impaired sequencing of fine-motor movements (Dodd, 1975; Henderson, Morris, & Frith, 1980; Seyfort & Spreen, 1979) and difficulties in processing sequential information (Hartley, 1982; Snart, O'Grady, & Dos, 1982) lend support to this assumption.

Early Parental Interaction

Several investigations of early parental interaction between mothers and their children with Down syndrome suggest that these mothers, like mothers of typically developing children, regulate their language and communicative strategies to fit the communication level of the child (Buckhalt, Rutherford, & Goldberg, 1978; Maurer & Sherrod, 1987; O'Kelley-Collard, 1978; Peterson & Sherrod, 1982; Rondal, 1977). However, the mothers of children with

DS tend to use more control and directiveness during conversations than do the mothers of typically developing children (Breiner & Forehand, 1982; Cardoso-Martins & Mervis, 1985; Levy-Shiff, 1986; Smith & Hagen, 1984). Research also suggests that the dyadic interactions between mothers and their children with DS are more restrictive (i.e., lower responsiveness, less initiations, less eye contact, less preverbal vocalization) than in dyads involving typically developing children (Berger & Cunningham, 1983; Buckhalt et al., 1978; Kogan, Wimberger, & Bobbitt, 1969). Furthermore, Leifer and Lewis (1984) found that children with DS were significantly delayed in their conversational responses to maternal question types relative to typically developing children matched by age but were more advanced relative to children matched by linguistic stage.

Masel (1987) directly evaluated children's conversational response abilities and mothers' requesting patterns and responsivity. She found similarities between the children with DS and cognitively matched, typically developing children in correct responses to requests, ability to maintain synchrony (i.e., the bidirectional, transactional quality of dyadic interaction), and mothers' responsivity to their children's behaviors. There was, however, a greater variability among the children with DS on measures of response appropriateness, and correct responses to requests for information and acknowledgment and in the relationship between maternal requesting patterns and the children's consistency of correct responses. Taken together, this research reveals a great deal of similarity in conversational response abilities of children with DS compared to cognitively matched, typically developing controls, although the results do reflect some variability across the group of children with DS. Nevertheless, the early linguistic environment for children with DS appears to be supportive and not a factor in speech or language delays, which are nonetheless prevalent in this population (Miller, 1988).

Lexical Development

There are four issues relevant to **lexical acquisition** in children with DS: rate of comprehension of words, rate of production of words, existence of a gap between comprehension and production, and thematic and semantic roles. Generally speaking the comprehension of words has been rarely investigated. The production of first words has been found to vary from study to study because of different standards of comparison, such as mental age or MLU.

Vocabulary Comprehension. Cardoso-Martins, Mervis, and Mervis (1985) reported on the development of vocabulary comprehension among children with DS. The focus of their investigation was on children's understanding of object names. Six children with DS were matched on cognitive levels (i.e., Bayley, 1969), birth order, and sex with six typically developing children. The children with DS were 17 to 19 months of age, with developmental ages between 8 and 14 months. The matched controls were younger, averaging 9 months of age, but they had similar developmental age ranges (i.e., from 10 to 12 months). All the children were observed in a series of home visits for 14 to 21 months: audio recordings were made of the words produced at each visit. In addition, the researchers tested for comprehension by placing four objects in front of the child and asking her or him to select the designated item. If the child touched or picked up the correct item, she or he was considered to have comprehended the vocabulary item.

The results indicated that, at Piaget's (1957) sensorimotor stages 5 and 6, the children with DS comprehended significantly fewer object names than did the matched controls. Thus, the researchers concluded that the early vocabulary comprehension of children with DS lagged behind that of children with typical development, and that cognitive measures were an effective means of predicting actual vocabulary size.

Vocabulary Production. The production of vocabulary in children with DS has consistently been reported to lag behind mental age–matched controls. In a comprehensive review of the topic, Barrett and Diniz (1989) reviewed nine studies on the lexical development of children with DS and concluded: (1) there were no differences in vocabulary skills between children with DS and children with other retardation, (2) children with DS differed in rate of acquisition from typically developing children, and (3) the actual words acquired by the children with DS were very similar to those acquired by typically developing children, but simply acquired at a slower rate. Barrett and Diniz (1989) found that first words typically did not emerge in children with DS until 3 years of age or later. Rondal (1978, 1988) found that children with DS produced 20 words around 3½ to 4 years of age, at an MA of two years, or at sensorimotor stage 6, whereas typically developing children produced 20 words at age 16–18 months (Nelson, 1973).

Miller (1992b) argued that the measures used to determine MA can contribute to reported delayed vocabulary acquisition in children with DS. He recommended that nonverbal measures based on MA should be included with subjects matched on mean length of utterance (MLU). For example, Miller, Budde, Bashir, and LaFollette (1987) found that children with DS produced fewer different words than did nonverbal MA–matched children, but when compared to children matched by MLU, the children with DS produced significantly more different words.

Miller (1992b) further contended that socioeconomic status may also have contributed to differences in vocabulary acquisition in children with DS. Therefore, he selected children with DS along with a control group matched for MA and socioeconomic status (SES). Miller found no difference on vocabulary acquisition between the two groups. A replication study with another set of subjects revealed similar findings (Miller, 1992b). Miller concluded that adding SES as a matching variable reduced the variability between the groups.

In another investigation, Miller (1992b) documented the vocabulary size of children with DS from data obtained through language samples and from parental reports (i.e., the MacArthur Communicative Development Inventories; Fenson et al., 1993). Miller found that using the data from language samples yielded no differences on vocabulary size between the children with DS and typically developing children matched by MA and SES. However, from the parental reports, the children with DS exhibited smaller overall vocabularies after 17 months MA, compared to typical developing children with a chronological age of 17 months. Furthermore, although the vocabulary size was smaller, the children with DS did demonstrate a rapid acceleration of vocabulary. A rapid growth in vocabulary has been found in typically developing children around 16 to 18 months, when they acquire approximately 11 new words per month (Nelson, 1973). In Miller's sample of children with DS, a similar rapid growth occurred, only less extensively. Miller concluded that children with DS acquire vocabulary in a similar way to typically developing children, but at a much slower rate. He also stated that using parental report measures is an excellent index for determining early vocabulary development in children with DS.

Verbal Comprehension versus Verbal Production.   In a recent study, Caselli et al. (1998) reported on the relationship between verbal comprehension and production in children with DS. A sample of 40 children with DS, ranging in age from 10 to 49 months, was compared to a sample of 40 typically developing children, ranging in age from 8 to 17 months. The children were matched on number of words comprehended on the Italian MacArthur Communicative Development Inventory (Caselli & Casadio, 1995). Caselli et al. found, as expected, that chronological age was higher at higher levels of comprehension for the children with DS. However, an unexpected finding was that word production did not differ between the two groups when comprehension levels were equated. The lag between verbal comprehension and verbal production was the same between the two groups. A third finding indicated that children with DS produced a greater percentage of gestures than did matched, typically developing children. The gestures of the children with DS included more advanced symbolic communicative forms, more pretend gestures, and higher numbers of action gestures that involved the ability to perform symbolic transformations. Caselli et al. concluded that children with DS appeared to follow a different pattern of vocabulary and gestural development than typically developing children. During early stages of development in children with DS, gestural productions were similar to typically developing children, but later on, the numbers of symbolic gestures and actions continued to increase and were actually more advanced in the children with DS.

Thematic and Semantic Roles.   **Thematic and semantic relations** are meaningful relations or categories of perception, actions, and thought that are often related to early linguistic features (Chafe, 1970). Thematic and semantic relations are the early bridge between single-word productions and multiword utterances. Meaningful relations such as agents, patients, actions, states, negation, existence, recurrence, locatives, and datives become part of early meaningful exchanges (Bloom, Lightbown, & Hood, 1975). Regrettably, only a few studies have looked at thematic relations among children with DS.

Dooley (1976) reported on a longitudinal investigation of two children with DS: a boy, age 3;10 with an MA of 2;5 at the onset of the investigation, and a girl, age 5;2, with an MA of 2;11. The parents raised both children at home. Dooley recorded samples of spontaneous speech in the children's homes every 2 weeks for 12 months and reported on the first three and last three samples. Both children were found to master grammatical morphemes in an order similar to that of typically developing children. Dooley also found the basic thematic relations expected at the various MLU stages to all be present, including recurrence, nonexistence, agent and action, entity, attribute, and agent-action-object.

In another study, Layton and Sharifi (1979) used Chafe's (1970) model of semantic competence to investigate the early multiword utterances of nine children with DS (ages 7;4 to 12;2), and nine typically developing children (ages 2; 10 to 5; 4), who were matched by MA. They obtained a corpus of spontaneous utterances from each child. The results indicated that the differences between the groups were mostly quantitative and not qualitative. For instance, the children with DS produced more agent-action relations and fewer patient-process relations than did the matched controls. This finding suggests that the meanings conveyed by the children with DS were restricted to the here and now or limited to talking about objects and events that were immediately present in time and space.

These two studies suggest that children with DS acquire all the necessary thematic and semantic relations that occur in typically developing children at the multiword level, but the acquisition of their relations are considerably slower to develop and the frequency of use may be more limited.

Language and Syntax

Children with DS have consistently been shown to have unexplainable delays in their acquisition of receptive and expressive language and especially in syntax (Chapman, 1995; Fowler, 1995; Miller, 1992a). Research has documented that a large discrepancy occurs in these children between measured language skills and expected levels according to mental age. Fowler (1990) has reviewed this literature and summarized the findings into four areas.

1. The expressive language of children with DS tends to develop more slowly than other aspects of motor or cognitive development. This lag is evident in infancy and becomes greater as the individuals grow older. Furthermore, when individuals with DS have been compared to children with other

mental retardation, the individuals with DS were found to have more "language handicaps" (Evans, 1977; Johnson & Abelson, 1969).

2. Some children with DS reach the language level of a typically developing 6-year-old. However, no investigation has been able to predict which children will acquire this more mature language and which will level off at a lower level. Most children with DS do not move beyond the level of simple phrases found in typically developing 6-year-olds.

3. The most pronounced deficits in children with DS occur in grammatical-syntactic components of language, whereas the lexical domain and nonverbal areas seem to be strengths for these children.

4. Language learning by children with DS does not proceed at a constant pace, but rather seems to reach plateaus and spurts differently throughout the growth period. Much of the language learning by these children appears to take place before the age of 7 years.

Chapman, Schwartz, and Kay-Raining Bird (1991) reported on the comprehension skills of 48 children and adolescents with Down syndrome (ages 5;6 to 20;6 years) compared to a nonverbal, MA-matched control group (ages 2 to 6 years). Subjects' performances were compared on the Peabody Picture Vocabulary Test–Revised (Dunn & Dunn, 1981) and the Test of Auditory Comprehension of Language–Revised (Carrow-Woolfolk, 1985). Chapman et al. found no difference between the two groups on either test; however, as the group of subjects with DS got older and were retested, the mean age difference between the two tests increased significantly. Syntactic comprehension did not increase at the same rate as vocabulary comprehension. In other words, a clear difference began to develop between vocabulary and syntactic comprehension.

In another study, Fowler, Gelman, and Gleitman (1994) reported on four adolescents with DS (mean age, 12;3) and a control group of younger MLU matched controls (mean age 2;7). They collected language samples under naturalistic conditions and compared the two groups on thematic and semantic units, indices of complex syntax, and vocabulary. Fowler et al. found no differences in thematic and semantic units between the two groups. In fact, the children with DS performed as well, if not better, than the matched controls. Furthermore, on Scarborough's (1990) IPSyn measure of productive syntax, the two groups were again similar in Noun Phrase, Verb Phrase, negatives, and interrogative sentences. However, the sentence complexity score was significantly different, superior in the children with DS. Fowler et al. concluded that during the early stages of development, children with DS acquire language in a way similar to younger typically developing children.

Fowler et al. (1994) also reported on a single-subject, longitudinal investigation of a young girl with DS (age 51 months at the onset of the study). The girl was visited in the home once a month for an hour-long session until she was 89 months of age. Fowler et al. reported on the child's thematic and morphologic development across Brown's five stages. During stages I to III, the girl essentially acquired normal morphemes and thematic units. However, during stage III her progress slowed, with her MLU ceasing to increase for nearly 10 months. For the remainder of the investigation, the child acquired only one additional morpheme and did not master negatives and interrogative forms. Thus, a plateau occurred, with several of the earlier acquired grammatical morphemes still being used inconsistently as well.

More recently, Chapman, Seung, Schwartz, and Kay-Raining Bird (1998) reported on a group of 47 children and adolescents with DS (ages 5; 6 to 20; 6), matched by nonverbal MA with a control group of younger children (ages 2; 2 to 6; 1). Conversations and event narratives were obtained and scored by SALT (Miller & Chapman, 1993) analysis. Chapman et al. found that the subjects with DS performed less well on MLU, number of different words, number of total words, and number of words per minute. Furthermore, the group of children with DS omitted more grammatical function words (i.e., copulas, auxiliaries, modals, articles, prepositions, pronouns, adverbs, conjunctions, and infinitives) and more morphemes (i.e., plural nouns, possessives, third person marker, contracted auxiliary, copulas, present progressive, regular past, contracted 'm, and contracted 'll) than did the controls. Chapman et al. also reported that the subjects with DS accelerated their expressive vocabulary more rapidly with advancing age than they did their syntax. Chapman et al. concluded that a verbal production deficit occurred in the older children with DS.

Fowler (1995) reports that children with DS evidence conversational skills beyond their expressive language levels, despite the appearance that syntax is the greatest area of deficit for them. They engage in imaginative play and use appropriate conversational rules, such as turn taking, asking questions, and making repairs, that go far beyond their expected expressive language level (Baren-Cohen, Tager-Flusberg, & Cohen, 1992). Fowler suggests that one current explanation for this discrepancy is related to a basic difficulty for these children in perceiving speech and encoding incoming acoustic information into a representational format in memory that can readily be retrieved to serve recall, production, and comprehension. Although this explanation is only at the beginning stages, Fowler does report some evidence by Racette (1993), who found a significant correlation between a simple test of articulation and verbal memory in young adults with DS. Racette also found that phonological skills correlated significantly with the correct imitation of grammatical markers, which, according to Fowler, is an accurate index of language production. Crosley and Doweling (1989) also reported a direct relationship between phonological and syntactic development in children with Down syndrome.

In summary, the language skills of children with DS can be characterized into four areas. First, children with DS show syntactic production skills that lag behind their expected abilities. This lag appears to widen as they age. Second, language production skills in these children are inferior in relation to their cognitive abilities. Third, syntactic development (as measured by MLU) in children with DS is characterized by periods of fairly rapid growth similar to those of typically developing children (Miller, 1988), but with protracted plateaus, which are not typical of normal development (Chapman, 1995; Fowler, 1988; Fowler et al., 1994). Fourth, lexical acquisition in these children exceeds their syntactic development. Thus, children with DS appear to exhibit a specific deficit in language learning, with particular difficulty in language production.

Reading and Literacy

The literature surrounding reading skills and reading instruction among children and young adults with DS is extremely sparse. It has been suggested that reading cannot be achieved until the typically developing child has reached a cognitive level or language age of approximately a 6-year-old; and since many individuals with DS never reach this level, it was assumed that learning to read was not possible for them. Therefore, reading was not recommended. However, in the past decade, a trend toward more literacy-related goals has emerged for children with DS, with some measurable success (Stratford, 1985). Children with DS are now reading for pleasure and writing creative stories. Furthermore, preschool children with DS are being introduced to reading in regular programs (Lorenz, Sloper, & Cunningham, 1985) and, interestingly, reading has been found to facilitate their communication skills and increase their acquisition of expressive morphosyntactic rules. Being able to read has also expanded employment opportunities into areas where reading and writing are necessary requisites for employment.

Several researchers have documented reading among very young children with DS (Buckley, 1995; Greene, 1987; Norris, 1989). For example, Buckley (1995) reported on a child, Digby, who learned to read at 25 months of age, long before he was able to speak his first word. Digby read the words or flashcards and pointed to the correct object or picture. Buckley also describes the early reading of four other children with DS who began to read between 28 and 41 months of age. One of these children, Daniel, used his reading to improve his expressive language skills. For example, after reading several single words and speaking at the one-word level, Daniel learned to read two-word phrases first, which subsequently carried over to the production of two-word spoken utterances. Three months later he learned to read three-word phrases, which again transferred to three-word spoken utterances. By 42 months of age, Daniel could read 66 words and was regularly producing many two to three-word combinations.

Unfortunately, there are few reported studies comparing the reading and cognitive skills among preschool-age children with DS and chronological or cognitive age-matched peers. All the studies have been done with school-age children (see Table 6-1).

Table 6-1. Four studies on reading and cognitive skills among children with Down syndrome

	Cossu et al. (1993)	Byrne et al. (1995)	Fowler et al. (1995)	Kay-Raining Bird & McConnell (1994)
Subjects	DS = 10 (11:4 yrs) Control = 10 (7:9 yrs)	DS = 24 (8:2 yrs) Av Readers = 42 (7:3 yrs) Poor Readers = 32 (7:1 yrs)	DS = 33 (17–25 yrs) ·Novice (n=12) ·Emerging (n=10) ·Developing (n=6) ·Skilled (n=5)	DS = 10 (9:6 yrs) Controls = 10 (4:7 yrs)
Matching Variable	Sight Words (stress/nonstress; real/nonwords)	Reading (British Ability Scales Word Reading subtest. Elliott, 1993)	N/A	PPVT-R
Word Attack			Novice-worst Emerging-3rd Developing-2nd Skilled-best	DS > control
Word Identification		AV Readers-best Poor Readers = DS	Novice-worst Emerging-3rd Developing-2nd Skilled-best	DS > control
Word Comprehension			Novice-worst Emerging-3rd Developing-2nd Skilled-best	
Segment Word				DS > control
Segment Syllable				Both Groups Equal
Segment Phoneme	DS Worse			Both Groups Equal
Letter Identify				DS > control
Phoneme Deletion	DS Worse		6:0 yr Level all subjects	
Phoneme Synthesis	DS Worse			
Spelling	DS Worse	AV Readers-best Poor Readers-2d DS-3rd		
Receptive Vocabulary			Novice-worst Emerging-3rd Developing-2nd Skilled-best	Matching Variable
Receptive Language		Controls-1st Poor Readers-2nd DS-3rd	Novice-worst Emerge = Developing Skilled-best	
Cognitive			Novice-worst Emerge = Developing Skilled-best	

(continues)

Table 6-1.   Continued

	Cossu et al. (1993)	Byrne et al. (1995)	Fowler et al. (1995)	Kay-Raining Bird & McConnell (1994)
Arithmetic		Controls-1st Poor Readers-2nd DS-3rd	Novice-worst Emerging-3rd Developing Skilled-best	
Memory (Vis-Aud)		Controls-1st Poor Readers-2nd DS-3rd	5:0 yr level for all subjects	

Three of the four relevant studies contained matched control groups (Byrne, Buckley, MacDonald, & Bird, 1995; Cossu, Rossini, & Marshall, 1993; Kay-Raining Bird & McConnell, 1994), whereas the fourth (Fowler, Doherty, & Boynton, 1995) investigated children with DS across four different reading levels. Various reading and cognitive skills were examined in all four studies. For example, in the Cossu et al. (1993) study, children with DS were matched to younger controls based on sight-word reading of normally stressed and non-stressed words and a second set of real and nonreal words. Both groups performed equally well on the sight-word tasks. However, on other phoneme awareness elements of reading, such as segmenting words by phonemes, deleting phonemes, and synthesizing phonemes, the children with DS performed less well than did the controls. According to Cossu et al., this finding suggests that the children with DS demonstrated proficient word recognition skills, as determined by the matching variables, despite making a poor showing on phoneme awareness skills. Thus, for this group of individuals, phoneme awareness was not a necessary prerequisite for reading.

Byrne et al. (1995) used the British Ability Scales Word Reading subtest (Elliott, 1983) to compare two control groups with 8-year-old children with DS: one control group consisted of younger children with average reading skills, and the second group consisted of younger children with poor reading skills. On the word identification tasks, the poor reading group and the children with DS performed quite similarly, whereas the average readers performed the best, as expected (see Table 6-1). In contrast, the poor reading group performed better than did the children with DS on standardized measures of literacy, language, and memory, with the average readers performing the best (see Table 6-1). According to Byrne et al., these findings can be interpreted to mean that the children with DS appeared to have an advanced reading level compared to their language and cognitive abilities. Thus, as a group, there appears to be a dissimilarity between reading achievement and language/cognitive abilities in children with DS.

Fowler et al. (1995) investigated reading skills among a group of young adults with DS (ages 17 to 25 years) and compared their reading skills with various other cognitive measures. The subjects were divided into four reading levels: novices (who decoded less than 2 words), emerging readers (who decoded 3 to 10 words), developing readers (who decoded 11 to 29 words), and more skilled readers (who decoded more than 29 words). As can be seen in Table 6-1, most of the subjects were either at the novice or emerging reading levels (i.e., 22 out of 33 subjects). Fowler et al. found that as a group, most subjects relied on sight-word reading and lacked decoding skills. In fact, lack of decoding skills appeared to restrict the reading ability for most subjects. There was, however, a relationship between phoneme awareness and decoding skills, in that the individuals with better phoneme awareness were also the better decoders. Fowler et al. also found that verbal short-term memory (STM) was related to reading success; that is, the greater the STM, the better the overall reading skill. Taken together, the results of the Fowler et al. study demonstrate a good deal of variability in reading skills among individuals with DS.

In the fourth study, Kay-Raining Bird and McConnell (1994) used receptive vocabulary scores to match children with DS (mean age, 9;6) to a much younger group of typically developing children (mean age, 4;7). Interestingly, the children with DS performed better than the younger controls on word attack, word identification, letter identification, and word segmentation skills. Both groups, however, performed equally well on syllable and phoneme segmentation. Kay-Raining Bird and McConnell also found that word and syllable segmentation abilities correlated significantly with word attack skills for the children with DS; however, for the younger controls, MLU and word segmentation correlated with letter identification, and MLU and rhyming skills correlated with word identification. Therefore, the two groups approached reading using quite divergent strategies.

Imaginary Companions

Based on clinical experience and anecdotal comments, this author has observed a number of children and young adults with DS interacting with imaginary companions. On two occasions, these interactions have become so consuming that the parents of the youngsters with DS sought medical and psychiatric help. Important issues are the expected prevalence of the phenomenon, how typical it is, its purpose, and what, if any, positive effects the imaginary companions may have on the individual's social-communicative skills.

In the general literature, imaginary companions have been discussed extensively. Vostrovsky (1895) was first to assign a "stabilizing" role to children's imaginary friends. Later writings, however, suggested that imaginary companions were an indication of a deep psychological pathology (cf. Singer & Singer, 1990). Preschool children between 3 and 5 years of age are most frequently reported to have imaginary companions (Breckenridge & Vincent,

1960; Nagera, 1969), with recent research focusing on the companions' creative and functional purposes (Manosevitz, Fling, & Prentice, 1977; Meyer & Tuber, 1989; Taylor, Cartwright, & Carlson, 1993).

Typically developing children with imaginary companions have been reported to be more social and less shy, have more real friends, be more active, and participate more in family-related activities (Manosevitz, Prentice, & Wilson., 1973; Manosevitz et al., 1977; Taylor et al., 1993). Imaginary companions appear to serve a variety of functions. For example, Manosevitz et al. (1973) found that imaginary companions were a means for coping with frustration, lessening feelings of loneliness, acting out forbidden behaviors, and teaching the child new or challenging skills. Jalongo (1984) identified different attributes among imaginary companions. They were supportive/playful, inconsiderate/impolite, docile/submissive, and generally the result of an unusual or novel experience. Harter and Chao (1992) suggest that the major function of imaginary companions is to assist the child with issues of mastery and competence. They note that boys tend to create more competent companions (therefore engendering feelings of greater competence through identification), whereas girls tend to create companions less competent than themselves (someone whom they can care for, teach, or help with a skill).

Little research has been reported on imaginary companions among children with DS. Nontheless, over the past several years, this author has found several children with DS to have at least one, and sometimes many, imaginary companions.

CASE STUDY: JACK

A young male student with DS, Jack, who was 14 years old, had several imaginary companions and refused to interrupt his conversations with his companions when his parents tried to talk with him. He had both male and female companions. Jack's imaginary companions took on many different roles. For example, one companion needed Jack's assistance to accomplish things, whereas one of the female companions frequently explained rules to Jack. When Jack was trying to learn something or establish a new rule in his life, he would comment, "She says to do it this way," speaking out loud about his companion.

Jack's mother reported that when the boy was verbally communicating with his imaginary companions, his level of language complexity and speech intelligibility improved. She also reported that he clearly used more logic during these interactions.

At one point, Jack's parents were concerned about whether he was attempting to escape from reality and viewed his imaginary companions as the sign of a serious psychological disorder. Jack was seen by a psychiatrist who prescribed medical treatment to alleviate the problem; however, the medica-

tion had a serious side effect on Jack's physical condition and his temperament, so his parents stopped it. Since then they have applied a behavioral management approach to lessen the situation: they set rules as to when and where Jack may converse with his imaginary companions. In general, this tactic seems to have worked. There are times, however, when Jack's imaginary companions still control the situation.

The role of imaginary companions in children with DS is not dissimilar to what is found among younger, typically developing children. However, it is still not known how many children with DS have imaginary companions, whether males with DS have different types of companions than females, and how long the imaginary relationships last. Do they persist, for example, into adulthood? Do the companions play an important role in facilitating the development of reasoning skills and higher language skills in children with DS? If imaginary companions improve the child's communication skills, should they be included in the therapy situation to teach improved interaction skills? These are important questions, which need further exploration.

INTERVENTION

Speech and language intervention programs for children with DS have changed over the years from highly structured behavioral approaches (Cole, 1995; Guess, Sailor, & Baer, 1974; McLean, 1976) to more naturalistic or milieu teaching approaches (Yoder, Kaiser, & Alpert, 1991; Yoder & Warren, 1993; Weismer, 2000). Emphasis has also shifted, in recent years, from speech intelligibility to more communication-based intervention. However, communication-based intervention may not always be the recommended approach for working with children with DS (Dodd et al., 1994). Currently, the approach to intervention for children with DS is the same as that recommended for children who are cognitively normal but who have specific language impairments (SLI) (Bricker, 1993; Weismer, in press). This is because the sequences of linguistic skills (e.g., vocabulary and syntactic rules) acquired by children with DS follow a similar order to those acquired by children with specific language impairments, although the children with DS may acquire the skills at a slower rate or over a more protracted time period. One possible difference, then, between the outcomes of the two populations is that the expectation of success may not be as rapid nor as far reaching for the children with DS as for the children with SLI. Children with DS acquire and maintain new communicative skills more slowly than children with SLI and tend to reach a plateau at around a 6-year language level (Fowler, 1988). Language intervention approaches used with children with SLI are generally quite effective for children with DS. There are, however, several additional worthwhile intervention strategies that empirically have proven useful for children with DS and should be used to augment the general language approach.

Oral-Motor Training

Since many children with DS present poor oral-motor strength, less coordination, and limited muscle range, it is recommended that training in these areas be introduced early in the child's development (Beckman, 1990). Exercises that help to strengthen the range of motion for the lips, tongue, and jaw are critical to adequate oral-motor development and the possible improvement of phonetic or speech production. In addition, lip-stretching exercises, proper chewing, introducing a variety of food textures, and proper breathing techniques are also important for improving oral-motor function (Beckman, 1990). It is suggested that these exercises should be ongoing, beginning when the child is first introduced to semisolid foods and continued on a regular schedule until she or he is well into school.

Speech Intelligibility

Intervention addressing speech intelligibility needs to be one of the primary goals for children with DS. Without intervention, Horstmeier (1987) reports that speech intelligibility in children with DS does not appear to improve with advancing age. Swift and Rosin (1990) suggest a three-stage sequence for improving speech intelligibility: paralinguistic, early linguistic, and late linguistic. In the prelinguistic stage, activities should include the use of amplification systems such as hearing aids, use of manual communication (Abrahamsen, Cavallo, & McCluer, 1985; Layton & Savino, 1990), oral-motor training, and parent training to facilitate communication. Then, in the early linguistic stage, Swift and Rosin (1990) suggest such activities as structured sound play, drill, scripts, carrier phrases, augmentative communication systems, computers (Meyers, 1984), and oral-motor work. The late linguistic stage is characterized by drill, scripts, repair strategies, and pairing graphic symbols to verbal productions.

Kumin, Councill, and Goodman (1995) have also suggested the use of pacing boards to facilitate speech intelligibility. A pacing board consists of a series of dots (either black dots or color coded dots related to initial, medial, and final sounds) placed across a cardboard sheet. Depending upon the age and need of the child, there may be as few as 3 or as many as 10 dots placed across the board. The professional uses the board to help the child identify and produce initial and final sounds of simple words, individual syllables from bisyllabic and trisyllabic words, and, later, different words from simple and complex sentences. For example, the child is taught to touch a dot each time she or he says a syllable in a multisyllabic word. The advantage of the pacing board is that it provides both a visual and a tactile cue. It also provides the child with structure and the necessary pacing for the proper articulatory movements of sounds, syllables, and words in sentences.

Dodd et al. (1994) have reported children with DS to be quite inconsistent in their speech production; therefore, one of their recommended goals is to establish a consistency of speech and word productions. To accomplish this, they trained parents to focus on phonological skills and consistency of word production in preschool age children with DS. The results were quite promising, with the children's phonological skills improving in relation to the parents' interactional communication skills.

Manual Communication

Several professionals have advocated the early introduction of manual communication (signing) for children with DS (Abrahamsen et al., 1985; Layton & Savino, 1990). The argument for using manual communication is that early communicative needs are not being met with these children because they lack the oral expressive skills necessary for verbal communication. They may understand the meaning of words, but they cannot produce them. As noted earlier, first words typically do not emerge in children with DS until 3 years of age or later. Furthermore, many children with DS have such severe oral-motor difficulties that oral communication becomes a life-long struggle. In that case, manual signing provides an important opportunity to early expression. It allows the child access to an early communication system that essentially is not otherwise possible.

CASE STUDY: BOBBY

Layton and Savino (1990) introduced a manual communication system to a young boy with Down syndrome. Bobby was 3;10 when he was first seen at a university clinic for therapy. At that time he had poor verbal imitative skills, and poor oral-motor control, had not gone through the typical babbling stage, had no consonant sounds but a few vowels, and was essentially nonverbal. An imitative oral-stimulation, naturalistic language intervention approach was introduced, but was found to be unsuccessful. He would neither imitate nor attempt to produce any words. Signing was introduced as an assistive system so that Bobby could communicate with his parents and teachers. On the very first day, Bobby learned the sign for "french fries." He and his father then went to McDonald's, where Bobby generalized the sign and requested, by signing, an order of "french fries." When he arrived home, Bobby's mother asked what he had done, and Bobby immediately signed, "french fries."

Bobby's sign vocabulary increased dramatically over the next few weeks and months, but oral words still failed to develop, in spite of a strong Total Communication approach, whereby Bobby was encouraged continuously to speak and sign his wants, needs, labels, questions, and so forth. Bobby achieved a sign vocabulary of approximately 150 words by age 4;10. After this, he began to acquire an oral-expressive vocabulary that reached about 12 words. Still, the number of oral words did not increase until his expressive sign vocabulary had reached approximately 400, at 5;10. At that time, his oral vocabu-

lary increased dramatically, with his use of signs dropping out almost completely. In fact, Bobby became a totally verbal child. Bobby had received therapy for five university terms, or approximately 2 years. He returned to the clinic approximately 2 years after his last session, when he was age 7;8, for a follow-up evaluation. The only sign Bobby could remember was the "name sign" for this author. At the time of the follow up, Bobby's expressive language was nearly age appropriate. He had a sentence-length equivalent to that of a 7-year-old, an MLU of 7.68, and an overall 94 percent correct production of morphosyntactic rules. Clearly, Bobby's early sign training provided him with an initial communication system and most likely helped to facilitate oral communication. It is possible that Bobby may have learned to talk without ever being exposed to signs, but that initial opportunity to communicate would not have been there had he not learned to sign. He could have gone months or years without any consistent or elaborated means of communicating.

In a related study, Kouri (1989) reported on a young (age 2;8) female. B.V. B.V. initially produced only 8 consonant-vowel (C-V) words. She participated in an 8-month child-directed individual-treatment program that incorporated a Total Communication approach twice a week for 40 minutes each. At the end of the program, B.V. had a total of 1,634 word productions, of which 278 were signed imitations, 90 simultaneous signed-plus-spoken imitations, 409 spoken imitations, 139 spontaneous signs, 58 spontaneous simultaneous signed-plus-spoken words, and 92 spontaneous spoken words. Most of the words that B.V. initially signed were later spoken. Kouri (1989) concluded that the use of sign with B.V. clearly supported her later production of spoken language.

Together these two studies suggest that the use of manual communication (signing) can facilitate early communicative opportunities and may support the later production of spoken words.

Teaching Reading

As noted earlier, introducing reading to children with DS can be an important therapeutic goal. Buckley (1995) and Oelwein (1995) detailed several suggestions on how to teach reading to children with DS. Both these authors present important guides. Oelwein's guides are in much greater detail and available in a softbound book, whereas Buckley presents an excellent summary on how to teach reading to these children. Buckley and her colleagues (Buckley, Emslie, Haslegrave, Le Prevost, & Bird, 1993) also published a book that goes beyond reading to discuss the relationship of language and reading development among children with DS. All three sources are excellent references for parents and professionals and include clear steps on how to introduce reading to children with DS. Some general guidelines for teaching reading to young children with DS, adapted from these references, include:

1. Begin to introduce reading in a naturalistic setting even before the child has learned to speak words. Use environmental print (e.g., labels, community icons) to help the child develop initial symbol awareness.

2. Read books with predictable themes. Predictable books are those with a repetitive theme, rhymes, or familiar sequences, such as number sequences, days of the week, or the alphabet (Katims, 1991).

3. Reading the stories is important. According to Morrow (1989), the adult can help a child gain meaning by prompting a response, scaffolding responses to model the intents, answering questions, relating responses to real experiences, and acknowledging and responding to the child's comments. Scaffolding refers to interactions in which the adult supplies a response the child cannot supply or provides support to help the child to answer.

4. Teale and Sulzby (1987) found that children are more likely to read a story that has been heard several times. Typically developing children have been found to increase their language and to respond more appropriately after multiple readings (Morrow, 1988). Although no similar findings have been reported for children with DS, we have observed similar behaviors in our clinical experience with young children with DS. We encourage reading and immediately rereading the same story while incorporating many of Morrow's (1989) suggestions. This, we have found, is an effective tool for increasing dialogue with the child, improving responses, and increasing her or his interest in books.

5. Begin to introduce words from a whole-word, sight-reading approach. Young children with DS seem to do better at memorizing the entire word rather than reading with an analytic or letter/syllable "sounding-out" approach. Do, however, introduce the letters of the alphabet, especially the lower-case forms. This is important for later segmentation skills and future writing.

6. Do not attempt to have the child read two-word combinations until she or he has acquired some 25 to 50 sight words. First sight words should be highly functional, such as the child's name, names of family members, favorite food items, toys, and so on.

7. Buckley (1995) strongly urges that initial learning needs to be errorless. This is the best way to build success and to establish self-confidence since it is difficult for the child with DS to correct mistakes. Children with DS appear to shut down and resist taking risks. If the child does not know the word, provide prompts and guide her or him through the whole word.

Many relevant strategies for teaching reading are available in Kaderavek and Sulzby (2000). These suggestions are all useful for children with DS.

Direct Learning and Rehearsal

Over the years, working with children with DS has taught this author two important strategies: most children with DS need some direct training on a skill, and rehearsing old information is critical to their maintenance of acquired skills. Direct learning is an important step in the acquisition of most skills, whether it be learning to produce appropriate oral-motor skills, producing a new sound, learning a vocabulary word or a new linguistic concept, reading a new word, or practicing how to tell a story. Most of these children need some direct instruction on what is expected, followed with some drill and practice. A good approach is initially to teach outside the natural context, but then immediately contextualize the task back into typical situations. Thus, the child learns what is expected and then is given the opportunity to practice it in meaningful contexts.

Maintaining already acquired skills requires a rehearsal of what had been previously learned. Children with DS frequently forget skills that have not been fully established. It is as though those skills that have not been fully mastered are susceptible to fading. Rehearsing, or going back over previously learned skills, helps to refresh what previously had been learned and to strengthen memory. For example, an older student with DS had difficulty discriminating between a quarter and a nickel. He needed to know the difference between coins for his job, yet to him, the coins were visually the same. After several lessons, he learned through visual and auditory strategies to differentiate between the two coins. He could consistently identify both coins in real-life experiences and in direct clinical activities. His consistency was highly accurate and continued for several weeks. However, after dropping the activity and going on to another needed area, the two coins were introduced a couple of weeks later and he again confused them. Training was reintroduced, and after a few trials his old strategies resurfaced and he successfully discriminated the two coins. However, 3 weeks later, he again had trouble telling the two coins apart in a real-life situation. Thus, real-life and decontextualized training were introduced. Currently, the student has no difficulty discriminating between the two coins in all situations, but periodic rehearsal will continue.

CASE STUDY: GEORGE

George was first seen at the University clinic when he was age 3;9. He had previously received speech-language and physical therapy services in another state. George did not produce any spontaneous words when he first arrived. He did try to imitate or repeat words produced by familiar adults. In one anecdote, George's mother explained that he had asked if a vehicle was a big truck by using a rising intonation within a nonsense word. George was initially a child with a lot of smiles, but somewhat opposing. It was difficult to establish a rapport with him because when he refused to attempt a task, one could not tell whether he was not capable of it or just resisting the requests made by the clinician.

The language intervention approach used was mostly child centered, with a minor emphasis on articulation. A number of play routines were incorpo-

rated into the language session so that George could anticipate the language and initiate requests. For example, when the child was handed the cracker container, it was expected that he would be unable to open it and would have to say, "open," or "help." Later on, unexpected events were substituted for expected ones so that George, in reaching for the juice container, might find it empty or filled with styrofoam chips. The clinician would wait to hear George's comments or requests.

When George was 3;11, formal testing was attempted. He received a receptive vocabulary age on the Peabody Picture Vocabulary Test–Revised (PPVT-R), (Dunn & Dunn, 1981) of 2;4; an expressive vocabulary age on the Expressive One-Word Picture Vocabulary Test (EOWPVT), (Gardner, 1981) of 2;10; a receptive language age on the Sequenced Inventory of Communication Development–Revised (SICD-R), (Hedrick, Prather, & Tobin, 1984) of 2;4; and an expressive language age (SICD) of 3 years. Approximately 1 year later, when George was age 4;9, he was tested again. He received a receptive vocabulary age (PPVT-R) of 3;11 and an expressive vocabulary age (EOWPVT) of 3;2. Thus, over 1 year's time, his receptive and expressive vocabulary increased by nearly 1 year.

When George was age 4;3, his spontaneous word combinations were recorded for 30 minutes during five different occasions over 2 months. The results indicated that George had many two-word utterances in the action plus object form (e.g., "open it," "play playdough," "fix it"); pronoun + verb + object (e.g., "I wanna play Ernie's shoe," "I do it," "I did it," "I go get books," "I can't get it out"); negatives (e.g., "I can't," "No open," "No, I open," "I working not go well"); attributes (e.g., "two buses," "all blue ones," "green monsters," "make some big worms"); questions (e.g., "where's Tracia go?" "what's that?"); possessives (e.g., "I wanna play Ernie's shoe," "Bert's plane," "Cookie Monster has two bears"); be-forms (e.g., "The girl is sad," "Ernie is swinging," "Ernie is reading book," "she is happy"); and locatives (e.g., "put in there," "climb up the wall," "fall down," "right in there," "Bert in plane"). He also used the following pronouns: I, it, you, some, he, that, she. These word combinations would suggest that George was at the linguistic stage of typically developing 3-year-olds: he was about 1 year behind in expressive language compared to his chronological age.

George moved following his 5th birthday. At the beginning of the next school year, he entered a regular kindergarten classroom where he was fully included. He received continued speech-language therapy, physical therapy, and special assistance from an educational specialist. He remained in that classroom for 2 years, and his language skills continued to improve. He also was introduced to reading, and at the end of the 2nd year of kindergarten he was reading at a level comparable to that of his peers. He entered first grade in a fully included program, where he again improved in language and reading. At the end of that year, George's school system recommended that he not receive support services since he was performing at grade level in all academic areas and, therefore, did not qualify for special help. George's parents fought hard for the continued services since it was apparent that his progress was the result of the support he had been receiving. They felt that if those services were discontinued, George would fall behind his peers. Fortunately, George's parents were successful in convincing the school district of their belief, and he continued to receive special services in a fully included classroom.

SUMMARY

In many ways children with DS are both different from, and typical of, most children. They are individuals with varied personalities, strengths, and weaknesses. It is difficult to group them under one physical, behavioral, or communicative pattern because each has a different personality, means of communication, and individual learning strategies. To try and group them together runs the risk of underestimating the individual strengths and capabilities of these children. One purpose of this chapter is to demonstrate the unique qualities of each individual child with DS. On the other hand, there are common characteristics among these children that should not be overlooked, such as frequent middle ear problems, frequent hypotonia, oral motor difficulties, and poor expressive syntax. These characteristics make intervention with these children both a challenge and an intriguing experience. It is hoped that this chapter has identified some of the challenges and provided strategies on how to work with children with Down syndrome.

APPENDIX 6

Resources

National Down Syndrome Congress
1800 Dempster Street
Park Ridge, IL 60068-1146
708-823-7550
1-800-232-NDSC

ARC/Edward I. and Fannie L. Baker
International Resource Center for Down Syndrome
Keith Building, Suite #514
1621 Euclid Avenue
Cleveland, OH 44115
216-621-5858
1-800-899-3039
Fax: 216-621-0221

National Down Syndrome Society
666 Broadway
New York, NY 10012
1-800-221-4602

Research and Resources
Room 465 Waisman Center
University of Wisconsin-Madison
1500 Highland Ave
Madison, WI 53705-2280
608-263-5192

Internet Addresses

Down syndrome pages:

http://www.nas.com/downsyn'
http://ic.net/~defrain/defrain.html
http://members.carol.net/~ndsc/
http://www.nads.org/
http://www.ndss.org/

Association for Retarded Citizens (ARC)
http://fohnix.metronet.com/~thearc/welcome.html

References

Abrahamsen, A., Cavallo, M., & McCluer, J. (1985). Is the sign advantage a robust phenomenon? From gesture to language in two modalities. *Merrill-Palmer Quarterly, 31,* 177–209.

Baird, P. A., & Sadovnick, A. D. (1988). Life expectancy in Down syndrome adults. *Lancet, 2,* 1354–1356.

Baken, R. J. (1987). *Clinical measurement of speech and voice.* Boston: College Hill Press.

Balkany, T. J., Downs, M. P., Jafek, B. W., & Krajicek, M. J. (1978). Otologic manifestations of Down's syndrome. *Surgical Forum, 29,* 582–585.

Balkany, T. J., Mischke, R. E, Downs, M. P., & Jafek, B. W. (1979). Small ears in Down's syndrome: A helpful diagnostic aid. *Journal of Pediatrics, 82,* 845–847.

Baren-Cohen, S., Tager-Flusberg, H., & Cohen, D. (Eds.). (1992). *Understanding other minds: Perspectives from autism.* New York: Oxford University Press.

Barrett, M., & Diniz, F. (1989). Lexical development in mentally handicapped children. In. M. Beveridge, G. Conti-Ramsden, & I. Leudar (Eds.), *Language and communication in mentally handicapped people* (pp. 73–95). New York: Chapman & Hall.

Bayley, N. (1969). *Bayley Scales of Infant Development.* San Antonio: Psychological Corporation.

Beckman, D. (1990). *Oral motor interventions.* Longwood, FL: Author.

Beeghly, M., Weiss-Perry, B., & Cicchetti, D. (1990). Beyond sensorimotor functioning: Early communicative and play development of children with

Down syndrome. In D. Cicchetti & M. Beeghly (Eds.), *Down syndrome: A developmental perspective* (pp. 329–367). New York: Cambridge University Press.

Benda, E. E. (1960). *The child with mongolism.* New York: Grune & Stratton.

Berger, T., & Cunningham, C. C. (1983). Development of early vocal behaviors and interactions in Down syndrome and nonhandicapped infant-mother pairs. *Developmental Psychology, 19,* 322–331.

Blackman, J. (1983). Down syndrome. In J. A. Blackman (Ed.), *Medical aspects of developmental disabilities in children birth to three* (pp. 91–95). Iowa City: University of Iowa Press.

Blanchard, I. (1964). Speech pattern and etiology in mental retardation. *American Journal of Mental Deficiency, 68,* 612–617.

Bloom, L., Lightbown, P., & Hood, L. (1975). Structure and variation in child language. *Monographs of the Society for Research in Child Development, 40*(2).

Bodine, A. (1974). A phonological analysis of the speech of two Mongoloid (Down syndrome) boys. *Anthropological Linguistics, 16,* 1–24.

Breckenridge, M., & Vincent, E. (1960). *Physical and psychological growth through adolescence.* Philadelphia: Saunders.

Breiner, J., & Forehand, R. (1982). Mother-child interactions: A comparison of a clinic-referred developmentally delayed group and two non-delayed groups. *Applied Research in Mental Retardation, 3,* 175–183.

Bricker, D. (1993). Then, now, and the path between: A brief history of language intervention. In A. Kaiser & D. Gray (Eds.), *Enhancing children's communication: Research foundation for intervention* (pp. 11–34). Baltimore: Brookes.

Buckhalt, J. A., Rutherford, R. B., & Goldberg, K. E. (1978). Verbal and nonverbal interaction of mothers with their Down syndrome and nonretarded infants. *American Journal of Mental Deficiency, 82,* 337–343.

Buckley, S. (1995). Teaching children with Down syndrome to read and write. In L. Nadel & D. Rosenthal (Eds.), *Down syndrome: Living and learning in the community* (pp. 158–168). New York: Wiley & Sons.

Buckley, S., Emslie, M., Haslegrave, G., Le Prevost, P., & Bird, G. (1993). *The development of language and reading skills in children with Down's syndrome.* Portsmouth, U.K.: University of Portsmouth.

Byrne, A., Buckley, S., MacDonald, J., & Bird, G. (1995). Investigating the literacy, language and memory skills of children with Down's syndrome. *Down's Syndrome: Research and Practice, 3,* 53–58.

Cadman, D., Shurvell, B., Davies, P., & Bradfield, S. (1984). Compliance in the community with consultants' recommendations for developmentally handicapped children. *Developmental Medicine and Child Neurology, 26,* 40–46.

Cardoso-Martins, C., & Mervis, C. B. (1985). Maternal speech to prelinguistic children with Down syndrome. *American Journal of Mental Deficiency, 89,* 451–458.

Cardoso-Martins, C., Mervis, C. B., & Mervis, C. A. (1985). Early vocabulary acquisition by children with Down syndrome. *American Journal of Mental Deficiency, 90,* 177–184.

Carrow-Woolfolk, E. (1985). *Test for Auditory Comprehension of Language–Revised.* Allen, Tex.: DLM Teaching Resources.

Caselli, M., & Casadio, P. (1995). *Il primo vocabolario del bambino.* Milano, Italy: Franco Angeli.

Caselli, M., Vicari, S., Longobardi, E., Lami, L., Pizzoli, C., & Stella, G. (1998). Gestures and words in early development of children with Down syndrome. *Journal of Speech-Language-and-Hearing Research, 41,* 1125–1135.

Chafe, W.L. (1970). *Meaning and the structure of language.* Chicago: University of Chicago Press.

Chapman, R. (1995). Language development in children and adolescents with Down syndrome. In P. Fletcher & B. MacWhinney (Eds.), *The handbook of child language* (pp. 641–662). Oxford, U.K.: Blackwell.

Chapman, R., Schwartz, S., & Kay-Raining Bird, E. (1991). Language skills of children and adolescents with Down syndrome: I. Comprehension. *Journal of Speech and Hearing Research, 34,* 1106–1120.

Chapman, R., Seung, H., Schwartz, S., & Kay-Raining Bird, E. (1998). Language skills of children and adolescents with Down syndrome: II. Production deficits. *Journal of Speech, Language, Hearing Research, 41,* 861–873.

Chuang, M., & Layton, T. (1992). *Play behavior in Chinese toddlers.* Unpublished manuscript. University of North Carolina at Chapel Hill.

Cicchetti, D., & Stroufe, L. (1976). The relationship between affective and cognitive development in Down's syndrome infants. *Child Development, 47,* 920–929.

Cole, K. (1995). Curriculum models and language facilitation in the preschool years. In M. Fey, J. Windsor, & S. Warren (Eds.), *Language intervention: Preschool through the elementary years* (pp. 39–60). Baltimore: Brookes.

Cooley, W. C., & Graham, J. M. (1991). Down syndrome—An update and review for the primary pediatrician. *Clinical Pediatrics, 30,* 233–253.

Cossu, G., Rossini, F., & Marshall, J. (1993). When reading is acquired but phonemic awareness is not: A study of literacy in Down's syndrome. *Cognition, 46,* 129–138.

Cronk, E., & Annerén. G. (1992). Growth. In S. Pueschel & J. Pueschel (Eds.), *Biomedical concerns in persons with Down syndrome.* Baltimore: Brookes.

Crosley, P., & Doweling, S. (1989). The relationship between cluster and liquid simplification and sentence length, age, and IQ in Down's syndrome children. *Journal of Communication Disorders, 22,* 151–168.

Cunningham, C. C., & Sloper, T. (1977). Parents of Down's syndrome babies: Their early needs. *Child: Care, Health, and Development, 3,* 325–347.

Cunningham, C. C., Morgan, P. A., & McGucken, R. B. (1984). Down's syndrome: Is dissatisfaction with disclosure of diagnosis inevitable? *Developmental Medicine and Child Neurology, 26,* 33–39.

Dahle, A. J., & Baldwin, R. L. (1992). Audiologic and otolaryngologic concerns. In S. M. Pueschel & J. K. Pueschel (Eds.) *Biomedical concerns in persons with Down syndrome* (pp. 69–80). Baltimore: Brooks.

Dahle, A. J., & McCollister, F. P. (1986). Hearing and otologic disorders in children with Down syndrome. *American Journal of Mental Deficiency, 90*, 636–642.

D'Arcy, E. (1968). Congenital defects: Mothers' reactions to first information. *British Medical Journal, 3*, 796–798.

Dodd, B. J. (1975). Recognition and reproduction of words by Down's syndrome and non–Down's syndrome retarded children. *American Journal of Mental Deficiency, 80*, 306–311.

Dodd, B. J. (1976). A comparison of the phonological system of mental age matched normal, severely subnormal and Down's syndrome children. *British Journal of Disorders of Communication, 11*, 27–42.

Dodd, B. J., & Iacono, T. (1989). Phonological disorders in children: Changes in phonological process use during treatment. *Journal of Disorders of Communication, 24*, 333–351.

Dodd, B. J., & Leahy, J. (1989). Disordered phonology and mental handicap. In M. Beveridge, I. Leuder, & C. Conti-Ramsden (Eds.), *Language and communication in mentally handicapped people* (pp. 33–56). London: Chapman Hall.

Dodd, B. J., McCormack, P., & Woodyatt, G. (1994). Evaluation of an intervention program: Relation between children's phonology and parents' communicative behavior. *American Journal of Mental Retardation, 98*, 632–645.

Doherty, W. J., & Baird, M. A. (1986). Developmental levels in family-centered medical care. *Family Medicine, 18*, 153–156.

Dooley, J. F. (1976). *Language acquisition and Down's syndrome: A study of early semantics and syntax.* Ph.D. dissertation, Harvard University, Cambridge, Mass.

Down, J. L. (1866). Observations on an ethnic classification of idiots. *London Hospital. Clinical Lectures and Reports, 3*, 259–262.

Duncan, P. M. (1866). *A manual for the classification, training and education of the feeble-minded, imbecile and idiotic.* London: Longmans, Green & Co.

Dunn, L., & Dunn, L. (1981). *Peabody Picture Vocabulary Test–Revised.* Circle Pines, Minn.: American Guidance Service.

Elliott, C. D. (1983). *British Ability Scales.* Windsor, U.K.: NFER-Nelson.

Engler, M. (1949). *Mongolism.* Bristol, U.K.: John Wright.

Esquirol, J. E. D. (1938). *Des maladies mentales considerees sous les rapports medical, hygienique et medico-legal* [Mental illness considered by the medical, health, and medical-legal reports]. Paris: Bailliere.

Evans, D. (1977). The development of language abilities in mongols: A correlational study. *Journal of Mental Deficiency Research, 21*, 103–117.

Fein, G. (1981). Pretend play in childhood: An integrative review. *Child Development, 52*, 1095–1118.

Fenson, L., Dale, P. S., Reznick, J. S., Thal, D., Bates, E., Hartung, J. P., Pethick, S., & Reilly, J. S. (1993). *MacArthur Communicative Development Inventories: User's guide and technical manual.* San Diego: Singular Publishing Group.

Fowler, A. (1988). Determinants of language growth in children with Down syndrome. In L. Nadel (Ed.), *The psychobiology of Down syndrome* (pp. 217–245). Cambridge, Mass.: MIT Press.

Fowler, A. (1990). Language abilities in children with Down syndrome: Evidence for a specific syntactic delay. In D. Cicchetti & M. Beeghly (Eds.), *Children with Down syndrome: A developmental perspective* (pp. 302–327). New York: Cambridge University Press.

Fowler, A. (1995). Linguistic variability in persons with Down syndrome: Research and implications. In L. Nadel & D. Rosenthal (Eds.), *Down syndrome: Living and learning in the community* (pp. 121–131). New York: Wiley.

Fowler, A., Doherty, B., & Boynton, L. (1995). The basis of reading skill in young adults with Down syndrome. In L. Nadel & D. Rosenthal (Eds.), *Down syndrome: Living and learning in the community* (pp. 182–196). New York: Wiley.

Fowler, A., Gelman, R., & Gleitman, L. (1994). The course of language learning in children with Down syndrome. In H. Tager-Flusberg (Ed.), *Constraints on language acquisition: Studies of atypical children* (pp. 91–140). Hillsdale, N.J.: Erlbaum.

Gardner, M. (1981). *Expressive One-Word Picture Vocabulary Test.* Novato, Calif.: Academic Therapy.

Gayton, W. F., & Walker, L. (1974). Down Syndrome: Informing the parents. *American Journal of the Disordered Child, 127,* 510–512.

Gibson, D. (1981). *Down's syndrome: The psychology of mongolism.* New York: Cambridge University Press.

Greene, K. (1987). Involving parents in teaching reading: A project with nine children with Down's syndrome. *Mental Handicap, 15,* 112–115.

Griffiths, M. I. (1976). Development of children with Down's syndrome. *Physiotherapy, 62,* 11–15.

Guess, D., Sailor, W., & Baer, B. (1974). To teach language to retarded children. In R. Schiefelbusch & L. Lloyd (Eds.), *Language perspectives: Acquisition, retardation, and intervention* (pp. 529–564). Baltimore: University Park Press.

Hadadian, A., & Merbler, J. (1995). Parents of infants and toddlers with special needs: Sharing views of desired services. *Infant-Toddler Intervention, 5*(2), 141–152.

Harter, S., & Chao, C. (1992). The role of competence in children's creation of imaginary friends. *Merrill-Palmer Quarterly, 38*(3), 350–363.

Hartley, X. (1982). Receptive language processing by Down syndrome children. *Journal of Mental Deficiency Research, 26,* 263–269.

Hays, M., Layton, T., & Hooper, C. (1991). *Voice quality of children with Down syndrome based on glottal characteristics.* Paper presented at the American Speech-Language and Hearing Association convention, Atlanta.

Hedrick, D., Prather, E., & Tobin, A. (1984). *Sequenced Inventory of Communication Development*. Seattle: University of Washington Press.

Henderson, E. E., Morris, J., & Frith, U. (1980). The motor deficit in Down's syndrome children: A problem of timing? *Journal of Child Psychology and Psychiatry, 22*, 233–245.

Hollien, H., & Copeland, R. H. (1965). Speaking fundamental frequency characteristics of mongoloid girls. *Journal of Speech and Hearing Disorders, 30*, 344–349.

Horstmeier, D. (1987). Communication intervention. In S. Pueschel, C. Tingey, J. Rynders, A. Crocker, & D. Crutcher (Eds.), *New perspectives on Down syndrome* (pp. 134–156). Baltimore: Brooks.

Igrashi, M., Takahashi, M., Alford, B. R., & Johnson, P. E. (1977). Inner ear morphology in Down's syndrome. *Acta Otolaryngology, 83*, 175–181.

Ingram, D. (1976). *Phonological disability in children*. New York: Elsevier.

Jalongo, M. R. (1984). Imaginary companions in children's lives and literature. *Childhood Education, 60*(3), 166–171.

Johnson, R. C., & Abelson, R. B. (1969). Intellectual, behavioral, and physical characteristics associated with trisomy, translocation, and mosaic types of Down's syndrome. *American Journal of Mental Deficiency, 73*, 852–855.

Kaderavek, J., & Sulzby, E. (2000). Emergent literacy issues for children with language impairments. In L. Watson, E. Crais, & T. Layton (Eds.), *Handbook of early language impairment in children: Assessment and intervention*. Albany: Delmar.

Katims, D. (1991). Emergent literacy in early childhood special education: Curriculum and instruction. *Topics in Early Childhood Special Education, 11*(1), 69–84.

Kay-Raining Bird, E., & McConnell, L. (1994). *Language and literacy relationships in children with Down syndrome*. ASHA presentation paper, New Orleans.

Kogan, K., Wimberger, H., & Bobbitt, R. (1969). Analysis of mother-child interaction in young mental retardates. *Child Development, 40*, 799–812.

Konstantareas, M. M. (1989). After diagnosis, what? Some of the possible problems around diagnostic assessments. *Canadian Journal of Psychiatry, 34*, 549–553.

Korsch, B. M., & Negrete, V. F. (1972). Doctor-patient communication. *Scientific American, 227*, 66–74.

Kouri, T. (1989). How manual sign acquisition relates to the development of spoken language: A case study. *Language, Speech, and Hearing Services in Schools, 20*, 50–62.

Krakow, J., & Kopp, C. (1983). The effects of developmental delay on sustained attention in young children. *Child Development, 60*, 108–118.

Kumin, L, Councill, C., & Goodman, M. (1995). The pacing board: A technique to assist the transition from single word to multiword utterances. *Infant-Toddler Intervention, 5*, 293–303.

Layton, T., & Savino, M. (1990). Acquiring a communication system by sign and speech in a child with Down syndrome: A longitudinal investigation. *Child Language Teaching and Therapy, 6,* 59–76.

Layton, T., & Sharifi, H. (1979). Meaning and structure of Down's syndrome and nonretarded children's spontaneous speech. *American Journal of Mental Deficiency, 83,* 439–445.

Leifer, J. S., & Lewis, M. (1984). Acquisition of conversational response skills by young Down syndrome and nonretarded young children. *American Journal of Mental Deficiency, 88,* 610–618.

Lejeune, J., Turpin, R., & Gautier, M. (1959). Le mongolisme, premier exemple d'abérration autosomique humaine. *L'Année Génétique, 2,* 41–49.

Levy-Shiff, R. (1986). Mother-father-child interactions in families with a mentally retarded young child. *American Journal of Mental Deficiency, 91,* 141–149.

Lind, J., Uvorenski, V., Rosberg, G., & Partanen, L. (1970). Spectrographic analysis of vocal response to pain stimuli in infants with Down syndrome. *Developmental Medicine and Child Neurology, 12,* 478–486.

Lorenz, S., Sloper, T., & Cunningham, C. (1985). Reading and Down's syndrome. *British Journal of Special Education, Research Supplement, 12,* 65–67.

Manosevitz, M., Fling, S., & Prentice, M. (1977). Imaginary companions in young children: Relationships with intelligence, creativity, and waiting ability. *Journal of Child Psychology and Psychiatry, 18,* 73–78.

Manosevitz, M., Prentice, M., & Wilson, F. (1973). Individual and family correlates of imaginary companions in preschool children. *Developmental Psychology, 8*(1), 72–79.

Mans, L., Cicchetti, D., & Stroufe, L. (1978). Mirror reactions of Down's syndrome infants and toddlers: Cognitive underpinnings of self-recognition. *Child Development, 49,* 1247–1250.

Martin, F. N., George, K. A., O'Neal, J., & Daly, J. A. (1987). Audiologists' and parents' attitudes regarding counseling of families of hearing-impaired children. *Asha, 29,* 27–33.

Masel, K. (1987). *Mother-child interaction in Down syndrome and normally developing children.* M.A. thesis, University of North Carolina at Chapel Hill.

Maurer, H., & Sherrod, K. B. (1987). Context of directives given to young children with Down syndrome and nonretarded children: Development over two years. *American Journal of Mental Deficiency, 91,* 579–590.

McLean, J. (1976). Articulation. In L. Lloyd (Ed.), *Communication assessment and intervention strategies* (pp. 325–370). Baltimore: University Park Press.

McWilliam, P. J., Winston, P., & Crais, E. (1996). *Practical strategies for family-centered intervention.* San Diego: Singular Publishing Group.

Meyer, J. R., & Tuber, S. (1989). Intrapsychic and behavioral correlates of the phenomenon of imaginary companions in young children. *Psychoanalytic Psychology, 6*(2), 151–168.

Meyers, L. (1984). Unique contributions of microcomputers to language intervention with handicapped children. *Seminars in Speech and Language: Augmenting Language Skills with Computers, 5,* 23–24.

Michel, J. F., & Carney, R. J. (1964). Pitch characteristics of mongoloid boys. *Journal of Speech and Hearing Disorders, 29,* 121–125.

Miller, J. (1988). Developmental asynchrony of language development in children with Down syndrome. In L. Nadel (Ed.), *Psychobiology of Down syndrome* (pp. 167–198). Cambridge, Mass.: MIT Press.

Miller, J. (1992a). Development of speech and language in children with Down syndrome. In J. Y. Lott & E. McCoy (Eds.), *Clinical care for persons with Down syndrome* (pp. 167–198). Cambridge, Mass.: MIT Press.

Miller, J. (1992b). Lexical development in young children with Down syndrome. In R. Chapman (Ed.), *Processes in language acquisition and disorders* (pp. 202–216). St. Louis: Mosby.

Miller, J., Budde, M., Bashir, A., & LaFollette, L. (1987). *Lexical productivity in children with Down syndrome.* Paper presented at the Annual Convention of the American Speech-Language and Hearing Association, New Orleans.

Miller, J., & Chapman, R. (1993). *Systematic Analysis of Language Transcriptions (SALTI): Version 3.0.* University of Wisconsin-Madison, Language Analysis Laboratory, Waisman Center.

Montague, J. C., Brown, W. S., & Hollien, H. (1974). Vocal fundamental frequency characteristics of institutionalized Down syndrome children. *American Journal of Mental Deficiency, 78,* 414–418.

Montague, J.C., & Hollien, H. (1973). Perceived voice quality disorders in Down syndrome children. *Journal of Communication Disorders, 6,* 76–87.

Morrow, L. (1988) Young children's responses to one-to-one story readings in school settings. *Reading Research Quarterly, 23,* 89–107.

Morrow, L. (1989). The effect of small group story reading on children's questions and comments. In S. McCormick & J. Zutell (Eds.), *Cognition and social perspectives for literacy research and instructions* (pp. 77–96). (38th Yearbook of the National Reading Conference, pp. 77–96). Chicago, Ill.: National Reading Conference.

Motti, F., Cicchetti, D., & Stroufe, L. (1983). From infant affect expression to symbolic play: The coherence of development in Down syndrome children. *Child Development, 54,* 1168–1175.

Nagera, H. (1969). The imaginary companion: Its significance for ego development and conflict solution. *The Psychoanalytic Study of the Child, 24,* 165–196.

Nelson, K. (1973). Structure and strategy in learning to talk. *Monographs of the Society for Research in Child Development, 38*(1–2).

Norris, H. (1989). *Teaching reading to help develop language in very young children with Down's syndrome.* Paper presented at the National Portage Conference, Peterborough, U.K.

Novak, A. (1972). The voice of children with Down syndrome. *Folia Phoniatrica, 24,* 182–194.

Oelwein, P. (1995). *Teaching reading to children with Down syndrome: A guide for parents and teachers.* Bethesda, Md.: Woodbine House.

O'Kelley-Collard, M. (1978). Maternal linguistic environment of Down syndrome children. *Australian Journal of Mental Retardation, 5,* 121–126.

Pentz, A. L. (1987). Formant amplitudes of children with Down syndrome. *American Journal of Mental Deficiency, 92,* 230–233.

Peterson, G. A., & Sherrod, K. A. (1982). Relationship of maternal language to language development and language delay of children. *American Journal of Mental Deficiency, 86,* 391–398.

Piaget, J. (1957). *The language and thought of the child.* New York: World Publishing Company.

Polani, P. E. (1976). Causative factors in Down's syndrome. *Physiotherapy, 62*(1), 2–5.

Power, P. W. (1989). Working with families: An intervention model of rehabilitation nurses. *Rehabilitation Nursing, 14,* 73–76.

Pueschel, S. M. (1991). The person with Down syndrome: Medical concerns and educational strategies. In I. T. Lott & E. E. McCoy (Eds.), *Down syndrome: Advances in medical care* (pp. 55–59). New York: Wiley-Liss.

Pueschel, S. M., & Murphy A. (1976). Assessment of counseling practices at the birth of a child with Down's Syndrome. *American Journal of Mental Deficiency, 81,* 325–330.

Quine, L., & Pahl, J. (1986). First diagnosis of severe mental handicap: Characteristics of unsatisfactory encounters between doctors and parents. *Social Science Medicine, 22,* 53–62.

Racette, K. (1993). *Phonological bases of memory in normal preschoolers and young adults with Down syndrome.* Master's thesis, Bryn Mawr College, Bryn Mawr, Pa.

Rondal, J. A. (1977). Maternal speech in normal and Down's syndrome children. In P. Mittler (Ed.), *Research to practice in mental retardation: Vol. 2. Education and training* (pp. 193–266). Baltimore: University Park Press.

Rondal, J. A. (1978). Developmental sentence procedure and the delay-difference question in language development of Down's syndrome children. *Mental Retardation, 16,* 169–171.

Rondal, J. A. (1988). Language development in Down syndrome: A life-span perspective. *International Journal of Behavioral Development, 11,* 21–36.

Rosin, M. Swift, E., Bless, D., & Vetter, D. (1988). Communication profiles of adolescents with Down syndrome. *Journal of Childhood Communication Disorders, 12,* 49–64.

Scarborough, H. S. (1990). Index of productive syntax. *Applied Psycholinguistics, 11*(1), 1–21.

Schwartz, D. M., & Schwartz, R. H. (1978). Acoustic impedance and otoscopic findings in young children with Down's syndrome. *Archives of Otolaryngology, 104,* 652–656.

Seguin, E. (1846). *Le traitment moral, l'hygience et l'education des idiots* [The moral treatment, hygiene and education of idiots]. Paris: Bailliere.

Seyfort, B., & Spreen, O. (1979). Two-plated tapping performance by Down's syndrome and non–Down's syndrome retardates. *Journal of Child Psychology and Psychiatry, 20,* 351–355.

Singer, D. G., & Singer, J. L. (1990). *The house of make-believe: Children's play and the developing imagination.* Cambridge, Mass.: Harvard University Press.

Smith, L., & Hagen, V. (1984). Relationship between the home environment and sensorimotor development of Down syndrome and nonretarded infants. *American Journal of Mental Deficiency, 89,* 124–132.

Snart, F., O'Grady, M., & Dos, J. P. (1982). Cognitive processing by subgroups of moderately mentally retarded children. *American Journal of Mental Deficiency, 86,* 465–472.

Springer, A., & Steele, M. W. (1980). Effects of physicians' early parental counseling on rearing of Down Syndrome children. *American Journal of Mental Deficiency, 85,* 1–5.

Stoel-Gammon, C. (1981). Speech development of infants and children with Down's syndrome. In J. K. Darby (Ed.), *Speech evaluation in medicine* (pp. 341–360). New York: Grune & Stratton.

Stratford, B. (1985). Learning and knowing: The education of Down's syndrome children. In D. Lane & B. Stratford (Eds.), *Current approaches to Down's syndrome* (pp. 22–56). New York: Praeger.

Strauss, D. & Eyman, R. (1996). Mortality of people with mental retardation in California with and without Down syndrome, 1986–1991. *American Journal on Mental Retardation, 100,* 643–653.

Strazzula, M. (1953). Speech problems of the mongoloid child. *Quarterly Review of Pediatrics, 8,* 268–273.

Strome, M. (1981). Down's syndrome: A modern otorhinolaryngological perspective. *Laryngoscope, 91,* 1581–1594.

Swift, E., & Rosin, P. (1990). A remediation sequence to improve speech intelligibility for students with Down syndrome. *Language, Speech, and Hearing Services in Schools, 21,* 140–146.

Taylor, M., Cartwright, B., & Carlson, S. (1993). A developmental investigation of children's imaginary companions. *Developmental Psychology, 29*(2), 276–285.

Teale, W., & Sulzby, E. (1987). Literacy acquisition in early childhood: The roles of access and mediation in storybook telling. In D. Wagner (Ed.), *The future of literacy in a changing world* (pp. 111–130). New York: Pergamon Press.

Telle, D. W. (1984). Otitis media with effusion during the first three years of life and development of speech and language. *Pediatrics, 74,* 282–287.

Unger, J., Zelazo, P., Kearsley, R., & O'Leary, K. (1981). Developmental changes in the representation of objects in symbolic play from 18 to 34 months of age. *Child Development, 52,* 186–195.

Vostrovsky, C. (1895). A study of imaginary companions. *Education, 15,* 383–398.

Weinburg, B., & Zlatin, M. (1970). Speaking fundamental frequency characteristics of five and six year old children with mongolism. *Journal of Speech and Hearing Research, 13*, 418–425.

Weismer, S. (in press). Language intervention for children with language impairments. In L. Watson, E. Crais, & T. Layton (Eds.), *Handbook of early language impairment in children: Assessment and intervention.* Albany: Delmar.

Westby, C. (1980). Assessment of cognitive and language abilities through play. *Language, Speech and Hearing Services in School, 11*, 154–168.

Whiteman, B. C., Simpson, G. B., & Compton, W. C. (1986). Relationship of otitis media and language impairment in adolescents with Down syndrome. *Mental Retardation, 24*, 353–356.

Wolraich, M. L., & Siperstein, G. N. (1983). Assessing professionals' prognostic impressions of mental retardation. *Mental Retardation, 21*, 8–12.

Yoder, P., Kaiser, A., & Alpert, C. (1991). An exploratory study of the interaction between language teaching methods and child characteristics. *Journal of Speech and Hearing Research, 34*, 155–167.

Yoder, P., & Warren, S. (1993). Can developmentally delayed children's language development be enhanced through prelinguistic intervention? In A. Kaiser & D. Gray (Eds.), *Enhancing children's communication: Research foundations for intervention* (pp. 35–62). Baltimore: Brookes.

Traumatic Brain Injury in Young Children

Jean L. Blosser, Ed.D., CCC-SLP
Interim Associate Provost
University of Akron, Ohio
and
Roberta DePompei, Ph.D.
Professor, School of Communicative Disorders
University of Akron, Ohio

Key Terms

acquired brain injury (ABI)
closed head injury
head injury
intentional injuries
mild traumatic brain injury
moderate traumatic brain injury

open head injury
severe traumatic brain injury
shaken baby–sudden impact
traumatic brain injury (TBI)
unintentional injuries

Overview

"A time was established for each of us to complete our earthly education. Some spirits would come only to be born, to give experience to others and then to quickly pass out of this world"—Eadie, 1992, p. 96.

In the world of traumatic brain injury, there are children who survive and become the best they can be over time; and there are children who live only for a short period of time, but who teach us valuable lessons as they touch our hearts and spirits. This chapter is about those children who continue to develop and learn after sustaining brain injury. But it is dedicated to those children who were intentionally injured and who died, leaving us to share their stories in the hopes that other little people will not be harmed.

The purpose of this chapter is to help the reader understand the epidemiology of acquired and traumatic brain injury, define three assessment phases applicable to the affected population, and describe the interrelationship between assessment and intervention as it focuses on communication skills in this population.

WHO ARE THESE CHILDREN?

Each year approximately 1 to 2 million children and adolescents sustain central nervous system injuries as the result of falls, motor vehicle crashes, sports injuries, assaults, or abuse. Many survive their injuries (some of which appear to be minor) but begin a lifetime of altered development, growth, language acquisition, and learning. This section will report incidence and causes, describe the brain injury, outline the unique characteristics of brain injuries and other problems affecting young children, and discuss developmental issues that influence assessment and intervention.

Incidence and Causes in Younger Children

It is difficult to secure accurate statistics on infants and preschool children who sustain brain injury. Data collection is problematic because hospitals and other agencies that treat infants and young children have not developed systematic or universal guidelines that provide uniform methods for record keeping. Estimates of occurrence from studies that used dozens of diagnostic codes indicated numbers that ranged from 1 of every 40 (National Head Injury Foundation, 1989) to 1 of every 550 (Kraus, Fife, Cox, Ramstein, & Conroy, 1986) of all children. Kraus et al. (1986) reported the specific injury rate of the newborn to 4-year age range as 1 in every 667 children.

Infants and young children appear to be at high risk for death and disability after brain injury. The prognosis for children under the age of 2 is less favorable than for children who are injured during the school-age years (Kaiser, Rudenberg, Frankhauser, & Zumbel, 1986). This finding may be related to two issues. First, the brain of a child in the newborn to 2-year age range is in a period of rapid growth and is particularly vulnerable to this type of injury. Skull strength is less before the sutures between the bones close, and there is less protection when a blow is sustained. Differences in brain structure and physiology, including large head size in relation to body size and blood vessel fragility, can also contribute to severe injury (Dobbing & Smart, 1974; Raimondi & Hirschauer, 1984).

Second, infants who are abused are frequently not seen immediately following injury or at all. Opportunities for medical or rehabilitative intervention often are not provided to these children. They may be lethargic and noncommunicative for long periods of time and may have language learning problems when they enter school.

Additionally, many young children sustain a blow to the head and are seen in emergency departments or physicians' offices, where immediate treatment is provided but long-term follow-through is not indicated. These types of visits often are not recorded or counted in trauma records, and physicians' office records are not easily accessed. Because of the underreporting of mild to moderate injuries and the lack of reporting of many shaken baby incidents, Savage (1994) suggested that brain injuries to young children may be significantly underreported.

Some recent data can provide a picture for causes of brain injury in our nation. The information that follows is compiled from data issued by:

- Arizona Department of Health Services (Arizona Department of Health and Morrison Institute for Public Policy, 1994), which compiled injury information on children age newborn–19 years for the period 1989-1992.

- Ohio Head Injury Incidence Reporting Pilot, completed by the Ohio Head Injury Program and Advisory Council (1994), which compiled data regarding trauma injuries from the period 1991–1992.

- National Pediatric Trauma Registry (1996; DiScala, Osberg, & Savage, 1997), which maintains an ongoing record of trauma to children from 80 children's hospitals across the United States. This registry is continually updated with incidence and cause information. The data from this source represents 12,433 cases, age newborn to 4 years of age, from a total of 45,702 cases (ages newborn to 19) in the registry.

For children in the newborn to 4-year age category, the following information regarding causes is available:

- *Falls:* Two broad categories exist for injury-related falls: (1) those that occur when falling from one level to another (e.g., from a bed, ladder, or playground equipment), and (2) those that occur on a level surface (e.g., by slipping or being pushed or shoved). Falls in the home and community represented about 50 percent of the injuries in this age range and were more often falls from one level to another.

- *Occupant in transportation vehicle:* Motor vehicle crashes or crashes with motorcycles, bicycles, or all terrain vehicles represented about 20 percent of the injuries for this age range. Lack of restraints (seat belts) and helmets was commonly reported as contributing to the severity of the injuries, with those who were not wearing restraints twice as likely to suffer an incapacitating injury as those who were wearing them.

- *Pedestrian:* About 12 percent of all children in this age range were reported to have been involved in pedestrian–motor vehicle accidents.

- *Assault/Abuse/Violence:* Intentional injuries, such as beating, gunshot wounds, stabbings, and blunt trauma to the head, accounted for 11 percent of all injuries in this age range. (An additional 5 to 7 percent of injuries are reported in the "other" category and may or may not also represent intentional types of injuries.) The category of assault/abuse/violence is cause for considerable concern as it represents intentional injury to infants and young children.

National statistics indicate that twice as many males as females are injured. This information is repeated in the state statistics and is consistent with data reported for all age ranges. Table 7-1 is a report of accident scene data from the National Pediatric Trauma Registry. The primary locations for injuries of children this age are at home and on the road. Ewing-Cobbs, Duhaime, and Fletcher (1995) provided a complete discussion of epidemiological and outcome issues in young children, to which the reader is referred for additional information.

Intentional versus Unintentional Injury

There are two categories of injuries to children, intentional and unintentional. **Unintentional injuries** result from unavoidable accidents, whereas **intentional injuries** result from others making choices that will harm children. It may be assumed that injuries resulting from motor vehicle crashes are intentional if the use of alcohol, lack of restraints, and risk taking are involved. However, the category of abuse, assault, and violence implies intentional force employed against another in every case. There is a growing concern about the number of children who suffer physical abuse. It should be noted that many of these children sustain brain injury that may result in a long-term disability.

Reports of child abuse and neglect in this country are increasing annually (Savage, 1995). Large numbers of children, especially those under 1 year of age, are severely shaken and impacted against a surface and sustain massive brain damage. It should be noted that it is the impact against any surface that is of concern rather than the shaking alone. Thus, the term shaken **baby–sud-**

Table 7-1. Scene of Injury by Age (Years)

	< 1yr N=228 %	1–4 yrs N=2,600 %
Home	58.8	56.8
Road	24.1	29.6
School	0.9	0.9
Recreational Area	2.2	3.7
Other	14.0	8.9
Total	100	100

Reprinted by permission from National Pediatric Trauma Registry (1996). *Children and adolescents with disability due to traumatic injury: A data book.* Boston, Mass.: Research and Training Center in Rehabilitation and Childhood Trauma.

den impact has been used to portray the mechanism of the injury more completely (Bruce & Zimmerman, 1989; Duhaime et al., 1987).

Savage (1995) provided a number of facts regarding shaken baby–sudden impact syndrome. They include:

- In 1986 there were 1.5 million reported cases of child abuse/neglect.
- In 1991 there were 1.9 million reported cases of child abuse/neglect.
- Child abuse is the leading cause of death in children under 1 year of age.
- Two-thirds of the abused infants suffer traumatic brain injury (20,000 per year).
- Shaken baby–sudden impact syndrome is the most common diagnosis in hospital pediatric intensive care units.
- The most common presenting complaints in the syndrome include lethargy, decreased muscle tone, respiratory arrest, irritability, seizures, and vomiting.

Savage (1994) conducted a study of perpetrators of abuse affecting 22 children between the ages of 3 months and 18 months. The majority of infants less than 6 months of age were injured by their mothers by nonviolent means (e.g., near-drowning, suffocation, smothering). The majority of children over 6 months of age were injured by a male (e.g., father, boyfriend) by violent means, such as hitting, shaking, or throwing.

Health care and education professionals must become more aware of the symptoms and diagnostic methods for identifying shaken baby–sudden impact syndrome. The delayed onset of neurological symptoms hours after the shaking episode can cause confusion in early detection. Diagnosis is further complicated by the child's inability to describe or explain what has happened or where it hurts. Parents are often reluctant to seek medical attention and do not wish to admit a child has been shaken, or they may be unaware that their child was shaken. Shaking a child is usually not an isolated experience; it is often preceded or followed by other types of abuse. It is essential that the public be made aware of the consequences of this behavior.

BRAIN INJURY DEFINED

A number of terms are used in the literature to describe injury to the brain. These terms are sometimes used synonymously, but they have different meanings. Because different terms are employed, some confusion can be created. Following is a listing of the most commonly used terms.

- **head injury:** damage to any part of the head. This is a broad term that encompasses injury from internal accidents such as stroke or external forces such as a blow to the head. Head injury can imply injury to the face, scalp, skull, or brain (Jones & Lorman, 1989).

- **open head injury:** brain tissue is penetrated from the outside, as with an obvious wound to the head such as a gunshot wound or a crushing of the skull. The injury tends to result in localized (focal) damage and somewhat predictable impairments according to localization and degree of damage (Jennett & Teasdale, 1981; West, Wehman, & Sherron, 1992).

- **closed head injury:** no open wound to the head. Damage is caused by a blunt blow to the head or an acceleration/deceleration of the brain within the skull. This injury results in more diffuse brain damage than open head injuries, with resultant variable and unpredictable consequences (Vogenthaler, 1987).

- **traumatic brain injury (TBI):** "an acquired injury to the brain caused by an external force, resulting in total or partial functional disability or psychosocial impairment, or both, that adversely affects a child's educational performance. The term applies to open or closed head injuries resulting in impairments in one or more areas, such as cognition; language; memory; attention; reasoning; abstract thinking; judgment; problem solving; sensory, perceptual, and motor abilities; psychosocial behavior; physical functions; information processing; and speech. The term does not apply to brain injuries that are congenital or degenerative, or brain injuries induced by birth trauma." ("Definition of traumatic brain injury," 1992, p. 189).

- **acquired brain injury (ABI):** a more general term, which includes both traumatic and non-traumatic injuries to the brain. Savage (1993) outlined the following causes for ABI: open or closed head injury; anoxic injuries caused by such events as anesthetic accidents, hanging, choking, or near-drowning; infections such as encephalitis or meningitis; strokes; tumors; metabolic disorders such as insulin shock and liver or kidney disease; and toxic encephalopathy resulting from lead poisoning, mercury, crack cocaine, and other chemical agents.

Figures 7-1 and 7-2 are diagrams showing how Savage (1993) suggested that ABI and TBI are interrelated, yet distinct.

In addition to terminology used to describe the type of injury to the brain, brain injuries are also described in terms of severity, as follows:

- **mild traumatic brain injury:** a very brief, or no, loss of consciousness occurs at the time of the injury. Signs of injury may include nausea, vomiting, headache, lethargy, or irritability. Infants and small children often do not lose consciousness as readily as older children and adults. They sometimes are considered to have mild injuries when, in truth, more severe damage has occurred (Michaud, Rivira, Grady, & Reay, 1992).

- **moderate traumatic brain injury:** a possible loss of consciousness of up to 24 hours. Infants and toddlers with moderate TBI may have skull fractures or contusions (bruises) of the brain. Some damage may be identified on computerized tomography or magnetic resonance imaging.

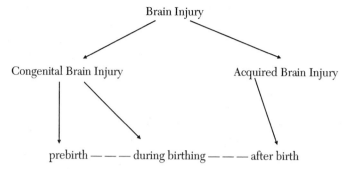

Figure 7-1.   Continuum of possible brain injuries. Reprinted from Blosser, J.L. & DePompei, R. (1992). A proactive model for treating communication disorders in children and adolescents with traumatic brain injury. *Journal of Communication Disorders,* 2(2), 52–65, with permission from Elsevier Science.

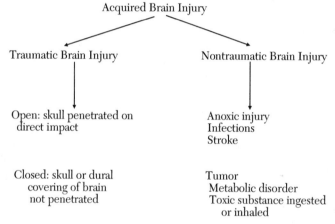

Figure 7-2. Differentiation of acquired brain injury and traumatic brain injury. Reprinted from Blosser, J.L. & DePompei, R. (1992). A proactive model for treating communication disorders in children and adolescents with traumatic brain injury. *Journal of Communication Disorders,* 2(2), 52–65 with permission from Elsevier Science.

- **severe traumatic brain injury:** unconsciousness for more than 24 hours is common. Multiple physical, cognitive-communicative, social, and behavioral problems can arise, and special considerations in the home or preschool are often required as a result.

THE PATHOPHYSIOLOGY OF BRAIN INJURY

Specific and detailed information regarding the pathophysiology of brain injury and the impact of this injury has been discussed in detail by Pang (1985),

Beukelman and Yorkston (1991), Rosenthal, Griffeth, Bond, and Miller (1990), and Graham (1999). The reader is referred to these resources for complete information.

Briefly, the mechanism of injury is as follows: The brain is surrounded by cerebrospinal fluid and encased in a bony skull, which provides protection (Figure 7-3). When a TBI occurs, the force of the acceleration/deceleration moves the brain rapidly within the skull. This movement can result in several types of damage.

Coup-contrecoup: Figure 7-4 shows that damage can be localized (focal) to the area at the point of impact (coup). A second focal injury (contrecoup) can occur as the brain bounces from the point of impact to the opposite side of the skull.

Diffuse axonal shearing: Because the brain floats in cerebral spinal fluid, it moves slightly more slowly than the skull. As the brain sits on the spinal cord, much like a flower on a stem, twisting and swirling movements can produce a forcing together of tissues, a pulling apart of tissues, and a tearing or shearing of axonal fibers (Figure 7-5). These movements can result in widespread (diffuse) damage.

While both types of injury are problematic, in particular the diffuse axonal damage (DAF) can be a major contributor to the overall delay in cognitive development in small children. Ylvisaker (1993) indicated that outcomes from DAF can include slowdown in processing of information, difficulty alerting, attention problems, slowed and more labored gait or speech, fatigue, and difficulty integrating information and organizing responses. This type of injury also forms the basis for understanding the uniqueness of the injury from one child to another, as no two children will suffer identical diffuse damage.

When a TBI occurs there is the potential for considerable damage, some temporary and some permanent. The differences in the type of injury, the areas of

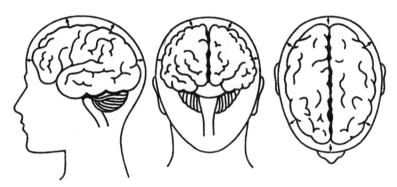

Figure 7-3.   Normal brain position within the skull as viewed from the side, front, and top. From Jones, C. & Lorman, J. (1994). *Traumatic Brain Injury: A Guide for Patient and Family*. Stow, Ohio: Interactive Therapies Inc.

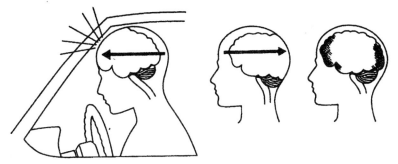

Figure 7-4. Multiple injuries to the brain: Injury occurring at the point of impact and opposite of point as the brain bounces within the skull. From Jones, C. & Lorman, J. (1994). *Traumatic Brain Injury: A Guide for Patient and Family.* Stow, Ohio: Interactive Therapeutics Inc.

the brain affected, and the diffuse versus focal nature of the injury account for the vast variability of preserved ability in some children and new challenges as a result of the acquired disabilities in others. In no population is this injury so challenging as in the newborn to 5-year age group. As the brain is still developing and myelination is incomplete, injury to children in this age range can interfere permanently with the normal acquisition of language, cognitive, and social skills. Several investigators (Mahoney, D'Souza, & Haller, 1983; Raimondi and Hirschauer, 1984) have suggested that infants and toddlers are especially vulnerable to the effects of TBI and that their age is not an advantage in outcome following TBI. Ylvisaker (1993) suggested that this age group may not "rebound" as previously thought and that language development may be seriously affected. Wolcott, Lash, and Pearson (1995) suggested that the idea that "the

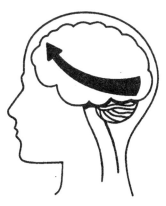

Figure 7-5. Rotational injury to nerve fibers in the brain results as the brain is twisted within the skull. From Jones, C. & Lorman, J. (1994). *Traumatic Brain Injury: A Guide for Patient and Family.* Stow, Ohio: Interactive Therapeutics Inc.

younger the child when injured, the better the recovery" is a myth, and indicated that the brain's ability to rewire itself is more limited in the younger population than once thought. They suggested that while previously learned skills may be intact, the ability to learn new information may be a common problem. Other authors (Ewing-Cobbs, Miner, Fletcher, & Levine, 1989; Klonoff, Low, & Clark, 1977; Levin, Culhane, & Mendelsohn, 1993) have suggested that outcome is often worse in young children than in adolescents and adults.

CHARACTERISTICS OF THIS POPULATION

This population is the only category among those established by the Individuals with Disabilities Education Act of 1990 that is defined by its etiology and not by characteristic behaviors of the disability (Savage, 1997). The specific guidelines provided to qualify for services under the TBI category suggest a number of problems that may exist. However, these problems may exist in any combination, and there are none that must be present in order to qualify for special education services.

There are three important issues to consider when discussing the characteristics of this population: the specific impairments that can emerge after injury, the developmental issues surrounding these children, and the differentiating characteristics.

Specific Impairments That Can Occur

When a preschooler is injured, a variety of physical, social, behavioral, and communicative problems can emerge. The primary areas that may be affected include the following.

Physical Impairments.   The child may have a severe physical motor involvement that results in hemiplegia, or he or she may exhibit deficits in fine motor control that will affect motor development during the first few years of life. Motor control problems can affect the development of adequate speech production, and dysphagia (swallowing and feeding problems) may also result from the injury. Additionally, visual or auditory perceptual problems can occur as a result of traumatic brain injury. Therefore, physical, gross motor, fine motor, vision, and hearing evaluations are essential to the evaluation and treatment of these children.

Communication Disorders.   Communication skills are used to learn and function appropriately in home, school, and community life. These language skills typically develop rapidly at the preschool level. It is often the inability to use adequate language skills in learning and social environments that interferes with successful interactions. Difficulty with communication sometimes leads to a loss of friends, misunderstandings, or poor performance on school tasks. Potential problems with both speech and language should be considered in this population.

Expressive Speech Problems.　Children may exhibit difficulty in formulating phonemes, words, or sentences following TBI. A child may exhibit poor motor planning (apraxia) or muscle control (dysarthria), resulting in unintelligible speech production. Characteristics may include:

- slurred production of words
- drooling
- difficulty swallowing
- hoarse or nasal voice quality
- slowed rate of speech due to motor control difficulty
- increased rate of speech due to reduced self-inhibition and poor self-monitoring skills
- loss of the ability to use verbal speech due to paralysis of the vocal mechanisms

Expressive Language Problems.　There is little empirical information that delineates expressive language difficulties following TBI in the preschool population. Chapman (1995, 1997) suggested that narrative discourse abilities may be a problem after TBI and that the development of these skills may need to be emphasized in treatment. Ewing-Cobbs, Miner, Fletcher, and Levin (1989) reported on expressive and receptive language in infants and preschoolers following closed head injury. Their findings indicated that expressive language, which develops rapidly during the preschool years, appeared to be substantially disrupted in children less that 6 years of age at the time of the head injury. Behaviors that may indicate problems include:

- difficulty remembering a desired word
- problems developing and using new vocabulary
- difficulty with hyperverbal or nonstop talking
- inability to learn or maintain new sentence structures
- inability to learn or increase narrative discourse skills

Receptive Language Problems.　The child with a TBI may have difficulty understanding what is said and may exhibit problems in developing age-appropriate listening skills. Problems may include:

- difficulty following simple directions
- poor recognition of vocabulary
- inability to act after one statement is made—may require multiple repetitions

- difficulty processing auditory information (rate, amount, complexity) at age-appropriate levels
- lack of attention in teaching situations

Cognitive-Communicative Impairments. Cognitive-communication is a combination of the ability to use language and underlying skills such as attention, memory, self-awareness, problem solving, and reasoning to communicate effectively. Underlying skills that may not develop adequately include the following.

Attention. The child's ability to maintain awareness long enough to respond to a stimulus may be affected. Children may have poor vigilance and be unable to sustain attention adequately to complete a task of appropriate length for their age. (Note that the emphasis is on completion of a task rather than maintaining attention for a specified amount of time without task completion.) Dividing attention in the presence of two stimuli may also be a problem. Moreover, the child may not respond in a conversation because the topic was lost in a distracting environment.

Slowed Processing. The child may exhibit a decreased rate for processing what is said and may require additional time to understand. The child also may take a longer than expected amount of time to formulate a response.

Inappropriate Social Interactions. A young child may not learn the pragmatic language skills that are essential for the development of self-awareness. This inability may be demonstrated as difficulty with turn-taking, sharing, rule following, or playing cooperatively. Children with TBI may not be able to organize their thoughts to say what is on their mind, which makes them appear nonresponsive or disinterested.

Memory. The ability to employ short-term memory (information is briefly retained but not stored) and recall what was asked long enough to act on it is often impaired in children with TBI. Long-term memory (information that is stored and can be recalled when needed) can be a problem as well. However, empirical data regarding difficulty with memory in preschoolers after TBI is not provided in the literature. Stimulation for both short- and long-term memory skills should be provided, as with many other preschool populations in which memory skills may be affected (Bleile, 1997; Noonan & Siegel-Causey, 1997).

Inability to Problem Solve. Children may be unable to organize their thoughts to solve problems without much more direction than was needed prior to the injury.

Any of these problems can emerge in unusual combinations in this preschool population. As the majority of information about the characteristics of the preschool population after injury is anecdotal and subject to concerns about other influencing factors, such as environment, socio-economic status, and variability in developmental norms, additional empirical research is needed to further delineate specific characteristics.

Emotional Problems.   Emotional problems can develop after TBI in children. There is very little empirically based evidence regarding very young children and how these problems emerge or what can be done to intervene. O'Shannick (1999) discussed pharmagological intervention for children who are depressed, anxious, aggressive, or self-injurious. Certainly, more empirical information regarding emotional problems in infants and toddlers is needed. Developmental aspects of the preschooler must also be considered.

Developmental Issues

Preschool children are in a period of especially rapid change, during which they progress from complete dependence on others to independent mobility, self-assertion, communication through spoken language, and social interaction. Areas of functioning such as sensory, motor, language, emotional, behavioral, and social interaction are highly interdependent on one another during this developmental period. Consequently, the interruption of functioning in one area is likely to result in difficulty in others and may jeopardize the developmental course of the child (Lehr & Savage, 1991). Several developmental factors must be considered when a child sustains a TBI:

First, the injury can impact the developing brain. Considerable neurophysiological change occurs in the normally developing brain of a preschooler. When a brain injury impacts that developmental process, the ability of the brain to accommodate to the injury must always be considered. Young preschool children have little previously learned information on which to rely in new learning situations. According to Savage (1995) preschoolers have some of the worst recovery records and most difficulty in adapting to brain injury because they have no base of experience from which to draw and because the brain itself is in such an early stage of development.

Second, long-term effects may be cumulative. The injury can, and does, interfere with long-term capacity to develop. Therefore, a possible cumulative effect of impairments must be considered. For example, a 4- or 5-year-old may have developed an adequate vocabulary for his or her age prior to the injury. At the time of testing of vocabulary after the injury, the child may be able to rely on previously learned information and score within normal limits on the assessment. Thus, it may be assumed that the child's language capabilities are not impaired. However, as the child progresses into first or second grade, demands on vocabulary development and the retention of new information may increase and the child may begin to falter. It may take years to recognize the relationship of the brain injury and the decreased learning capacity.

Finally, there may be a delayed onset of disability. Because an injury may affect parts of the brain that are in the process of developing or are not expected to be fully functioning for years to come, it is possible for the effects of the injury not to be apparent for many years after the time of injury (Lehr & Savage, 1991). Various developmentalists, such as Piaget (Furth, 1970) have outlined developmental stages for children. It is possible that a preschooler with TBI will not reach the next developmental stage. It can be years later when a child who was injured during the preschool years first demonstrates an inability to use organizational skills or deductive reasoning. Because so much time has elapsed between the injury and the onset of difficulty, parents and educators may not realize the connection between the earlier TBI and a lack of performance years later.

Differences between Children with TBI and Children with Other Disabilities

When infants and children with brain injury are compared to children with disabilities resulting from congenital problems, some clear differences emerge. First, the onset of a brain injury is sudden. The child was, in most cases, growing and developing age appropriate skills prior to the injury. The family was not learning over time to live with a child who had special needs. Instead, they were suddenly forced to deal with unanticipated alterations in a typically developing child of a nature that can affect the entire family for a lifetime.

Second, a wider range of disability is possible in a child with TBI. After the injury, children can exhibit decreased physical abilities, difficulty with language development, alterations in learning potential, and increased inappropriateness in social interactions. The disabilities can also exist in unusual combinations that are not anticipated and are therefore often not understood or quickly related to the TBI.

Third, the severity of the injury is not necessarily related to the severity of the disability, nor can it predict what the long-term outcome will be. Many children sustain severe injuries yet recover with few long-term problems. On the other hand, some children with mild to moderate injuries may have significant problems with language learning, memory, or behavior control, which may result in lifelong challenges.

Fourth, the potential for dramatic changes in the child exists. There is little information available regarding the speed with which changes can take place in the preschool population. However, it has been reported anecdotally that children with TBI have the potential to change skill levels rapidly. For example, after a brain injury, a child may not have the ability to walk and may be placed in a classroom for children who are orthopedically challenged. Other children in this type of class may never have the potential to walk, yet a child with TBI may recover walking skills sooner than anticipated and no longer belong in such an orthopedically focused environment. This alteration in skill level is often surprising to family, teachers, and other professionals alike.

ONGOING ASSESSMENT AND INTERVENTION

Assessment and intervention are interrelated and must be ongoing as the youngsters progress through medical treatment to increased participation in daily activities. There are three distinct treatment phases that are applicable to this group of children. Phase I is carried out while the child is still recovering medically from the injury. Phase II is conducted after the child is medically stable and is ready to begin receiving habilitative intervention services. Phase III focuses on ongoing assessment and intervention as the child increases participation in daily living and learning activities. The underlying goals for all three phases are the same:

1. to determine the child's and family's strengths and needs at the specific point in time

2. to establish goals for intervention that are appropriate for the child's and family's needs at that time

3. to identify information that professionals should provide for family members so as to increase their understanding of the child's disabilities and needs

4. to identify specific intervention approaches that caregivers and service providers can use to help the child gain important skills and improve functional performance

5. to prepare the caregivers and service providers for their roles in the treatment process

The assessment findings during each of these phases should lead to concrete recommendations for developing a long-term intervention plan.

Phase I

Immediately following a traumatic brain injury, assessment and treatment of the child generally focus on medically related aspects of care and on stabilizing the child's physical condition. The events that have occurred and the confusing medical atmosphere often frighten families. Thus, the family's level of understanding about traumatic brain injury and immediate needs for information and guidance should also be assessed during this time period. Family members should be provided, in a clear and concise manner, with important information about what has happened to their child. Such counseling can serve as the foundation for the long-term intervention plan developed for the child. Hosack and Rocchio (1995) and Blosser and DePompei (1994) have suggested that the following topics be discussed with families:

- the nature and extent of the injury and the child's status (including how the brain functions)
- the contents of medical reports and medical evaluations, including computed tomography (CT) scans and other laboratory results
- the roles and responsibilities of each health care worker and service provider who becomes involved with the child's treatment
- the course of treatment generally followed
- potential problems that may result from the injury
- recommended strategies for becoming involved in the care of the child
- necessary steps the family can take to access services and prepare for future stages of treatment
- ethical, legal, and financial aspects related to the injury
- resources that might provide support and additional information following discharge

Children may demonstrate a wide range of behaviors in Phase I, including a continuum from unconsciousness to adequate communication skills. It is important for the family to know the extent of the damage to the brain, the area of the brain injured, the likelihood of seizure activity, the extent of motoric involvement, and medications the child is taking. When developing an intervention plan it is essential to determine physical care needs that might affect treatment, such as respiratory, swallowing, or motor control problems. (Ylvisaker, 1999, provided an excellent review of assessment and intervention for swallowing, motor, or oral motor problems after TBI.) All these health-related factors will have an impact on the child's functioning after the injury and can influence intervention decisions. Professionals who are treating the child during this time period should seek answers to the following questions:

- What is the child's overall medical status?
- Does this child demonstrate feeding, chewing, or swallowing problems?
- Are there standardized tests that should be administered at this time to determine communication performance capabilities and needs?
- What is the quality of the child's communicative interaction with parents and other family members; with service providers?
- Does the child engage in age-appropriate play and interactions?
- Considering this child's medical condition, how do his or her communication skills compare to those of children of a similar age group?
- Are there any medical treatments that will affect the quality of the child's performance (technological equipment or medication)?
- Taking everything into consideration, how can the child's overall performance be characterized? This description should address cognitive skills,

communication skills, social interaction, physical mobility, behavior, and medical condition.

Questions that professionals should ask the caregivers about the child's communication skills at this time are:

- How would you describe your child's communication skills at this time?
- What differences do you see in your child's ability to communicate now versus how he or she communicated prior to the injury?
- How does your child respond to your attempts to talk and play with him or her?

CASE STUDY: AMY

Amy, age 3, was struck by a car in front of her home. She was hospitalized for 8 weeks. Her parents maintained a vigil by her bedside throughout the entire stay. During this time, Amy was able to respond to simple questions with single words and identify familiar objects. She played quietly with familiar toys in her bed. She was unable to follow simple instructions to play games that had previously been fun for her.

Amy's parents were confused by her actions. The doctors kept insisting that Amy was improving, so her parents expected her to communicate and interact as she had always done. Thus, they began to demand more complex communication from Amy.

Amy's parents were provided with information about problems that could potentially occur following a traumatic injury. Amy's speech and language development and play skills prior to the injury were discussed. Her parents were provided with strategies for stimulating language and interaction without creating stress and frustration for themselves or for Amy. Regular reviews of her progress were scheduled.

Amy's communication continued to develop more slowly than expected. However, her parents responded with greater patience and decreased frustration. They naturally integrated prompts and cues into their interactions with Amy. This resulted in greater success during communication exchanges for both Amy and her parents. Her parents felt that they were better able to understand Amy's needs and respond in a supportive manner.

Phase II

The second phase of treatment focuses on determining the child's functional strengths and needs in a broad range of areas, including cognition, communication, social-emotional, physical, and behavioral domains. Assessment efforts should result in a unique profile of the child that can serve as a focus for discussion during intervention planning.

Professionals charged with assessing young children with TBI may have two reactions. First, they may fear that they lack the capability or tools to complete an appropriate assessment. Indeed, many professionals have no experience in the identification and assessment of children with TBI. In addition, assessment instruments have not yet been designed and standardized specifically for this population. Second, some professionals may attempt to assess the child with TBI using the same frame of reference that is used for assessing other children with more common disabilities. In this case, professionals often find that assessment results do not make sense because they do not fit an expected mold.

For these reasons, it is suggested that the assessment team take time to critically review their current assessment approaches to determine if they are appropriate and applicable for children with TBI. The instruments and procedures selected should sample a broad range of skill areas, provide opportunities for the child to demonstrate skills in natural contexts, and enable examiners to develop a descriptive profile characterizing the child's performance. It is recommended that assessment procedures include activities that facilitate observation of the young child's ability to take part in social and daily routines, acquire and recall new information, learn rules of age-appropriate games, and recall simple vocabulary. Weak performances in skill areas such as these may signal the presence of cognitive-communicative problems. A knowledge of developmental norms in all of the targeted domains is helpful to guide the assessment team's analysis of findings.

To summarize, the assessment of young children with TBI should be guided by the following: (a) knowledge of the characteristics of children with traumatic brain injury; (b) knowledge of typical development of preschoolers; and (c) critical analysis of assessment procedures to determine if they are appropriate for assessing this particular child. Assessment of young children with TBI requires ingenuity, resourcefulness, and collaboration among many professionals and other people who know the child.

Current literature in the areas of early intervention, traumatic brain injury, and special education provides an excellent basis for the team's discussion about assessment procedures (Crais, 1993, 1995; Ewing-Cobbs et al., 1995; Gillette, 1996; Weber, Behl, & Summers, 1994). Several assessment procedures can serve as a focus for team discussion.

Standardized Assessment Instruments. No standardized tests have been developed specifically for assessing children with a TBI. Professionals should consider using available instruments that have been developed for assessing cognitive functioning in the preschool population. The Bayley Scales of Infant Development–Second Edition (Bayley, 1993) permit a global characterization of development and can help professionals identify specific problem areas. Developmental scales such as the Portage Guide to Early Education (Bluma et al., 1976) and the Vineland Adaptive Behavior Scales (Sparrow, Balla, & Cicchetti, 1984) can provide insights into social, emotional, language, motor, and self-help skills. For very young children (8 to 24 months), the Communication and Symbolic Behavior Scales (CSBS), (Wetherby & Prizant, 1993), can be used to profile the child's behaviors across communication, symbolic and constructive play, and book interaction skills. The MacArthur Communicative Development Inventories (MCDI), (Fenson et al., 1993), can be used to look at production vocabulary and early syntactic information in 8- to 30-month-old children. The younger version (8-16 months) includes both production and comprehension, common gestures, social games, play imitation of parents, and some symbolic play items. In addition, the MCDI is a standardized measure that utilizes parent report and therefore can be viewed as a tool for systematic observation of the child by family members (discussed subsequently).

As with other preschool populations, caution should be exercised when administering and interpreting results of standardized tests such as those listed here. These instruments were not specifically designed for the preschooler with TBI. The results cannot provide information about how the child would function under natural circumstances; however, the astute professional can use findings to supplement data obtained via other assessment approaches. One advantage of standardized tests is that they often consist of subtests that focus on specific areas of concern.

Professionals should seek information about the extent of the injury, including the degree, type, and distribution of tissue damage. This information can contribute to the team's understanding of the potential deficits that might be present. Segments of standardized tests as well as informal testing procedures that are designed to evaluate specific cognitive and communication behaviors can then be selected and administered as part of a comprehensive testing protocol.

Functional Assessment Procedures. These assessment approaches permit a practical analysis of the child's functional skills in various environmental contexts. Functional assessment techniques require the assessment team to perform continuous observations of the child in diverse environments with changing expectations and demands. Four applicable functional assessment procedures are: (1) interviews or surveys of family members and other important people in the child's world; (2) systematic observation by the family; (3) systematic observation by service providers in varying contextual situations within the healthcare and education settings; and (4) curriculum-based assessment.

Interviews and Surveys. Interviews and surveys are viable means for obtaining information about a child's functional abilities. These techniques can be used to obtain valuable information about the child's preinjury status and medical history (relevant to the injury), as well as current behaviors. The types of interview questions that professionals can ask family members are described in subsequent sections.

Systematic Observation by Family. Direct observation is often the most useful means for understanding the child. The contexts of the home, community, and play environments provide much opportunity for determining children's strengths and needs. Observation within these diverse contexts helps foster a better understanding of the child's special needs on the part of family members. It also encourages the infusion of intervention approaches into the home setting. However, parents and other caregivers will not be able to provide quality information unless they are provided with structured guidance and assistance for completing observations. During the assessment phase, time should be allocated for interviewing key family members and discussing with them how to conduct observations to obtain information about the child.

Systematic Observation by Health Care and Education Service Providers. Observing the child with TBI during play or learning activities in day-care or preschool situations can yield worthwhile information about how he or she is functioning. Interaction in play is generally nonthreatening and unobtrusive. Therefore, play offers a great opportunity for constructing a profile of the child's strengths and needs (Weber et al., 1994). Play scales developed by Westby (1980), Linder (1994), Fewell (1984), and Fewell and Rich (1987), as well as the play components from the CSBS (Wetherby & Prizant, 1993), can be used as formats for observing the child's performance in play. Scales such as these provide a basis for characterizing and profiling a child's behaviors so that the assessment team can deduce an age range that correlates with cognitive, language, social-emotional, and sensorimotor achievements. These results can then be used to derive recommendations for an intervention plan. Abilities that are present during play may signal the degree of the child's readiness to learn specific types of information or skills. In addition, family members and service providers can develop perceptions about useful intervention strategies (Weber et al., 1994). When provided with proper guidance, family members can also learn to gather and report data about the child's functioning during play at home. Observations made during play afford professionals and families opportunities for creating a profile of the child's strengths and needs in the following skill areas: play, cognitive functioning, language functioning, sensorimotor functioning, and social-emotional functioning. Emerging skills in each area can also be identified.

Curriculum-based Assessment. Early childhood curricula provide an excellent point of reference for exploring children's strengths and needs because they represent skills and behaviors that must be mastered in home and preschool environments. Sample available curricula include the Assessment, Evaluation, and Programming System (AEPS), (Bricker, 1993, 1996), and the Carolina Curriculum for Infants and Toddlers with Special Needs (Johnson-Martin, Jens, Attermeier, & Hacker, 1991). Both instruments can also be utilized by both professionals and family members for systematic observation of the child.

Selection and Interpretation of Assessment Procedures. During Phase II, it is important to determine the child's strengths and needs in a broad range of skill areas. When selecting assessment procedures and reviewing evaluation results, assessment team members should answer the following questions:

- What segments of our assessment protocol are appropriate for assessing this child, considering the information we have received about the nature of injury and services provided to date?
- Does the child have adequate motor control for respiration, phonation, and articulation?
- Can the child maintain attention for completion of age-appropriate tasks?
- During interaction and play situations, is the child able to appropriately communicate his or her intent?
- What receptive and expressive communication/language skills does the child demonstrate?
- Do the child's responses to instructions or questions appear slower than expected considering the child's age and the situation?
- Are the child's pragmatic language skills appropriate for the situational context?
- Taking everything into consideration, how can the child's overall performance be characterized? This description should include cognitive skills, communication skills, social interaction, physical mobility, and behavior.

The assessment team should encourage family members to participate meaningfully in the assessment process by providing them with specific instructions and guidelines for observing the child's behaviors in various situations. Their input can be obtained by asking questions such as the following:

- Can you describe typical ways your child communicated prior to the injury?
- What changes have you noticed in your child's communication since the injury?
- If you give your child one, two, or three things to do, can he or she complete the directions? Does he or she need clues or assistance from you?
- Is your child's vocabulary growing? Can you provide examples of new and big words that your child has recently used?
- How does your child communicate when playing with other children?
- If your child wanted you to [get him or her a drink, buy a toy for him or her at the store], how would he or she let you know? Does he or she do so differently than he or she would prior to the injury?

CASE STUDY: ALLEN

Allen was 2 years old when he was severely assaulted by his mother's boyfriend. His right side was paralyzed. Consequently, his motor control for speech was impaired. Day-care workers and Allen's mother reported that his speech and language development had been progressing typically prior to the injury. He was placed in foster care after discharge from the hospital. At 3 months post-injury, Allen was observed to struggle during physical activities. He was able to follow simple one-step directions, but his vocabulary development appeared to be arrested. He withdrew from other children during play activities, and he demonstrated little initiative for new learning.

The intervention goals established during this phase were as follows:

1. determine a simple, effective communication system that Allen and his foster parents can use to communicate with one another (based on his motor, sensory, and cognitive abilities)

2. help Allen's foster family understand how to utilize opportunities for presenting new vocabulary and stimulating language

3. identify vocabulary that will help Allen successfully access people and items in his environment

4. help the family understand and respond to his communication attempts

5. provide the family with strategies for developing Allen's oral-motor skills

6. keep Allen's natural mother informed of progress, needs, and suggestions in case Allen is returned to her home

Phase III

Assessment should lead to selecting specific intervention strategies for teaching new skills or changing behaviors. The least intrusive procedures are often the most effective for young children. It is recommended that assessment and treatment strategies be integrated into the child's daily living and learning activities. Caregivers, teachers, and other service providers must become an integral part of the assessment and intervention process. This will lead to long-term intervention and follow-up.

Family members, educators, and others can play a major role in intervention. They must learn to: (a) recognize that the child is experiencing difficulty; (b) relate the difficulty to the underlying deficit; and, (c) know what to do to provide assistance, when to provide the assistance, and how to provide it (Blosser & DePompei, 1994).

To successfully incorporate family members and others into the intervention program, the environment and individuals encountered within that environment must also be the subject of assessment. Blosser and DePompei (1994) refer to this phase of assessment as "scanning and analyzing the environment." Thus, in addition to participating as team members to help analyze the child's behaviors, the caregivers within the environment and the characteristics of the environment must themselves also be analyzed.

Environmental assessments should be made in the home, community, and preschool environments. Conducting an environmental assessment does not necessarily imply on-site observation. Although this may be the preferable method, it is not always a realistic option. Therefore, alternative techniques of obtaining information may be implemented, such as questionnaires, surveys, phone calls, group discussions, videotapes, and anecdotal reports.

The environmental analysis is comprised of three steps. First, the professionals and caregivers identify the demands and expectations that will confront the child in various situations. Demands may be created by elements or people in the environment. Examples of environmental elements that pose unique demands and expectations for children include rules, routines, expectations for communication, space allocations, time allocations, visual and auditory distractions, changing contexts for interaction, and various forms of work materials. The purpose of an environmental assessment is to produce a profile of the most important factors around which treatment goals and objectives can be formulated. The success of the intervention process will be partially dependent on creating more favorable environmental conditions for communication.

Children encounter many people in their environments. It is imperative to begin with a clear understanding of the communication partners the child will encounter—who they are, what they understand about TBI, how they communicate and interact with the child, and their potential for participating in intervention. Each of these people display unique manners and styles of communication during interactions with the child, including variations in rate and quality of speech, word choice, organization of conversations, method of providing directions, responsiveness to the child's queries, and recognition of the child's problems.

In the second step of scanning and analyzing the environment, the professionals and caregivers must decide if the demands and expectations or communicative interaction manners and styles facilitate successful interactions or pose obstacles to success for the child. For example, a child who has difficulty understanding complex communication will have difficulty understanding his or her parent's instructions to perform a task. This may lead to frustration, which in turn may result in punishment. Blosser (1990) developed a communication style identification chart for assessing significant communicators' mannerisms and style of communication. The results can be used as a basis of discussion for formulating concrete recommendations (Blosser & DePompei, 1992, 1994, 1995; Neidecker & Blosser, 1993).

In the third step of the environmental scan, the professionals and family work together to specify the opportunities in the daily routine that can be seized for implementing intervention strategies. This will help identify the most appropriate times throughout the day for initiating instruction or interacting with the child to gain the maximum benefit.

Each of these dimensions must be explored in order to develop a relevant intervention plan. The influence of environmental factors is frequently overlooked and not considered when planning treatment programs for young children with TBI. The next case study presents a planning format for gathering data about the child and the environment. It can be used for team review and analysis and to support planning efforts. Information can be supplied by family members, health care professionals, rehabilitation professionals, and education team members. The composite picture then can be sorted and discussed during team planning meetings. If organized systematically in a report or outline format, the information can be used as a guide for development of the Individualized Family Service Plan (IFSP) or Individualized Education Plan (IEP), or for periodic, ongoing case review and discussion in subsequent meetings. The findings can serve as a framework for further assessment and intervention planning.

CASE STUDY: JOHN

John, age 4 years, was injured after falling from a sliding board at preschool. He was hospitalized in the local hospital for 3 weeks. He then was transferred to a pediatric rehabilitation facility in a neighboring state for 6 months because, due to the extent of his medical needs, his parents were unable to care for him in the home. His parents were expected to continue intervention procedures in the home following his discharge from the rehabilitation facility. John's parents and 6-year-old brother were excited to have him return home. They were looking forward to resuming a normal routine. Within 2 weeks, however, they realized that John's needs were still great. Although he had recuperated physically, there was still much that he needed to accomplish.

The following is an illustration of how an environmental scanning and analysis process was used to determine John's needs and recommend intervention strategies. Steps were taken to develop a comprehensive description of John's current status including medical, physical, communication, motor, social, emotional, and behavior skills. The professionals and family members determined that John's fine and gross motor movements were labored and his speech was unintelligible. Language production was limited to one- and two-word utterances. He seemed to have forgotten vocabulary and skills he had gained prior to the injury. His play was solitary, and he exhibited outbursts when he became frustrated or could not obtain toys or assistance. If distracted by noises and objects, he would lose interest in what he was doing.

The environmental demands and expectations that confronted John in various contexts were determined. The professionals and his parents concluded that his parents expected him to follow simple instructions, play with playmates who came to visit, and observe established routines for meals and bedtime. When they talked with John, his parents expected correct responses. There was much activity in the house, with the television on most of the time and toys scattered throughout.

The mannerisms and style of the significant people in John's environment were analyzed to determine the positive or negative impact on his performance. The analysis included John's parents, siblings, teacher, and caregivers. John's mother was an energetic person, who talked continuously as she moved around him in the course of caretaking and her daily activities. His father was slower paced, did not talk much, and enjoyed reading. His brother used many voices as he engaged in role-playing games. He liked to spend time with John and was very inquisitive about what had happened to him. Finally, John's teachers were attentive and caring but had had little experience with children with special needs.

This information was synthesized to determine the demands, expectations, and interpersonal interactions that may represent strengths for John. Several environmental elements and people who could provide positive opportunities for success for John were identified. John's mother and teachers showed interest in providing stimulation. His mother was creative in her attempts to help John resume home life, and requested ideas for helping. His teachers were trying hard to understand John's needs and individual styles of learning. John's father provided a calming influence and was willing to read to him, and his brother seemed to know how to engage John in interactive play.

The information was also synthesized to determine those demands, expectations, and interpersonal interactions that may pose obstacles for John. Everyone agreed that the two different adult communication styles exhibited by John's parents could be problematic because John had to constantly shift between the two, trying to match his communication attempts to the different demands. His mother worried that she was overstimulating him, while his father wondered if he was providing enough stimulation.

Specific intervention strategies were discussed and agreed on based on the results of the analysis. Various interactive communication strategies were suggested to be used by his different partners. John's mother was encouraged to slow her rate of speech; position herself closer when talking directly to John; use simple, short sentences when talking; and remove distractions during rest time. Recommendations to John's father included reading simple books and varying his voice and intonation when reading key words. It was also suggested that he encourage John to point to pictures that match words. John's brother was encouraged to play "quiet games" with John such as cards and blocks, help John remember the names of toys, and talk about actions while engaged in play. John's teachers were encouraged to help him feel a bigger part of circletime activities by helping him contribute the simple words that he could use. They were encouraged to help him use "survival words" (short words that could help him signal his needs, such as "no," "more," "juice," "potty," "help," and the names of his favorite toys), and to help him develop different ways to get his needs met (e.g., through eye gaze, gestures, vocalizations, and word approximations as well as words and word combinations).

Guidelines for Environmental Scans. The types of questions that can guide the professional through the environmental scan and analysis such as the one developed for John are as follows:

- What environmental situations does this child participate in daily within the home, community, or school situation?

- What are the demands and expectations held for the child in each of the primary situations (contexts)?
- Is the child able to meet these expectations? If not, why not, and how is the inability characterized?
- What problems could arise when the demands and expectations of the environment exceed the child's skill level?
- What assistance or modifications would be necessary to enable the child to meet the demands and expectations?
- What solutions to the problems that arise can be proposed to help maintain this child in each particular environmental situation?
- How can the demands and expectations be altered to better match the child's capability?
- Who are this child's primary communication partners within each of these environmental contexts?
- What are the communication mannerisms and style exhibited by each of the primary communication partners?
- Is the child able to understand and respond positively to the communication partners' mannerisms and styles? If not, what is the nature of the mismatch?
- What modifications can communication partners make in order to facilitate successful interactions and promote positive learning?
- What communication strategies should communication partners learn in order to facilitate improvement and promote success for the child?
- What opportunities do the daily routines offer for implementing key intervention strategies?

Creating a Strong Assessment Team

Children who sustain a traumatic brain injury often pass through numerous service delivery settings, including medical, rehabilitation, and school. Therefore, cooperation among personnel from a wide number of disciplines and agencies is essential for planning and implementing appropriate intervention.

It is important to provide needed information to key personnel who will function on the TBI assessment team, including family members. This will ensure that each member has an opportunity to gain in-depth understanding of the cognitive-communication, learning, physical, social, psychological, and behavioral characteristics that are often associated with traumatic brain injury. In addition, it will provide a forum for personnel to discuss their perceptions of the obstacles or opportunities that exist for the child. A successful alignment of team goals and expectations is critical to effective treatment.

SUMMARY

Intervention goals and treatment strategies for young children with TBI should be based on factors that will lead to the greatest potential improvement for the child and family. In the context of communication, this means that the skills selected for development must be important for improving the child's ability to function successfully in home and learning situations. There are two areas of focus for intervention that should be considered: providing direct service to the child, and providing indirect service by altering the expectations of the environment and the communication behaviors of the child's significant communication partners.

References

Arizona Department of Health, and Morrison Institute for Public Policy. (1994). *Arizona's child and adolescent injury data book.* Phoenix: Arizona Department of Health Services, Office of Women's and Children's Health.

Bayley, N. (1993). *Bayley Scales of Infant Development* (2nd ed.). San Antonio: Psychological Corporation.

Beukelman, D. R., & Yorkston, K. (1991). *Communication disorders following traumatic brain injury: Management of cognitive, language, and motor impairments.* Austin, Tex.: Pro-Ed.

Bleile, K. (1997). Language intervention with infants and toddlers. In L. McCormick, D. Loeb, & R. Schiefelbusch (Eds.), *Supporting children with communication difficulties in inclusive settings* (pp. 307–334). Needham Heights, Mass.: Allyn & Bacon.

Blosser, J. (1990). *Making your SLP program relevant to educational needs.* Luzerne County Schools Inservice Day, Scranton, Penna.

Blosser, J., & DePompei, R. (1992). A proactive model for treating communication disorders in children and adolescents with traumatic brain injury. *Clinics in Communicative Disorders, 2*(2), 52–65.

Blosser, J. L., & DePompei, R. (1994). *Pediatric traumatic brain injury: Proactive interventions.* San Diego: Singular Press.

Blosser, J., & DePompei, R. (1995). *Let's talk and listen today! Calendars of daily activities for developing language and listening skills.* Phoenix: ECL Publications.

Bluma, S., Shearer, M., Frohman, A., & Hilliard, J. (1976). *Portage guide to early education.* Portage, Wisc.: Cooperative Education Service Agency 12.

Bricker, D. (ED.). (1993). *AEPS Measurement for birth to three years.* Baltimore: Brookes.

Bricker, D. (ED.). (1996). *AEPS Measurement for three to six years.* Baltimore: Brookes.

Bruce, D. A., & Zimmerman, R. A. (1989). Shaken impact syndrome. *Pediatric Annals, 18*, 482–494.

Chapman, S. (1997). Cognitive-communication abilities in children with closed head injury. *Journal of Speech-Language Pathology, 6,* 50–58.

Chapman, S. (1995). Discourse as an outcome measure in pediatric head-injured populations. In S. Broman & M. E. Michel (Eds.), *Traumatic head injury in children* (pp. 95–116). New York: Oxford University Press.

Crais, E. (1993). Families and professionals as collaborators in assessment. *Topics in Language Disorders, 14*(1), 29–40.

Crais, E. (1995). Expanding the repertoire of tools and techniques for assessing communication skills of infants and toddlers. *American Journal of Speech-Language Pathology, 4*(3), 47–59.

Definition of traumatic brain injury. 57 *Federal Register* 189 (1992, Sept. 29).

DiScala, C., Osberg, S., & Savage, R. (1997). Children hospitalized for traumatic brain injury: Transition to postacute care. *Journal of Head Trauma Rehabilitation, 12*(2), 1–10.

Dobbing, J., & Smart, J. L. (1974). Vulnerability of developing brain and behavior. *British Medical Bulletin, 30,* 164–168.

Duhaime, A. C., Gennarelli, T., Thibault, L., Bruce, D., Marguiles, S., & Wiser, R. (1987). The shaken baby syndrome: A clinical, pathological, and biomechanical study. *Journal of Neurosurgery, 66,* 409–415.

Eadie, B. J. (1992). *Embraced by the light.* Placerville, Calif.: Gold Leaf Press.

Ewing-Cobbs, L., Duhaime, A., & Fletcher, J. M. (1995). Inflicted and noninflicted traumatic brain injury in infants and preschoolers. *Journal of Head Trauma Rehabilitation, 10*(5), 13–24.

Ewing-Cobbs, L., Miner, M. E., Fletcher, J. M., & Levin, H. S. (1989). Intellectual, motor, and language sequelae following closed head injury in infants and preschoolers. *Journal of Pediatric Psychology, 14,* 531–547.

Fenson, L., Dale, P., Reznick, S., Thal, D., Bates, E., Hartung, J., Pethick, S., & Reilly, J. (1993). *MacArthur Communicative Development Inventories.* San Diego: Singular Publishing.

Fewell, R. (1984). *Play Assessment Scale* (4th ed.). Unpublished ms., University of Washington, Seattle.

Fewell, R., & Rich, J. S. (1987). Play assessment as a procedure for examining cognitive, communication, and social skills in multihandicapped children. *Journal of Psychoeducational Assessment, 2,* 107–118.

Furth, H. (1970). *Piaget for teachers.* Englewood Cliffs, N.J.: Prentice-Hall.

Gillette, Y. (1996). Early intervention in communication development: A model for professionals consulting with families. In M. Smith, & J. Damico (Eds.), *Childhood language disorders* (pp. 300–324). New York: Thieme Medical Publishers.

Graham, D. I. (1999). Pathophysical aspects of injury and mechanisms of recovery. In M. Rosenthal, E. Griffeth, J. Kreutzer, & B. Pentland (Eds.), *Rehabilitation of the adult and child with traumatic brain injury* (pp. 19–41). Philadelphia: Davis.

Hosack, K. R., & Rocchio, C. A. (1995). Serving families of persons with severe brain injury in an era of managed care. *Journal of Head Trauma Rehabilitation, 19*(2), 57–65.

Jennett, B., & Teasdale, G. (1981). *Management of severe head injuries.* Philadelphia: Davis.

Johnson-Martin, N., Jens, K., Attermeier, S., & Hacker, B. (1991). *Carolina curriculum for infants and toddlers with special needs* (2nd ed.). Baltimore: Brookes.

Jones, C., & Lorman, J. (1989). *Head injury.* Stow, Ohio: Interactive Therapeutics.

Jones, C., & Lorman, J. (1994). *Traumatic brain injury: A guide for patient and family* (rev. ed.). Stow, Ohio: Interactive Therapeutics.

Kaiser, G., Rudenberg, A., Frankhauser, I., & Zumbuhl, C. (1986). Rehabilitation medicine following severe head injury in infants and children. In A. J. Raimondi, M. Chous, & C. DiRocco (Eds.), *Head injuries in the newborn and infant* (pp. 263–279). New York: Springer-Verlag.

Klonoff, H., Low, M. D., & Clark, C. (1977). Head injuries in children: A prospective five year follow-up. *Journal of Neurology, Neurosurgery, and Psychiatry, 40*, 1211.

Kraus, J. F., Fife, D., Cox, P., Ramstein, K., & Conroy, C. (1986). Incidence, severity, and external causes of pediatric head injury. *American Journal of Public Health, 140*, 687–694.

Lehr, E., & Savage. R. (1991). Community and school integration from a developmental perspective. In J. S. Kreutzer & P. Wehman (Eds.), *Community integration following traumatic brain injury* (pp. 301–309). Baltimore: Brookes.

Levin, H. S., Culhane, K. A., & Mendelsohn, D. (1993). Cognition in relation to magnetic resonance imaging in head-injured children and adolescents. *Archives of Neurology, 50*, 897.

Linder, T. (1994). *Transdisciplinary play-based assessment.* Baltimore: Brookes.

Mahoney, W. J., D'Souza, B. J., & Haller, J. A. (1983). Long term outcome of children with severe head trauma and prolonged coma. *Pediatrics, 71*, 756.

Michaud, L. J., Rivira, F. P., Grady, M. S., & Reay, D. T. (1992). Predictors of survival and severity of disability after severe brain injury in children. *Neurosurgery, 31*, 254–264.

National Head Injury Foundation. (1989, December). *Head injury update.* Presented at the National Head Injury Annual Symposium, Washington.

National Pediatric Trauma Registry. (1996). *Children and adolescents with disability due to traumatic injury: A data book.* Boston: Research and Training Center in Rehabilitation and Childhood Trauma.

Neidecker, B., & Blosser, J. (1993). *School programs in speech-language pathology: Organization and administration.* Boston: Allyn & Bacon.

Noonan, M. J., & Siegel-Causey, E. (1997). Special needs of young children with severe disability. In L. McCormick, D. Loeb, & R. Schiefelbusch

(Eds.), *Children with communication difficulties in inclusive settings* (pp. 405–432). Needham, Mass.: Allyn & Bacon.

Ohio Head Injury Program and Advisory Council. (1994). *Ohio head injury incidence reporting pilot.* Columbus: Ohio Rehabilitation Services Commission.

O'Shannick, G. (1999). Pharmacological intervention. In M. Ylvisaker (Ed.), *Traumatic brain injury rehabilitation: Children and adolescents* (pp. 53–59). Boston: Butterworth-Heineman.

Pang, D. (1985). Pathophysiological correlates of neurobehavioral syndromes following closed head injury. In M. Ylvisaker (Ed.), *Head injury rehabilitation: Children and adolescents* (pp. 3–70). San Diego: College Hill Press.

Raimondi, A. J., & Hirschauer, I. (1984). Head injury in the infant and toddler. *Child's Brain, 11,* 12–35.

Rosenthal, M., Griffeth, E., Bond, M., & Miller, J. D. (Eds.). (1990). *Rehabilitation of the adult and child with traumatic brain injury.* Philadelphia: Davis.

Savage, R. (1993, January 6). *Defining acquired/traumatic brain injuries* (Testimony to the U.S. Congressional Committee on Special Education). Washington: Author.

Savage, R. (1994, November). *Shaken baby-sudden impact syndrome.* Unpublished manuscript.

Savage. R. (1995, December). *Shaken baby-sudden impact syndrome.* Presentation to the Pediatric Task Force of the National Head Injury Foundation, San Diego.

Savage, R. (1997). Integrating rehabilitation and education services for school-aged children with brain injuries. *Journal of Head Trauma Rehabilitation, 12*(2), 11–20.

Sparrow, S., Balla, D., & Cicchetti, D. V. (1984). *Vineland Adaptive Behavior Scales.* Circle Pines, Minn.: American Guidance Service.

Vogenthaler, D. R. (1987). Rehabilitation after closed head injury: A primer. *Journal of Rehabilitation, 53*(4), 15–21.

Weber, C., Behl, D., & Summers, M. (1994). Watch them play, watch them learn. *Teaching Exceptional Children, 27*(1), 30–35.

West, M., Wehman, P., & Sherron, P. (1992). Applications for youth with traumatic brain injury. In P. Wehman (Ed.), *Life beyond the classroom: Transition strategies for young people with disabilities.* Baltimore: Brookes.

Westby, C. E. (1980). Assessment of cognitive and language abilities through play. *Language, Speech and Hearing Services in Schools, 11,* 154–168.

Wetherby, A., & Prizant, B. (1993). *Communication and Symbolic Behavior Scales* (1st ed.). Chicago: Riverside.

Wolcott, G., Lash, M., & Pearson, S. (1995). *Signs and strategies for educating students with brain injury: A practical guide for teachers and schools.* Houston: HDI Publishers.

Ylvisaker, M. (1993). *Assessment and treatment of traumatic brain injury with school aged children and adults.* Buffalo: EDUCOM.

Ylvisaker, M. (Ed.). (1999). *Traumatic brain injury rehabilitation: Children and adolescents.* Boston: Butterworth-Heineman.

Landau-Kleffner Syndrome: Acquired Childhood Aphasia

Melody Harrison, Ph.D., CCC-SLP
Associate Professor
University of North Carolina
Chapel Hill

Key Terms

acquired aphasia
auditory agnosia
electroencephalogram (EEG)
Landau-Kleffner syndrome
paroxysmal electroencephalogram
status epilepticus

Overview

Language delay in young children is not a rare occurrence. In the majority of these cases, the child either initiates language usage at a later than typical age or develops linguistic competency at a delayed rate. It has been estimated that between 2 and 3 percent of school-age children have language delays (Silva,

1980). However, very few children begin to develop language in a normal manner at the appropriate time, only to then rapidly lose their acquired language abilities. Among those who do, a causal agent or factor such as head trauma, tumor, or illness can almost always be identified. There is, however, a group of children with **acquired aphasia** who exhibit no discernible cause for the deterioration of their language abilities.

In the four decades since Landau and Kleffner (1957) described a syndrome of acquired aphasia with convulsive disorder and **paroxysmal electroencephalogram abnormalities** in children, more than 160 cases have been presented in the literature (Paquier, Hugo, Van Dongen, & Loonen, 1992). Although the prevalence and incidence of this condition are unknown, the ratio of males to females in the cases reported is two to one (Miller, Campbell, Chapman, & Weismer, 1984). Although it is generally assumed to be a very rare condition, **Landau-Kleffner syndrome** (LKS) has been described more frequently than any other type of acquired childhood aphasia, such as might occur following a traumatic brain injury or a tumor. The clinical features, although variable, have been well documented. LKS typically manifests itself between the ages of 18 months and 13 years, with onset usually occurring between 3 and 7 years (Sawhney, Suresh, Dhand, & Chopra, 1988; Tharpe & Olsen, 1994). Males are most often affected, accounting for 65 percent of the reported cases (Miller et al., 1984). Although the **electroencephalogram (EEG)** is invariably abnormal, clinical seizures do not occur in all children with LKS. That is, it may not be apparent to an observer that the child is experiencing abnormal EEG activity. Until the onset of symptoms, the child's language, cognitive, and psychomotor skills develop uneventfully. Seizures and aphasia are equally likely to be the first symptom of the syndrome. Inattentiveness to sound and loss of language abilities may be either sudden or gradual. A full 75 percent of the children have very sudden language loss, which sometimes progresses from a typical level of functioning to a postmorbid state within a few hours (Miller et al., 1984). The other 25 percent of cases experience gradual language regression over a course of months.

Children with LKS often give the impression of having developed a sudden-onset hearing loss; however, reliable behavioral evaluation of hearing can be difficult because of their problems in comprehending, attending to, and responding to the tasks involved in audiologic assessment. Depending on the degree of **auditory agnosia** present at the time of testing, hearing levels ranging from normal hearing to profound hearing loss may be documented with behavioral audiometry. In those cases when auditory evoked potentials have been obtained at the time of behavioral measures, the results have been consistent with normal peripheral hearing even when behavioral measures have suggested the presence of a hearing loss (Msall, Shapiro, Befour, Niedermeyer, & Capute, 1986; Penn, Friedlander, & Saling, 1990; Tharpe, Johnson, & Glasscock, 1991).

The language deficits associated with LKS affect both the receptive and the expressive domains. Difficulty with auditory comprehension is the first language-related symptom to appear, and may become so severe and pervasive as to prevent the comprehension of nonspeech sounds. Receptive language skills may regress from the ability to process oral communication competently, to a level of total unresponsiveness to language (Paquier et al., 1992). The receptive breakdown is followed by deterioration in expressive language. The expressive abilities of individuals in acute stages of the syndrome can also vary widely. These language dysfunctions may fluctuate, lasting anywhere from a day to several months or years, and may reappear numerous times throughout childhood. During periods of remission, the child's receptive and expressive language may improve significantly.

ETIOLOGY

In 1957, when they first described the syndrome, Landau and Kleffner hypothesized that the persistent convulsive discharges observed in the temporal lobe might cause the functional ablation of the primary cortical areas subserving language and result in language deficits. In spite of dozens of clinical reports of the syndrome, the etiology remains unknown. The relationship between the abnormal electrical activity, seizures, and aphasia is not understood, and the course of the disorder and ultimate prognosis for recovery are unpredictable. In the early 1990s, Landau (1992) called for an international, interinstitutional study of LKS. Noting the complete lack of epidemiological data for LKS in regard to infectious disease, toxins, nutrition, geography, or other environmental factors, Landau identified etiology as the number one question to be investigated in such an effort.

Despite the consistent pattern of EEG abnormalities, clinical examinations have not revealed any relevant, associated neurologic signs. The results of auditory evoked potentials, early neurologic examinations (other than language), and central nervous system function have also been found to be normal in children with LKS (Hirsch et al., 1990). Evaluation of the structural integrity of the brain has provided no consistent pattern of lesions or abnormality that could account for the symptoms expressed in the syndrome. In all but three reported cases of LKS, structural deficits were not detected by computed tomography (CT) scans, magnetic resonance imaging (MRI), or cerebral angiography. Otero, Cordova, Diaz, Garcia-Terval, and del Brutto (1989) presented a case of neurocysticerosis that was found deep in the left sylvian fissure in a child with symptoms of LKS. Another study reported the case of a 3-year-old boy whose seizures stopped and language improved after a temporal lobectomy with partial resection of a low-grade astrocytoma (Solomon, Carson, Pavlakis, Fraser, & Labar, 1993). The third case in which structural deficits were found was a 6-year-old girl with LKS secondary to inflammatory, demyelinating disease. In this case, the MRI showed small lesions in both the white matter of the left periventricular frontal lobe and in the right parietal centrum semiovale (Perniola, Margari, Buttiglione, Andruela, Simone, & Santostasi, 1993).

Although a consistent pattern of structural deficits has not been found, functional differences in metabolic activity have been exhibited by some children with LKS. Using positron emission tomography (PET), Maquet, Hirsch, Dive, Salmon, Marescaux, and Franck (1990) found functional differences in metabolic activity in the temporal lobes of five children with LKS. Cole et al. (1988) reported on a child with LKS and intractable, complex, partial seizures. Using PET to investigate metabolic activity, they found a 50 percent decrease in glucose utilization in the right temporal lobe, as compared to glucose utilization in the left temporal lobe. O'Tuama, Urion, Janicek, Treves, Bjornson, & Moriarity (1992) used single-photon emission computed tomography (SPECT) to investigate cerebral perfusion (the rate of flow of blood to tissue) as an indirect assessment of brain function in five patients with classic LKS symptoms. They found that asymmetric temporoparietal perfusion appears characteristic of LKS. The abnormal perfusion pattern occurs across the range of seizure behavior, appearing in children with seizures as well as those without. This characteristic pattern of perfusion is different from that found in other children with language disorders studied by this group. O'Tuama and colleagues concluded that their findings, in conjunction with the metabolic abnormalities described in the PET studies, may be indicative of central pathogenic features of the disorder. The relationship of the EEG abnormalities found in LKS and the metabolic patterns described in these studies deserves continued investigation.

A number of other etiologies have been suggested by a variety of investigators. Woorster-Drought (1971) suggested that LKS is the result of an autoimmune chronic encephalitis involving the temporal lobes; however, subsequent pathology reports on tissue from two patients who had undergone temporal lobectomies indicated no evidence of encephalitis. Holmes, McKeever, and Saunders (1981) proposed that the EEG abnormalities in childhood aphasia are not the cause of language abnormality but rather are an epiphenomenon of the underlying pathology of areas of the brain concerned with language function. The lack of correlation between the degree of abnormal EEG activity and degree of language impairment experienced by the child supports this argument. Some investigators have proposed that this syndrome has more than one etiology. Deonna, Beumanoir, Gaillard, and Assal (1977) described several clinically distinct subcategories of LKS and suggested that the variability in recovery among children with the syndrome could be a function of the differing pathogenesis. Despite the interest generated by this syndrome, the pathogenesis remains undefined 40 years after its initial description.

DIAGNOSTIC ISSUES

Until the onset of epilepsy or the rapid deterioration of language abilities, children with LKS follow a typical developmental course. Family and personal histories have not been found to be positive for patterns of either epilepsy or childhood language disorders. Differential diagnosis of LKS is based on the presence of two factors: an acquired aphasia that appears in conjunction with an abnormal, paroxysmal (showing the sudden onset of a seizure) EEG. The encephalographic disturbances are usually bilateral, and the temporal region is always involved. The EEG abnormalities, which are characterized by spikes, sharp waves, or spike-and-wave discharges, may be most significant during sleep (Shu-Xian, Xi-Ru, Chin, & Shou-Yu, 1989). This syndrome is classified among the epilepsies with both focal and generalized seizures (Genton et al., 1992).

The relationship between EEG abnormalities, seizures, and language deficits is confusing. Although up to 80 percent of children with LKS have seizures, about 20 percent experience deterioration in language abilities without accompanying seizures (Shu-Xian et al., 1989). Of those children who do develop seizures, approximately 40 percent experience seizures prior to developing aphasia, 40 percent develop seizures after the onset of aphasia, and 20 percent experience the simultaneous onset of seizures and aphasia (Rapin, Mathis, Rowan, & Gordan, 1977). A correlation between severity of seizure activity and severity of the aphasia has not been demonstrated. Moreover, individuals experiencing seizures may have them infrequently and often outgrow them by adolescence (Beaumanoir, 1985).

The occurrence of abnormal activity in an EEG that is recorded while the child is awake is not directly predictive of the course of accompanying aphasia. After the onset of LKS, the normalization of the EEG does not necessarily indicate that there will be an improvement in the aphasia in the near future. However, the observation that improvement in language function occurs only after the EEG has become normal strongly suggests that the aphasia is the result of a "functional disorganization of the cortex subserving speech. . . . the longer the period of epileptic discharges, the more the cortex is affected and the longer it takes to recover. After a long period of time, cortical disorganization may become irreversible" (Lerman, Lerman-Sagie, & Kivity, 1991, p. 259). Six patients with LKS were reviewed by Paquier et al. (1992), who reported that despite the varied clinical course of the syndrome and the unpredictable nature of the aphasia, the epilepsy and electroencephalographic abnormalities usually regressed or disappeared as the children aged.

PROGNOSIS

One of the several puzzling aspects of this syndrome is the variability in long-term outcome. The course of the aphasia is characterized by fluctuations in remissions and exacerbations. Reporting on nine children who had been followed for 10 or more years since the onset of LKS, Mantovani and Landau (1980) found that four had fully recovered language function, one experienced mild language dysfunction, and four others had moderate dysfunction. When the recovery of language function does occur, the residual deficits can vary from mild phonological disorders to receptive and expressive language difficulties significant enough to require placement in a special education class.

Recovery can take place either within days of onset of symptoms or over a period of years. Bishop (1985) reviewed 45 cases from the literature in which there was follow-up until the children reached an age of at least 12 years and suggested that the age of onset of symptoms may be a factor in prognosis in that the younger the age of onset, the poorer the prognosis for full recovery. Initially, this may seem counter to what is known about the relationship of brain plasticity to age. It has been shown that before approximately 5 years of age, the brain demonstrates a great deal of plasticity in language function. In cases of structural brain disease or trauma occurring prior to that age, the brain is capable of effectively shifting language function from the dominant hemisphere to the opposite side. If it is the case that the early onset of symptoms of LKS is predictive of a poor prognosis for the recovery of language function, there are at least two explanations for the failure of a functional shift; either the hemisphere that is dominant for language function is not compromised enough to force a shift or the dysfunction is bilateral. A hypothesis of bilateral involvement is supported by numerous reports of bilateral, abnormal EEG recordings (Gascon, Victor, Lombrosco, & Goodglass, 1973; Hirsch et al, 1990; Tuchman, 1994). Among the patients followed by Mantovani and Landau (1980), the four adults who attained full recovery experienced the onset of LKS symptoms between 5 and 9 years of age, slightly beyond the theorized maximum age of brain plasticity. Those whose symptoms began before the age of 5 years experienced residual language deficits. The long-term outcomes for these patients supports the observation by Bishop (1985) that age of onset is a key factor in prognosis.

COMMUNICATION

In their initial description of the syndrome, Landau and Kleffner (1957) described five children, each of whom had experienced typical acquisition of speech and language but subsequently developed aphasia. They hypothesized that "persistent convulsive discharge in the brain tissue largely concerned with communication, results in functional ablation of these areas from normal linguistic behavior" (p. 529). Numerous studies have documented the nature of the aphasia, which is almost always described as beginning with receptive language difficulties (Landau & Kleffner, 1957; Mantovani & Landau, 1980; Miller et al., 1986; Tharpe & Olsen, 1994). Most often, parents report that the children initially behave as if they have lost their hearing. They fail to respond to comments or requests and generally seem unable to understand language that had previously been easily comprehended. It is not unusual for children to fail a hearing evaluation at this juncture. Although they may be able to hear pure tone stimuli, they are incapable of understanding the verbal instructions regarding what the task is and how they are to respond. In their initial report, Landau and Kleffner emphasized the importance of obtaining a differential diagnosis from that of peripheral nerve deafness. The degree of receptive language involvement has been reported to vary widely. Receptive language skills may regress from the ability to competently process oral communication to a level of total unresponsiveness to language (Paquier et al., 1992). Some of the children are able to understand simple commands, whereas others appear to be unaware of spoken language. Worster-Drought (1971) reviewed the histories of 14 children with LKS and reported that some were able to follow simple oral commands whereas others were completely unresponsive to verbal stimuli. Although the term aphasia has been applied to this population, its use is problematic. Aphasia implies the loss of an intact language system; however, because many of the children are still developing language when they acquire LKS, it is possible that language acquisition is affected.

All reported cases of LKS involve receptive and expressive language to varying degrees (Tharpe et al., 1991). Typically, expressive language problems occur as a gradual increase in misarticulations and a decrease in sentence complexity. Depending on the length of the auditory agnosia, speech can deteriorate to the use of single words, jargon-like speech, or in some cases, total mutism. Some children express a variety of misarticulations, others have word retrieval problems or produce inappropriate paraphasias, and others exhibit expressive fluent aphasias. Mutism is also seen among children with LKS. Based on a review of the case studies published in the 30-year period following Landau and Kleffner's initial description, Miller et al. (1984) reported that communication problems reoccurred or persisted in 94 percent of the cases. In 80 percent of the children they studied, the disruption in language abilities persisted for longer than 6 months.

Some of the children with LKS are able to maintain a near-normal voice, whereas others develop atypical vocal qualities. Speech with a high fundamental frequency and lacking in normal inflection, similar to that of deaf children, was observed in some of the children studied by Miller et al. (1984).

Despite the significant receptive and expressive language disruptions that occur as a component of LKS, the children's literacy abilities often are far superior to their use of spoken language. Campbell and Heaton (1979) reported that the reading comprehension abilities of the children they saw were advanced in comparison to their levels of comprehension of oral language.

Denes, Balliello, Volterra, and Pelligrini (1986) reported on a 10-year-old boy who began to lose language at the age of 3 years. Beginning at 6 years of age, his mother taught him to match pictures with the written word. He was able to learn to read and write well enough to attend his local primary school. Denes and colleagues described an almost total dissociation of written and oral language. Although skills involving phonemic discrimination, identification, or production were completely absent, the boy displayed excellent comprehension and production of single written words. His lexical/semantic ability was clearly within normal limits; however, his comprehension and production of sentences was selectively impaired. In tasks requiring the use of free morphemes, such as articles and prepositions, his comprehension and production were highly impaired; however, in tasks using bound morphemes (such as "s," "ing"), his performance was similar to that of typically developing children of his age. The authors pointed out that his performance supports the hypothesis of Caramazza, Berndt, and Basili (1983), that producing and understanding function words requires some form of phonological coding and decoding.

Numerous other examples of literacy abilities among children with LKS can be found. Miller et al. (1984) described an 11-year-old who demonstrated deficits in auditory comprehension of spoken language but could match a written word with the appropriate picture. The preservation of reading, writing, and signing ability was observed in a patient with uncontrollable seizure behavior and acquired aphasia (Cole et al., 1988). Gordon (1990) observed that children with the syndrome respond best to language in a visual modality and suggested that schools can use that relative strength to provide them with a means of communication. Hirsch et al. (1990) reported on a boy who first experienced symptoms of LKS at age 4;5, yet was successfully taught to read at 9 years of age.

It should be noted, however, that among children who were in the process of acquiring reading and writing skills, these skills have been shown to deteriorate after the onset of symptoms (Harrison et al., in press; Hirsch et al., 1990; Rapin et al., 1977). Gordon hypothesized that skills that have been recently acquired or are in the process of acquisition have not been sufficiently embedded in long-term memory and are therefore vulnerable to any disturbance of function.

Other forms of visually represented language have also been successfully employed as a communication strategy. Tharpe and Olsen (1994) described a child who was diagnosed with LKS at 41 months. Within 1 year following enrollment in a total communication classroom, she had acquired more than 200 signs and her expressive sign language consisted of two- to three-word utterances. The fact that reading, writing, and the use of sign language may be relatively spared suggests that this is not a true aphasia but rather verbal auditory agnosia.

BEHAVIOR

Behavioral problems have frequently been described in children with LKS. Among the numerous behavioral issues associated with the syndrome are hyperactivity, aggressiveness, inattentiveness, temper tantrums, depression, and withdrawal (Beaumanoir, 1985; Gordon, 1990; Tharpe at al., 1991; White & Sreenivasan, 1987). Mantovani and Landau (1980) noted the prevalence of behavioral abnormalities among children with LKS and reported that in at least half the patients described in the literature, hyperactivity was present. Sawhney et al. (1988) reported on a 5-year-old boy who developed irritability, hyperactivity, and destructive behavior following the development of LKS.

Night terrors or nightmares (Genton et al., 1992; Shoumaker, Bennet, Bray, & Curless, 1974) and sleep disturbances (Kellerman, 1978) are also frequently mentioned as problems among children with LKS. A plausible explanation of such symptoms is that they may well be secondary to the confusion and frustration children experience when they become unable to understand and communicate with others. Mantovani and Landau (1980) hypothesized a more neurophysiologic basis for the behaviors, suggesting that these problems are a reflection of a primary disinhibition of the limbic system of the brain, which provides regulatory function of emotions and affect.

Although rare, psychotic behavior has been reported. Cole et al. (1988) described a patient who began to experience LKS symptoms at the age of 4½ years. At 13 years of age she was described as having strikingly poor social adjustment, and over the next 10 years her behavior deteriorated to such a degree that it was described as being similar to that of individuals with schizophrenia. Hirsch et al. (1990) reported on five children, one of whom experienced an initial onset of symptoms at age 6;3, and was described at age 10;9 as having intellectual deficits and psychotic behavior.

Because the expression of symptoms is highly variable, LKS is often misdiagnosed, at least initially, as autism, hearing loss, an emotional or behavioral disorder, or another type of acquired aphasia. The resulting management of the child may be inadequate or inappropriate.

TREATMENT

Both surgical and pharmacological management of the symptoms associated with Landau-Kleffner syndrome have been reported in the literature.

Surgery

Cole et al. (1988) reported on the surgical treatment of two patients with LKS. The first patient, a 7-year-old boy, exhibited a classic onset of LKS symptoms. Following a normal pregnancy and delivery, he walked and used his first word by 12 months. When he was 2 years old, his family reported that he began to have difficulty understanding spoken commands. They thought he was unable to hear. Following an adenoidectomy, the boy's understanding of language began to improve; however, at 4 years of age he again experienced difficulty understanding spoken language. Although seizures were never present, his expressive and receptive language abilities fluctuated widely over the next 3 years. When he was 6½ years old, an initial EEG showed epileptogenic (epilepsy-causing) activity from the left posterior temporal and parietal regions. At that time his Performance IQ was reported as 91, however his language abilities were reported to be between 2 and 3 years. At the age of 7 years he underwent a left temporal lobectomy. At the time of this surgery, the natural course of LKS was unclear and it was hoped that removal of the tissue producing continuous electrical abnormalities would improve his language functioning. In fact, immediately after the operation his communication abilities began to change rapidly. By the time of discharge the child was forming five- to seven-word sentences and his auditory comprehension was reported to have improved. He was enrolled in a special first grade class and received additional language therapy.

At reevaluation 10 months later, he was able to identify colors and name objects. He counted to 30 with two errors. A slight dysarthria was noted. Although language comprehension had improved, he continued to experience difficulty discriminating between words that sounded similar. Compared to the evaluation that occurred immediately after surgery, he was able to remember twice as many details from an orally presented story. An EEG revealed active epileptogenic discharges from the left mid- and posterior temporal regions. Unfortunately, shortly after the 10-month postoperative evaluation, both his language and EEG deteriorated. Not long after he was lost to further follow-up.

The other patient, a girl, followed a very different course, not only in the development of the syndrome but also in surgical outcome. Until she was 4½ years old she followed an unremarkable and typical developmental course. At that time her parents noticed that she began to hesitate in responding to oral directions and requests, and within 15 months, her language had regressed to complete verbal agnosia with mutism. An EEG showed spike activity; however, no other details are available from the initial report.

When she was 6 years old the child experienced her first seizure. An EEG showed bursts of generalized, multiple spike discharges, which were followed by slow waves. She was treated with an anticonvulsant and remained seizure free for 1 year; however, the verbal agnosia and mutism continued. The next year she once again began to have seizures, and she experienced eight generalized seizures and four episodes of generalized **status epilepticus** between the ages of 7 and 12 years. (Status epilepticus occurs when generalized seizures follow one another without the recovery of consciousness between attacks.)

When she was 12 years old, she began to have seizures that were described as complex, partial seizures characterized by staring, chewing, and automatic movements of the right hand. Although no formal measures were administered, at 13 years it was reported that verbal deficits were severe and that she used sign language and fingerspelling to communicate. Her behavior was described as withdrawn and uncooperative.

Over the next 10 years the girl experienced frequent complex partial seizures and infrequent generalized convulsions. As a 28-year-old adult she could read and write simple sentences and occasionally used sign language and fingerspelling to communicate. Although she continued to be mute, audiograms and brainstem auditory evoked potentials were consistent with normal hearing. Her score on the Peabody Picture Vocabulary Test–Revised (Dunn & Dunn, 1981) was at the 2;6-month level, and she was able to respond correctly to 38 of the first 40 items on the Token Test of Language Comprehension (DiSimoni, 1978).

At the age of 28 years, a portion of the left anterior temporal lobe was surgically removed in an attempt to control the complex partial seizures. One year after the surgery, the frequency of seizures had been reduced by 90 percent. Although neuropsychological testing demonstrated a continued severe disturbance of speech skills, her parents reported a qualitative improvement in her communication abilities.

In the late 1960s, Morrell and colleagues began to explore the benefits of a surgical procedure to eliminate the ability of cortical tissue to generate seizures while maintaining the physiologic integrity and normal cortical function of vital motor and language areas of the brain (Morrell, 1973; Morrell et al., 1995; Morrell & Hanberry, 1969; Morrell & Whistler, 1982; Morrell, Whistler, & Bleck, 1989). The procedure they developed was capable of selectively disrupting the horizontally running intracortical fibers, which are necessary to generate hypersynchronous eliptiform discharges, while sustaining minimal injury to the main cortical elements, which are vertically arranged and are the architectural building blocks of normal cortical functioning. In 1995, Morrell et al. reported outcomes on a clearly delineated subgroup of 14 children with Landau-Kleffner syndrome who met the following criteria and subsequently underwent subpial intracortical transection. The first criterion was that a striking discrepancy between verbal and nonverbal IQ scores must be shown, thus ruling out children with pervasive developmental delay or autism. The disorder had to have been electrophysiologically identified as having a unilateral origin of the EEG abnormality. In addition, the child had to have been without effective language for at least 2 years and had to have developed age-appropriate speech prior to the onset of the disorder, thus eliminating children with so-called developmental aphasia.

Following surgery, 7 of the 14 children (50%) recovered age-appropriate speech and language and were placed in regular classrooms. None of the 7 required speech-language services. Another 4 of the 14 (29%) demonstrated marked improvement. They were able to understand verbal instruction and were speaking, but they still received speech-language services. The language abilities of the other 3 children did not improve. Based on these results, this procedure appears to provide a viable treatment not previously used in the management of LKS.

Drug Therapy

Treatment with anticonvulsants is often undertaken to manage the seizure activity of children with LKS. The seizures, which may begin independently from the onset of aphasia, usually respond to treatment with anticonvulsants and have a good prognosis (Hirsch et al., 1990; Mantovani & Landau, 1980; Sawhney et al., 1988). Although most reports have found anticonvulsants to have no effect on the aphasic component of LKS, Deuel and Lenn (1977) suggested that antiepileptic treatment should be used, not merely to halt seizure activity but also to improve language functioning. They found that the addition of primidone (an anticonvulsive drug used in treating epilepsy) after seizure control was established can be effective in improving language function. Tharpe et al. (1990) reported improvement in responsiveness to sound in two patients following successful seizure control with anticonvulsants. Despite some reports of modest improvements in language ability following treatment with anticonvulsants, the current prevailing medical opinion is that their use, while effective for seizures, does not appear to have a significant effect on the accompanying aphasia (Paquier et al., 1992).

In 1991, there were only three reports of the use of corticosteroids in the treatment of LKS. As early as 1974, McKinney and McGreal reported the rapid recovery of language in three patients who were given steroids. Among six other patients, who did not receive corticosteroids, only one recovered. Four years later, Kellerman (1978) reported the recovery of a patient following treatment with prednisone; however, the effects of the drug were questioned because spontaneous remissions had occurred in this child both with and without the drug. In 1984, Van der Sandt–Koenderman, Smit, Van Dongen, and Van Hest reported remission, relapse, and an eventual spontaneous recovery following treatment with prednisone. However, the recovery was thought to be coincidental to the drug therapy. More recently, Lerman et al. (1991) reported on four patients who appeared to have made a full recovery of language function following treatment with corticosteroids. They suggested that timing the steroid treatment early after the onset of auditory agnosia and using the appropriate dosage are critical to outcome.

Education

Although many studies mention school placement and enrollment in speech-language therapy (Gordon, 1990; Paquier et al., 1992; Penn et al., 1990) and some provide suggestions for management (Tharpe et al., 1991; Tharpe & Olsen 1994), much less has been published regarding therapeutic/educational management than medical management. The following case study is presented to provide information regarding the assessment and management of a school-age child with LKS.

CASE STUDY: WILL

Will was placed in a residential school for the deaf at 9½ years of age after suffering lengthy, acute episodes of Landau-Kleffner syndrome starting from

7 years of age. After less than 1 year, the staff at the school became concerned that the placement was inappropriate and requested a multidisciplinary eval-uation so that recommendations for educational placement and strategies for learning could be made.

At the time of the assessment, Will was 11 years old. His prenatal and natal histories were unremarkable, and his developmental milestones were within normal range, except for language, which was delayed. By parent report, Will had an expressive vocabulary of approximately five words at 24 months of age. Initially, his language delay was thought to be due to chronic otitis media. Tympanostomy tubes were placed when he was 1 year old and again at age 2. Speech-language therapy was begun at 27 months of age but was terminated 8 months later.

Will first exhibited obvious signs of LKS at 7 years of age. His parents reported that he suddenly seemed unable to hear for a period of several days. He was seen by a physician who treated him for otitis media. Over the following 8 months, he experienced several more episodes of apparent sudden hearing loss and was treated for recurrent otitis media. By the following spring, the periods of hearing loss had increased in duration to more than several weeks each. During these episodes, Will was unable to understand speech. He was seen by a physician, who prescribed Ritalin in response to the child's increasing irritability and inability to concentrate; however, after approximately 6 months, the Ritalin was discontinued because there was no change in Will's behavior.

Hearing status: When Will experienced another period of apparent hearing loss at age 8;6, his parents had his hearing evaluated at a local hearing and speech center. Typanometry revealed normal middle ear function in both ears; however, Will could not be conditioned to respond to pure-tone auditory stimuli under headphones. The evaluation was terminated and, although another appointment was suggested, his family did not return. He continued to be unresponsive to sound. The following month, at the age of 8;7, he was seen by an audiologist and an otolaryngologist on the military base where his parents were living. The examination by the otolaryngologist revealed no physical abnormalities. The audiologist reported that Will's responses to behavioral testing were unreliable, and he was referred for electrophysiologic assessment. Click-evoked auditory brainstem response (ABR) wave latencies and latency-intensity functions were within normal limits bilaterally. At age 8;8, he was referred to a pediatric neurology clinic at a nearby university hospital.

An EEG obtained by the pediatric neurologist was abnormal, with frequent focal spike discharges in both central head regions. There was no seizure activity associated with the generalized discharges, nor was there a history of seizures. An MRI performed the same day revealed no abnormalities. A diagnosis of LKS was made on the basis of intermittent auditory agnosia with associated paroxysmal electroencephalogram (EEG). At the time of diagnosis Will was age 8;9. An EEG obtained 2 months later, at age 8;11, was also consistent with the EEGs of children with LKS.

Communication status: *During the third grade, Will's acute episodes of LKS increased in duration and severity. To compensate for his inability to comprehend oral language, Will and his teachers used a computer to communicate. This proved adequate until his reading and writing abilities began to deteriorate. From the ages of 8;11 to approximately 9;8, Will was unable to understand any oral language. His parents reported to the neurologist that his behavior was characterized by increased frustration and decreased self-esteem. His speech was marked by slurring, an abnormally slow rate, and monotone pitch.*

Beginning just prior to his 9th birthday and continuing until the age of 9;6, trials of several anti-seizure medications (i.e., Tegretol, Depakote, and Verapamil) were initiated, but all failed to improve his communication abilities. However, a trial of prednisone, prescribed at age 9;6, was followed by some improvement in both oral and written communication skills.

Despite the efforts of the teachers in the local public school, who used written communication via computer and longhand, academic work continued to be extremely frustrating for Will and increased his irritability. It was also noted by his teachers and parents that he was becoming inappropriately aggressive. With the support of the pediatric neurologist, his parents requested that he be evaluated for residential placement in a school for children with hearing loss. The need for intensive training in an alternative method of communication (signing) during acute episodes of LKS motivated this request. At the beginning of the fourth grade, Will was placed in a residential school for the deaf, where he completed the school year. At the beginning of the fifth grade his teachers at the residential school requested a consultation with the school psychologist. The teachers had two concerns: first, they were not convinced that placement at the school for the deaf was an appropriate means for Will's optimal educational and communication development; and additionally, they had observed that he had no friends at school. When Will was 11, a team evaluation at a multidisciplinary diagnostic center was requested by his parents and the professionals at the school to determine what educational placement and strategies would best fit his needs.

Prior to the assessment, a preassessment meeting was held to review Will's history and determine which assessment instruments and techniques should be used during the day-long evaluation. Will, who was 11 years old at the time of the evaluation, was not currently experiencing acute LKS symptoms and was able to understand simple directions and comments by members of the evaluation team. The team consisted of an audiologist, a speech-language pathologist, an educational specialist, and a school psychologist.

Results of Will's audiologic screening were consistent with those previously conducted when Will was not experiencing acute symptoms of LKS. Using standard procedures, his hearing was screened at 15 dB HL (i.e., hearing level) for the frequencies from 250 to 8000 Hz. He very cooperatively responded at this level to all frequencies except 8000 Hz, where responses were obtained at 20 dB HL, bilaterally. Speech reception thresholds of 10 dB HL were demon-

strated for both ears. Acoustic immittance results were also consistent with normal middle ear function, bilaterally. A previous audiological evaluation, also performed when Will was asymptomatic, provided additional speech discrimination information. At that time, he achieved a speech discrimination score of 88 percent at 60 dB in quiet. When 50 dB noise was introduced, his performance deteriorated to 60 percent. The lower speech discrimination score in noise is consistent with reports among children with LKS of increased difficulty in processing language when background noise is present (Tharpe & Olsen, 1994).

According to his parents, during periods of aphasia, communication was attempted through limited speech, written notes, gestures, and some sign. At these times, Will's speech could be understood inconsistently by family members, but not at all by others. When the acute symptoms of LKS were not present, Will was able to communicate in short, concrete sentences.

During the speech and language assessment Will almost never initiated communicative interactions. His responses were typically one or two words in length, but when prompted, he could respond in three- or four-word sentences. Throughout the day-long evaluation, his prosody and intensity were noted as abnormal. He spoke at a slow rate and in a monotone pitch. Vocal intensity was low, and the listener often had to lean forward and concentrate to hear Will or ask for repetition.

On the Arizona Articulation Proficiency Scale (Fudala, 1970), Will achieved a score of 98.5. He substituted /w/ for /l/, and /s/ was lateralized. Intelligibility was affected by low vocal intensity and abnormal prosody. When compared to children his chronological age, his performance on the Peabody Picture Vocabulary Test–Revised (PPVT), (Dunn & Dunn, 1981), was more than two standard deviations below the mean. The results of the Clinical Evaluation of Language Fundamentals–Revised (CELF-R), (Semel, Wiig, & Secord, 1987), indicated that he had moderate to severe deficits in receptive language. He performed poorly on subtests requiring the retrieval and comprehension of auditory information such as following oral directions and identifying semantic relationships. His strength in receptive language was his knowledge of syntactical rules in sentence structure. His performance on the sentence structure subtest was within normal limits. On the expressive portions of the CELF-R, Will had difficulty with the sentence formulation and sentence assembly subtests. His score on the sentence formulation subtest was more than two standard deviations from the mean, and on sentence assembly, more than one standard deviation from the mean.

Will's sign language vocabulary was minimal. As assessed by the Carolina Picture Vocabulary Test (Layton & Holmes, 1983), his vocabulary consisted of fewer than 20 nouns, 9 verbs (all of which were action verbs), and a few attributes.

In an effort to attain an ecological perspective, results from the team psychologist's evaluation were combined with results of observations of Will and an assessment performed several months earlier by the psychologist at the school for the deaf. The school psychologist noted that Will spent most of his time alone, seldom interacting or communicating with other students. He preferred to communicate with teachers and staff members, with whom he used speech. Will had difficulty understanding the teacher's signs and often asked her to fingerspell key words very slowly. He did not attempt to sign his responses. On the socialization portion of the Vineland Adaptive Behavior Scales (Sparrow, Balla, & Cicchetti, 1984), administered by the school psychologist when Will was age 10;3, his age-equivalent score was 4;7. Overall, he exhibited behavior indicating low self-esteem and immature socialization skills.

Achievement: The performance subtests of the Wechsler Intelligence Scale for Children, Third Edition (WISC-III), (Wechsler, 1989), were also administered by the school psychologist. Will's Performance IQ of 93 fell within the average range. Standard scores on the Peabody Individual Achievement Test–Revised (PIAT-R), (Markwardt, 1989), were in the average range, with the exception of recall of general information. Performance in that area was significantly below average. On the Wide Range Achievement Test–Revised (WRAT-R), (Jastak & Wilkinson, 1984), he attained standard scores in the average range for arithmetic, and in the low average range for reading and spelling. Will had the most difficulty in areas requiring auditory comprehension and was unable to understand some of the questions.

In contrast to Will's Performance IQ (93) on the WISC-III, his Verbal IQ of 75 fell into the borderline range of functioning. His lowest scores were on the Vocabulary and Comprehension subtests. He had difficulty with abstract verbal tasks such as identifying similarities between concepts and defining abstract vocabulary. His Verbal Comprehension Index score, which placed him in the lowest 5 percent, was consistent with his Verbal IQ. His performance on a related subtest, the Processing Speed Index, was more than two standard deviations below the mean. The subtests contributing to this index assess the ability to recall and process sequences of symbols, and Will's frequent lapses in attention may have affected his performance. The Freedom from Distractibility Index was in the low-average range, suggesting mild problems with attention and concentration.

On the Kaufman Brief Intelligence Test (K-BIT), (Kaufman & Kaufman, 1990), Will achieved a Vocabulary subtest standard score of 70, which is well below average. This was consistent with the Verbal IQ derived from the WISC-III (Wechsler, 1989) and the PPVT-R (Dunn & Dunn, 1981) score. In contrast, his performance on the Matrices subtest of the K-BIT (Kaufman & Kaufman, 1990) resulted in a standard score of 106, which is in the average range. The Matrices subtest is not timed, and all information needed to complete an item is presented on a single page. Since these items do not require sustained attention, processing speed, or sequential processing, Will's lapses in attention did not significantly affect performance on this subtest. His auditory comprehension, processing problems, and deficits in receptive and expressive language, however, affected his performance on the Vocabulary subtest. Overall, his verbal skills (as assessed by the WISC-III Verbal and K-BIT Vocabulary) were substantially lower than his visual-spatial and visual-motor skills (WISC-III Performance, K-BIT Matrices).

It had been reported that Will's ability to process written language had declined during the last acute episode of LKS; therefore, the focus of the educational assessment was reading comprehension and written expression. Although he was cooperative and worked diligently, Will had difficulty sustaining attention and distracted himself with associative off-task comments. He exhibited a high level of performance anxiety, repeatedly requesting feedback about his performance and asking whether or not items were timed. Portions of the Wechsler Individual Achievement Test (WIAT), (Wechsler, 1991), were administered and revealed a consistent academic profile for reading, writing, and mathematics. His relative strength was in spelling single words from dictation. Those scores reflected his visual retrieval skills and his grasp of the rules of phonics. In contrast, written expression, particularly the ability to generate ideas, was the most difficult for him. His vocabulary was basic and, even with prompting, ideation was concrete and tied to immediate personal experience. His strength in written expression was his knowledge of the rule-governed aspects of language, such as letter format and the use of complete sentences, appropriate capitalization, and punctuation.

Will's composite reading score placed him in the 13th percentile. In decoding written information, he attempted to apply rules of phonics. His errors reflected his lack of attention to detail. Similarly, his responses to questions regarding reading comprehension were affected by inconsistent attention to detail, although he was able to infer information from written material. His reading performance was adversely affected by his very limited vocabulary.

In mathematics, he was successful with problems that involved basic concepts and simple operations with whole numbers. He was able to perform addition, subtraction, and single-digit multiplication, and understood that division was the reverse operation of multiplication. He had not learned the multiplication tables, how to multiply two-digit numbers, or the procedures for long division. His conceptual grasp of the material was equivalent to his ability to perform computations.

Multidisciplinary assessment: *During the multidisciplinary assessment Will worked hard and concentrated to the best of his ability. At times he was impulsive when responding to questions and his attention seemed to wander frequently. There were other lapses in attention, during which Will was not focused on what he was doing or what the speaker was saying. It is important to note that these additional lapses appeared unrelated to his attention problems, high activity level, or poor impulse control. He seemed to momentarily "block out" conversation or his own train of thought. As a result, he missed parts of conversation and sometimes lost his place while solving problems. When this happened, he politely asked to have information repeated, which was a positive way to gain what he had missed. His inability to maintain focus may explain his difficulty completing tasks which required continual processing of new information. His relative strength in tasks in-*

volving an unchanging or familiar pool of information served to highlight the problem.

The multidisciplinary assessment of his skills facilitated the detection of patterns in Will's abilities across diverse tasks and enabled the team to develop a more complete set of recommendations that could be applied throughout the school day. Although his receptive language capabilities had improved, a constellation of behaviors that interfered with focusing attention continued to be present. These included impulsivity, lack of attention to detail, attention lapses, and a high level of activity.

Throughout the evaluation, tasks that required continuous processing of new information were the most difficult for him. Performance on language tests, particularly subtests requiring retrieval and comprehension of auditory information, revealed moderate to severe deficits. Errors in decoding text reflected inattention to detail and deficits in vocabulary. Reading comprehension was also affected by inconsistent attention to detail. Written expression was limited by concrete ideation, and a restricted vocabulary. In contrast, his skills in rule-governed aspects of language such as spelling, letter format, capitalization, and punctuation were much more advanced. His reliance on rules was not surprising, given his difficulty in processing new and changing information. His relative strengths were related to those tasks that assessed visual-spatial and visual-motor skills rather than verbal skills.

In addition to the learning/information processing issues, Will had experienced periods of hyperactivity, aggression, and withdrawal since the onset of LKS symptoms. At the time of evaluation, his self-esteem and socialization skills were assessed as being comparable to those of a 4- to 5-year-old. He had no friends, and was not involved in any group recreational activities. Similar behavioral issues have been reported in other cases of LKS (Beaumanoir, 1985; Mantovani & Landau, 1980; Sawhney et al., 1988; White & Sreenivasan, 1987).

Management plan: As a means to maintain and develop normal language and communication, it was recommended that Will be placed in a regular classroom with intensive support from the speech-language pathologist, the school psychologist, and the reading specialist. It was stressed that at least for the next few years, a well-coordinated team approach was necessary for this to be a successful placement. Furthermore, in the event that steroid therapy became less effective, a reassessment of his needs would be necessary. The need for visual presentation of information that had been presented orally to the class was also emphasized. Will's auditory processing difficulties were specifically addressed by a recommendation that he use an FM system. An FM system is a type of hearing aid that utilizes a wireless microphone worn by the teacher with a special receiver worn by the child. The microphone/transmitter sends its signal via an FM radio frequency, and the child's receiver is tuned to that frequency. Although an FM system cannot fully compensate for all of his attention and processing problems, presumably the reduction of background noise would facilitate his ability to process spoken language. The use of auditory trainers by children with LKS has been recommended by other clini-

cians (Tharpe & Olsen, 1994). Will's attention and processing difficulties were further addressed by the following recommendations made to his teachers and parents, all of which emphasized his need for visual support in processing auditory information.

1. Get his full attention before speaking.

2. Gain eye contact, and cue him by saying "stop and listen," or "ready?"

3. Supplement verbal material with visual information whenever possible.

4. Use short sentences and have him repeat directions.

5. Provide all assignments in writing.

6. Repeat the message if he does not respond, and model the appropriate response.

7. Grant preferential seating in the front and to the side of the classroom.

8. Have Will work for short periods of time, receive rewards after a successful performance, and take a short break before beginning a new task.

The team also recommended the use of brainstorming activities to increase Will's vocabulary and ideational fluency, and to encourage frequent writing activities. A specific suggestion was that he keep a personal journal.

In addition to academic difficulties, Will was experiencing a notable amount of difficulty with social interactions. To facilitate the development of interpersonal skills and provide appropriate outlets for his frustration, it was recommended that he participate in supervised recreational/sports activities. In order to most effectively develop and reinforce linguistic, pragmatic, and social skills, it was suggested that the psychologist and speech-language pathologist work in conjunction with the individuals directing the recreational activities.

SUMMARY

Will's story is, unfortunately, not atypical of that of many children with LKS. Despite effective medical management by a pediatric neurologist, the concern of his parents, and the cooperation of teachers in both his local public school and the residential school, he was unable to make adequate academic progress. In addition, his social isolation and immaturity appeared to be becoming increasingly problematic. Multidisciplinary analysis of the processing deficits that affect each child's ability to code and store verbal information in subtly different ways is ideal for identifying patterns of behavior and developing integrated remediation strategies across functional domains to maximize the processing and coding skills available to the child.

Although Landau-Kleffner syndrome is often simply described as an acquired childhood aphasia seen in conjunction with a paroxysmal EEG, it is a much more complex phenomenon than these two diagnostic components suggest. The cause of the disorder remains entirely unknown, and in fact, several investigators have suggested that there are multiple underlying factors rather than a single precipitating condition or insult. The prognosis of the syndrome is highly variable, not only in the severity and long-term outcome of the associated language disorder, but also as to whether seizures will be present, the severity and frequency of the seizures, the type of seizure activity, and the period of time during which the child will experience them. Thus, because of the variability in the course of the disorder, a prognosis for an individual child cannot be determined. Finally there is very little empirical evidence regarding the efficacy of various surgical, pharmacological, and therapeutic interventions. In spite of the more than 160 articles published on the topic, Landau-Kleffner syndrome has remained an elusive, but devastating, childhood language disorder. The need for a coordinated effort to identify an etiology, or etiologies, and to determine appropriate, effective treatment is clearly present. The relatively low incidence of the syndrome indicates the need for wide-ranging, collaborative, and multidisciplinary projects among a large number of medical centers. Without such an effort, the prospects for deriving definitive treatment information will remain dim.

References

Beaumanoir, A. (1985). The Landau-Kleffner syndrome. In Roger, Dravet, C., Bureau, M., Dreifuss, F., & Wolf, P. (Eds.), *Epileptic syndrome in infancy, childhood and adolescence* (pp. 181–191). London: John Libbey.

Bishop, D. (1985). Age of onset and outcome in acquired aphasia with convulsive disorder (Landau-Kleffner syndrome). *Developmental Medicine and Child Neurology, 27*(6), 705–712.

Campbell, T., & Heaton, E. (1979). An expressive program for a child with acquired aphasia: A case study. *Canadian Journal of Human Communication*, 89–102.

Caramazza, A., Berndt, R., & Basili, A. (1983). The selective impairment of phonological processing: A case study. *Brain and Language, 18*, 128–174.

Cole, A., Andermann, F., Taylor, L., Olivier, A., Rausmussen, T., Rabitaille, Y., & Spire, J. (1988). The Landau-Kleffner syndrome of acquired epileptic aphasia: Unusual clinical outcome, surgical experience and absence of encephalitis. *Neurology, 38*, 31–38.

Denes, G., Balliello, S., Volterra, V., & Pelligrini, A. (1986). Oral and written language in a case of childhood phonemic deafness. *Brain and Language, 29*, 252–267.

Deonna, T., Beumanoir, A., Gaillard, F., & Assal, G. (1977). Acquired aphasia in childhood with seizure disorder: A heterogeneous syndrome. *Neuropaediatrie, 8*, 263–273.

Deuel, R., & Lenn, N. (1977). Treatment of acquired epileptic aphasia. *Pediatrics, 90*, 959–961.

DiSimoni, F. (1978). *The Token Test for Children*. Chicago: Riverside Publishing.

Dunn, L. M., & Dunn, L. M. (1981). *Manual for the Peabody Picture Vocabulary Test–Revised*. Circle Pines, Minn.: American Guidance Service.

Fudala, J. (1970). *Arizona Articulation Proficiency Scale*. Los Angeles: Western Psychological Services.

Gascon, G., Victor, D., Lombrosco, C., & Goodglass, H. (1973). Language disorder, convulsive disorder and electroencephalographic abnormalities. *Archives of Neurology, 28*, 156–162.

Genton, P., Maton, B., Ogihara, M., Samoggia, G., Guerrini, R., Medina, M., Dravet, C., & Roger, J. (1992). Continuous focal spikes during REM sleep in a case of acquired aphasia (Landau-Kleffner Syndrome). *Sleep, 15*(5), 454–460.

Gordon, N. (1990). Acquired aphasia in childhood: The Landau-Kleffner syndrome. *Developmental Medicine and Child Neurology, 32*(3), 270–274.

Hirsch, E., Marescaux, C., Maquet, P., Metz-Lutz, M., Kiesmann, M., Salmon, E., Franck, G., & Kurtz, D. (1990). Landau-Kleffner syndrome: A clinical and EEG study of five cases. *Epilepsia, 31*(6), 756–767.

Holmes, G., McKeever, M., & Saunders, Z. (1981). Epileptiform activity in aphasia of childhood: an epiphenomenon? *Epilepsia, 22*, 631–639.

Jastak, S., & Wilkinson, G. (1984). *Wide Range Achievement Test – Revised*. Wilmington, Del.: Jastak Associates.

Kaufman, A., & Kaufman, N. (1990). *Kaufman Brief Intelligence Test*. Circle Pines, Minn.: American Guidance Service.

Kellerman, K. (1978). Recurrent aphasia with recurrent subclinical bioelectric status epilepticus. *European Journal of Pediatrics, 128*, 207–212.

Landau, W. (1992). Landau-Kleffner syndrome: An eponymic badge of ignorance. *Archives of Neurology, 49*, 353.

Landau, W., & Kleffner, F. (1957). Syndrome of acquired aphasia with convulsive disorder in children. *Neurology, 7*(8), 523–530.

Layton, T., & Holmes, D. (1983). *Carolina Picture Vocabulary Test*. Austin, Tex.: Pro-Ed.

Lerman, P., Lerman-Sagie, T., & Kivity, S. (1991). Effect of early corticosteroid therapy for Landau-Kleffner syndrome. *Developmental Medicine and Child Neurology, 33*(3), 257–266.

Mantovani, J., & Landau, W. (1980). Acquired aphasia with convulsive disorder: course and prognosis. *Neurology, 30*(5), 524–529.

Maquet, P., Hirsch, E., Dive, D., Salmon, E., Marescaux, C., & Franck, G. (1990). Cerebral glucose utilization during sleep in Landau-Kleffner syndrome: A PET study. *Epilepsia, 31*(6), 778–783

Markwardt, F. (1989). *Peabody Individual Achievement Test–Revised*. Circle Pines, MN: American Guidance Service, Inc.

McKinney, W., & McGreal, D. A. (1974). An aphasic syndrome in children. *Canadian Medical Association Journal, 110*(6), 637–639.

Miller, J., Campbell, T., Chapmen, R., & Weismer, S. (1984). Language behavior in acquired childhood aphasia. In A. Holland (Ed.), *Language dis-*

orders in childhood: Recent advances (pp. 57–99). San Diego, CA: College Hill Press.

Morrell, F. (1973). Multiple subpial transection for the surgical treatment of focal epilepsy. *Electroencephalographic Clinical Neurophysiology, 34,* 714. (Abstract) Psychological abstracts.

Morrell, F., & Hanberry, J. (1969). A new surgical technique for the treatment of focal cortical epilepsy. *Electroencephalographic Clinical Neurophysiology, 26,* 120.

Morrell, F., & Whistler, W. (1982). Multiple subpial transection for epilepsy eliminates seizures without destroying the function of the transected zone. *Epilepsia, 23,* 440–441. (Abstract) Psychological abstracts.

Morrell, F., Whistler, W., & Bleck, T. (1989). Multiple subpial transection: A new approach to the surgical treatment of focal epilepsy. *Journal of Neurosurgery, 71,* 629–630.

Morrell, F., Whistler, W., Smith, M., Hoeppner, T., de Toledo-Morrell, L., Pierre-Louis, S., Kanner, A., Buelow, J., Ristanovic, R., Bergen, G., Chez, M., & Hasegawa, H. (1995). Landau-Kleffner syndrome: Treatment with subpial intracortical transection. *Brain, 118,* 1529–1546.

Msall, M., Shapiro, B., Befour, P., Niedermeyer, E., & Capute, A. (1986). Acquired epileptic aphasia. *Clinical Pediatrics, 25,* 248–251.

O'Tuama, L., Urion, D., Janicek, M., Treves, T., Bjornson, B., & Moriarity, J. (1992). Regional cerebral perfusion in Landau-Kleffner syndrome and related childhood aphasias. *The Journal of Nuclear Medicine, 33,* 1758–1764.

Otero, E., Cordova, S., Diaz, F., Garcia-Tervel, I., & del Brutto, O. (1989). Acquired epileptic aphasia (the Landau-Kleffner syndrome) due to neurocysticercosis. *Epilepsia, 30*(5), 569–572.

Paquier, P., Hugo, R., Van Dongen, H., & Loonen, M. (1992). The Landau-Kleffner syndrome or acquired aphasia with convulsive disorder. *Archives of Neurology, 49*(4), 354–359.

Penn, C., Friedlander, R., & Saling, M. (1990). Acquired childhood aphasia with convulsive disorder (Landau-Kleffner syndrome). *South African Medical Journal, 77*(3), 158–161.

Perniola, T., Magari, L., Buttiglione, M., Andruela, C., Simone, I., & Santostasi, R. (1993). A case of Landau-Kleffner syndrome secondary to inflammatory demyelinating disease. *Epilepsia, 34*(3), 551–556.

Rapin, I., Mathis, S., Rowan, A. J., & Golden, G. G. (1977). Verbal auditory agnosia in children. *Developmental Medicine and Child Neurology, 19*(2), 192–207.

Sawhney, I., Suresh, N., Dhand, U., & Chopra, J. (1988). Acquired aphasia with epilepsy: Landau-Kleffner syndrome. *Epilepsia, 29*(3) 283–287.

Semel, E., Wiig, E., & Secord, W. (1987). *Clinical Evaluation of Language Fundamentals–Revised.* New York: Psychological Corporation.

Shoumaker, R., Bennet, P., Bray, R., & Curless, R. (1974). Clinical and EEG manifestation of an unusual aphasic syndrome in children. *Neurology, 24,* 10–16.

Shu-Xian, H., Xi-Ru, W., Chin, L., & Shou-Yu, H. (1989). Landau-Kleffner syndrome with unilateral EEG abnormalities: Two cases from Beijing, China. *Brain and Development, 11*(6), 420–422.

Silva, P. (1980). The prevalence, stability and significance of developmental language delay in preschool children. *Developmental Medicine Childhood Neurology, 22,* 768–777.

Solomon, G., Carson, D., Pavlakis, S., Fraser, R., & Labar, D. (1993). Intracranial EEG monitoring in Landau-Kleffner syndrome associated with temporal lobe astrocytoma. *Epilepsia, 34*(3), 557–560.

Sparrow, S., Balla, D., & Cicchetti, D. (1984). *Vineland Adaptive Behavior Scales.* Circle Pines, Minn.: American Guidance Service.

Tharpe, A., Johnson, G., & Glassock, M. (1991). Diagnostic and management considerations of acquired epileptic aphasia or Landau-Kleffner syndrome. *The American Journal of Otology, 12*(3), 210–214.

Tharpe, A., & Olsen, B. (1994). Landau-Kleffner syndrome: Acquired epileptic aphasia in children. *Journal of the American Academy of Audiology, 5,* 146–150.

Tuchman, R. (1994). Epilepsy, language, and behavior: Clinical models in childhood aphasia. *Journal of Child Neurology, 9,* 95–102.

Van der Sandt-Koenderman, W., Smit, I., Van Dongen, H., & Van Hest, J. (1984). A case of acquired childhood aphasia and convulsive disorder. Some linguistic aspects of recovery and breakdown. *Brain and Language, 21,* 174–183.

Wechsler, D. (1989). *Wechsler Intelligence Scales for Children* (3rd ed.). New York: Psychological Corporation.

Wechsler, D. (1991). *Wechsler Individual Achievement Test.* New York: Psychological Corporation.

White, H., & Sreenivasan, V. (1987). Epilepsy-aphasia syndrome in children: an unusual presentation to psychiatry. *Canadian Journal of Psychiatry, 32*(7), 599–601.

Worster-Drought, C. (1971). An unusual form of acquired aphasia in children. *Developmental Medicine and Child Neurology, 13,* 563–571.

Prenatal Substance Use and Its Impact on Young Children

Shirley N. Sparks, M.S., CCC-SLP
Associate Professor Emeritus
Western Michigan University
Kalamazoo
and
Santa Clara University
California

Key Terms

fetal alcohol syndrome (FAS)
fetal alcohol effect (FAE)
genotype
phenotype

genetics clinic
palpebral fissures
philtrum
teratogen

Overview

In an attempt to answer questions regarding drug exposure, this chapter will target the deleterious effects of prenatal exposure to two substances, alcohol and cocaine. The social and educational courses of children affected by exposure to alcohol can be frustrating and difficult, but somewhat predictable, and this chapter is written for those who must obtain a diagnosis and assess their language and behavior. The neurological and behavioral sequelae of prenatal cocaine exposure are also discussed, along with guidelines for assessment and intervention. Throughout this chapter the postnatal component of attachment with a caregiver, and its importance to eventual outcomes, will be explored and illustrated through actual cases. The following case study poses many questions related to early intervention efforts with young children exposed to alcohol and other drugs.

CASE STUDY: NATHAN

Linda, 36, the mother of 3-year-old Nathan, sat in the office of the drug rehabilitation counselor at one of the few residential treatment centers for substance-using women and their children. Nathan's day-care teacher was also present. The purpose of the meeting was to answer Linda's questions and to plan some "next steps" for Nathan. Linda recognized that Nathan had been having problems adjusting to his day-care environment. She alternated between denying that Nathan's problems were the result of her drinking during pregnancy and assuming that whatever was wrong with him was entirely her fault. During her 3 months at the treatment center, she had not taken advantage of the counselor's efforts to help her modify her parenting skills, nor had she taken the appropriate steps to see that Nathan would receive assessment and intervention services.

Linda had been brought up by parents who both had problems with alcohol use (therefore, she herself may have been affected by prenatal exposure). She reported that at one time she drank heavily with her husband. They had separated several times. She said she had stopped drinking in her 3rd month of pregnancy with Nathan, as soon as she found out she was pregnant. She said she did not drink at all after that except for one night after her grandmother died, when she drank half a bottle of gin and passed out. After Nathan was born, she resumed her drinking but was now committed to treatment and staying sober. She smoked but said that she used no other drugs. "Are Nathan's troubles the result of my drinking?" she asked.

What were Nathan's troubles? He appeared to be a serious little boy who was very watchful of his mother's whereabouts. Their strong attachment was obvious; his mother's disappearance during the conference was cause for Nathan to be anxious, and he banged on the door several times during the meeting. His teacher reported that he could not follow the classroom routine and that he stayed outside the circle activities but had nonetheless made progress in the few months he had attended the center. The teacher described Nathan as a child who knew no boundaries and was unwilling to abide by any rules. His language seemed delayed, though no formal testing had been done, nor had his hearing been checked. Even if cognitive, language, and behavioral deficits could be predicted from the amount that Linda drank during her pregnancy, what effect could Linda's current parenting contribute to Nathan's behavior now? For that matter, what might be the carryover effect of Linda's own parents' behavior?

ETIOLOGY AND PRENATAL ENVIRONMENT

The etiology of the specific effects of alcohol and cocaine will be discussed in detail later. However, certain principles and basic facts are necessary to gain a clear understanding of the etiology in prenatal drug exposure. In general, drugs taken by the mother reach the placenta via the uterine arteries. The placenta acts as a drug recipient and a drug-transferring organ. The factors that affect drug distribution in the mother will control the amount transferred to the fetus. The action of the drug depends upon its concentration at the receptor site(s). In both the woman and the fetus, body distribution of the substance is influenced by relative proportions of lean body mass, fat, and water and by the immaturity of the blood-brain barrier of the fetus. The drug must be metabolized by the liver and excreted by the kidneys in both mother and fetus. Drug metabolism by the fetal liver is less effective than in later life. Thus, what may not be an overdose to the mother can be an overdose to the fetus. The excretion of drugs is affected by the fact that the kidney in the fetus is also immature (Jones & Lopez, 1988).

Women (and men) who use one drug are very likely to use other drugs at the same time. Women who use crack cocaine during pregnancy are also likely to smoke cigarettes and drink alcohol (although many more women who drink alcohol do not use other drugs concurrently). The concurrent use of multiple drugs is known as "polydrug" use and makes it exceptionally difficult to determine the effects of any one drug on subsequent child development. The babies cited in most of the research in this chapter who were prenatally exposed are babies of polydrug users. It is impossible to say which of the effects are actually due to cocaine, which to alcohol, which to other substances used, and which to the combination. We tend to think of the legal drugs, alcohol and nicotine, as the "good drugs," and illegal drugs, such as cocaine, heroin, and phencyclidine (PCP), as the "bad drugs," although, as this chapter will show, prenatal exposure to alcohol can have more deleterious effects on the fetus than exposure to illegal drugs. Based on what we know about child development in general, the deficits exhibited by some infants and toddlers exposed to drugs may predict subsequent developmental problems. However, findings from the developmental literature indicate that even children who are impaired by their exposure to drugs in utero can, and should, be helped by concerted early intervention programs (Kronstadt, 1991).

POSTNATAL ENVIRONMENTS

Studies of normal language development suggest that children develop their need to communicate from interactions with a responsive caregiver, which in turn enables the child to develop an internal working model of a human relationship. A baby forms a life-long impression that he or she is emotionally attached to one or more specific persons who make him or her feel comfortable and important; that in their presence he or she can safely explore, enjoy, and profit from experiences; and that it is to their presence that he or she must return whenever frustrated or in trouble. Thus the development of trust and the message about what can be expected of the adults in one's world are shaped by caregiving and can be discerned in a child's behavior very early. We know that a secure child has a good chance of entering school ready to learn, to tolerate frustration, and to look for help from the teacher if a task proves too difficult (Schafer, 1991).

When the caregiver is dependent on a drug, the care these babies receive over the first few months of life is unpredictable. It even may diminish until it becomes nonexistent. Burns and Burns (1988) reported anecdotal accounts by mothers who use drugs of being unable to make themselves get out of bed in the morning to care for their crying babies. Their feeding practices show little sensitivity to the needs of the infant. Attempts by these mothers to interact with their children with toys often result in the play directed toward the mother's needs rather than those of her child. These mothers are described as immature women who demonstrate an abnormal degree of egocentrism in the way they go about parenting. They frequently view the birth of the child as a gift for themselves and continue to interpret the child's growth and development in terms of their own needs. In addition, it is not unusual for drug-dependent mothers to admit to child abuse, sometimes in a way that they seem oblivious to the seriousness of the abuse.

Behaviors of drug-using mothers that are particularly important to professionals are described as follows (Burns & Burns, 1988):

> They have a great deal of difficulty understanding their infants' communications, since these communications are at first mostly expressions of the child's needs rather than responses to the mother's neediness. These mothers interpret their infant's attempts to communicate as demanding and inappropriate; and consequently they reject or criticize these early efforts to interact. At a time when their infant desperately needs encouragement to persist in social interaction, a message of discouragement is encountered instead. Parenting is experienced by the infant as a negative influence, as though the infants' growth and development were in competition with or at the expense of the mother's welfare. (p. 162)

Furthermore, when we consider that the infant may also have been affected by the drug use prenatally and that both the infant and the principal caregiver come to the dyad at high risk for dysfunction in their interactions, the risk for dysfunction grows exponentially, and the prognosis for recovery is likewise diminished.

Schafer (1991) provides three models of human relationships that result from failure to develop this sense of security from caregiving that can be discerned in a baby's behavior by 12 to 18 months of age.

1. Ambivalence: Infants who are ambivalent seem to possess the inner hunch that other people possess what they need, but will part with it with great reluctance, perhaps only if tricked or forced. The basic message these babies give to their caregivers is, "I need you with me at all times, but I am never content with what you offer me."

2. Avoidance: Babies who are avoidant appear quite independent, for they have acquired the belief that it is never safe to explore anything new or challenging in the presence of another person and that the best way to live is to do everything alone. The basic message they give to their caregivers is, "I don't need you; please leave me alone."

3. Emptiness: The infant identified as empty has the belief that there exists no one special—that all human partners are interchangeable because they are all equally insignificant. Infants who feel emptiness often fall victim to a range of early disturbances, including failure to thrive, sleep disorders, and head banging. They also appear depressed or developmentally delayed.

All three groups arrive at school with very different strategies for learning than do children from secure homes, and they also differ from each other. Babies who are ambivalent reach the primary grades with a very low tolerance for frustration. Their way of asking for help is to whine or throw a tantrum. Teachers see them as helpless and tend to overprotect them. The babies who are avoidant also reach school with a low tolerance for frustration, but they are more aggressive and tend to single out ambivalent children as their prey. Their manner of relating to teachers is often provocative. Some teachers react to this with irritation and dislike; others may respond by becoming detached. However, either reaction tends to further reinforce the children's avoidant stance. The children labeled empty enter school exhibiting bizarre behaviors. They are often seen as delayed and tend to become consumers of the vast array of special services for children with special needs (Schafer, 1991).

Conducting research on the development of children affected by drugs is extremely problematic for a number of reasons, not the least of which is the effect of care giving. It cannot be overemphasized that the postnatal environment of the child is a vital influence on behavior and must be controlled for in any comparative study. Research studies that do not compare groups from the same home background are suspect. For example, if a group of children exposed to drugs from foster homes or homes where drugs are used are compared to a group of nonexposed children living in stable homes, the contributing factor of the home environment cannot be discounted, and the groups are not comparable.

ALCOHOL-RELATED BIRTH DEFECTS

Alcohol-related congenital disorders are now recognized as the leading known cause of mental retardation in the United States (Abel & Sokol, 1987). The anomalies related to maternal drinking during pregnancy range from a severe recognizable pattern called **fetal alcohol syndrome (FAS)** to a condition in which not all the physical or behavioral symptoms of FAS are displayed, called **fetal alcohol effect (FAE)**. Individuals born with FAS and FAE are born with organic brain disfunction (Streissguth, 1997). There is some controversy concerning whether there are two disorders, FAS and FAE, or whether FAS and FAE are actually the extremes of a continuum of a single condition, alcohol-related birth defect. Throughout this chapter, the term *alcohol-related birth defect* (ARBD) will be used to include both FAS and FAE unless a specific distinction between the two is necessary.

Etiology of Alcohol-Related Birth Defects

Alcohol can have a direct toxic effect on the rapidly developing cells of the embryo and fetus in many different ways, causing a whole spectrum of effects. Some of these effects are observable in the newborn baby (poor suckling ability, heart defects, low birth weight). Others, however, are detectable only within the framework of a given developmental stage or a specific environment. For example, hyperactivity is often more obvious when children learn to walk or when they are required to perform in structured settings; thus attentional and learning problems become more apparent at some stages or in some settings (Streissguth, 1997).

ARBDs, like disorders attributable to other drugs taken by the mother during pregnancy, have an environmental, rather than a genetic etiology. That is, the insult to the fetus occurs in the uterine environment during gestation after the **genotype** (the actual genetic makeup of the child) has been established at conception. Therefore, individuals with ARBD cannot pass on any traits of the disorders to their children through their genes. The genotype is not affected by prenatal alcohol, but the **phenotype** (the observable or measurable expression of genes) is affected during prenatal development. Etiology is clearly attributed to alcohol intake by the mother during pregnancy.

A **teratogen** is a substance capable of producing death, malformations, growth deficiency, or behavioral aberrations as a result of prenatal exposure (Wilson, 1977). A behavioral teratogen is a substance that produces behavioral deviations as a result of prenatal exposure (Vorhees & Butcher, 1982). Perhaps the best-known teratogen is thalidomide, which was found to cause major limb malformations in children whose mothers took it during early pregnancy. During a short period in the early 1960s, 20 percent of the mothers who received the drug during the critical exposure period of pregnancy produced babies with a degree of limb aberration, usually congenital absence of the limb (McBride, 1977). However, no known teratogens, including alcohol, have been shown to have a definite cause-and-effect connection with a specific type of abnormality. That is, the abnormality does not always appear when the teratogen is present, and when it does appear, the features are variable.

One reason that alcohol has been identified as a teratogen only recently is that not every woman who drinks heavily during pregnancy produces an affected child, and yet a woman who drinks very little may have an affected child. As Beck (1984) writes, society is of two minds about the risk of teratogens:

> If alcohol were any other powerful teratogen, it would have been banned as soon as it was linked with birth defects—as thalidomide was. Even if it were merely suspected of causing birth defects in concentrations as small as one part per billion—as dioxin is—the government would feel obliged to spend millions of dollars to protect people from contact with it. Even if it only damaged second-generation rats whose mothers were overdosed almost to death—as saccharin did—the government would require warnings to be posted. But because it's liquor that's killing the brain cells of unborn babies and distorting their growth, what we do is just hope that women who are pregnant or about to become pregnant will somehow get the message and act on it themselves. (p. 94)

Three factors must be considered in risks of teratogenicity:

1. Time of exposure: Organ systems have differing critical periods of development when cell division is most rapid, and it is then that they are most vulnerable to teratogens. The brain has a relatively long critical period characterized by a complex series of specific critical periods for its different sections. Malformations probably are produced by high concentrations of alcohol at specific periods during the first trimester, when embryonic development of the central nervous system is taking place. Growth may be most vulnerable to heavy drinking during the second and third trimesters. Neurological damage resulting in behavior disturbance and intellectual impairment may occur throughout pregnancy, by chemical and structural disruption of the central nervous system in the first trimester and, in the second and third trimesters, during the later period of cell division associated with rapid brain growth and functional organization (Rosett, 1979).

2. Dosage: The neurobehavioral effects of prenatal alcohol exposure show, in general, a dose response relationship; high levels of exposure are associated with large effects, while moderate levels of exposure are associated with more subtle effects. It is not clear whether the damage results from brief, high concentrations of alcohol at particular stages of development or whether FAS symptoms are caused by continuous consumption at low doses (McKim, 1991). (For an in-depth discussion of dose-related symptomotology, see Little and Wendt, 1991.) Some of the strongest predictors of later neurobehavioral deficits are binge drinking (five drinks or more on an occasion in the designated time period) and drinking in the period prior to pregnancy recognition (Streissguth, Sampson, & Barr, 1989).

3. Susceptibility of the fetus and of the mother: Perhaps the discrepancies in the studies of dosage can be attributed, in part, to differences in individ-

ual susceptibility. The mother's ability to detoxify alcohol is a possible factor in determining teratogenicity to her fetus, as is the susceptibility of an individual fetus to the teratogen.

Diagnosis of Fetal Alcohol Syndrome

Diagnosis of FAS must be done by a physician. The diagnosis can be made by a pediatrician with an interest in dysmorphology or by referral to a **genetics clinic**, a clinic that specializes in diagnosing a variety of genetic and prenatal disorders. Genetics clinics can be found by calling the local chapter of the March of Dimes, which often sponsors such clinics. Visits are usually free, covered by insurance, or billed on a sliding fee scale. It usually is not necessary to have a physician refer a patient. In some states, schools may refer and parents may self-refer.

When certain fetal alcohol effects cluster in a specific way, and in a way that is unique to alcohol, the resulting condition is called FAS. FAS involves a specific pattern of features that has not been associated with any other prenatal condition. FAS is diagnosed when children meet the following three criteria (Streissguth, 1997):

1. Growth deficiency, prenatally or postnatally, for height, weight, or both.

2. A specific pattern of minor anomalies that includes a characteristic face, generally defined as short **palpebral fissures** (eye slits), a flat midface, a short upturned nose, a smooth or long **philtrum** (the set of ridges running between the nose and the lips), and a thin upper lip. Clarren and Astley (1995) have developed computer models for defining the facial dysmorphology crucial in the diagnosis of FAS.

3. Some central nervous system (CNS) damage, including microcephaly, tremors, hyperactivity, fine or gross motor problems, attentional deficits, learning disabilities, intellectual or cognitive impairments, or seizures. Mental retardation and developmental delays also qualify as CNS criteria but are not necessary for diagnosis.

A diagnosis of FAS also requires some presumed history of significant prenatal alcohol exposure. However, in 1996, the Institute of Medicine (IOM, Stratton, Howe, & Battaglia, 1996) suggested two classifications of FAS: one with and one without confirmed maternal alcohol exposure.

Fetal Alcohol Effect

Since 1978, the term *fetal alcohol effects* (FAE) has been used to describe conditions that are presumed to be caused by prenatal alcohol exposure (Clarren & Smith, 1978) but do not follow the exact configuration of the three characteristics that uniquely identify FAS. Usually, children with FAE are of normal size and have some, but not all, of the facial anomalies and CNS dysfunctions associated with FAS (Streissguth, 1997). The IOM (IOM et al., 1996) suggested a five-category system to describe the spectrum of prenatal alcohol effects on offspring. Categories 1 and 2 are FAS with and without confirmed alcohol exposure. A category of "partial FAS" (Category 3) includes confirmed exposure; evidence of some components of the pattern of characteristic facial anomalies; and one of the following:

> (1) . . . growth retardation; (2) evidence of CNS neurodevelopmental abnormalities (including decreased cranial size at birth, structural brain abnormalities, including microcephaly, and neurological hard or soft signs, such as impaired fine motor skills, neurosensory hearing loss, poor tandem gait, poor eye-hand coordination); or (3) evidence of a complex pattern of behavior or cognitive abnormalities that are inconsistent with developmental level and cannot be explained by familial background or environment alone, such as learning difficulties; deficits in school performance; poor impulse control; problems in social perception; deficits in higher-level receptive and expressive language; poor capacity for abstraction or metacognition; specific deficits in mathematical skills; or problems in memory, attention, or judgment." (p. 4)

A team of researchers has presented conclusive evidence (Streissguth et al., 1991) that ARBD is a disorder that lasts a lifetime; there is a predictable, long-term progression of the disorder into adulthood, in which maladaptive behaviors present the greatest challenge to management. Those maladaptive behaviors include predictable language disorders.

Behaviors in Alcohol-Related Birth Defects

It is the neurobehaviors that are the most devastating to children and adults with FAS and FAE, and it is these that require the services of clinicians, educators, and health care providers. Some common behaviors in children, adolescents, and adults are summarized in Table 9-1. Of note is "indiscriminate attachment," which refers to uncommon friendliness to people in the child's environment who are strangers or toward whom friendly behavior would not be expected. Children with alcohol-related disorders are known to seek bodily contact—snuggling and hugging—when such behavior is not appropriate. Behaviors specific to age are discussed later in this chapter.

Assessment

Initial assessment may have two different goals, depending on the circumstances: (1) An ARBD is suspected and the information will be used to make a referral to establish the diagnosis, or (2) the child has been diagnosed as having an ARBD, and appropriate placement or establishing eligibility for service delivery is the goal. Assessment for determining therapy goals is excluded here.

Table 9-1. Common Characteristics of Children with Alcohol-Related Birth Defects

Hyperactive and distractible
Poor attention
Delayed motor development
Poor fine-motor development
Learning problems
Uninhibited behavior
Socially engaging—but poor social skills
Indiscriminate attachment
Can be depressed and withdrawn
Poor judgment; do not learn from past experience

Adapted from Streissguth (1990, 1997)

Tests used for assessment should be norm-referenced to compare a child to peers in order to certify for service. However, children with ARBD, particularly very young children, generally have short attention spans and their activity levels will not permit protracted testing. Thus, professionals will need to use a variety of methods for collecting information. Professionals who work with infants, toddlers, and preschoolers under the guidelines of the Individuals with Disabilities Education Act as amended in 1997 (IDEA97) have the advantage of an assessment team which includes the family. Assessment should include gathering information on the following topics.

Family Concerns, Priorities, and Resources. Children with ARBD live in either their family of origin or an adoptive or foster family. In the former, they are frequently raised in high-risk environments by mothers who continue to drink or struggle for sobriety and have few resources and little support. Thus, children with alcohol-related birth defects are at a higher than average risk for physical abuse, sexual abuse, and neglect (Giunta & Streissguth, 1988). In adoptive or foster families, parents may have more stability and resources but may be baffled by the child's behavior, whether or not they knew of the alcohol exposure when they gained custody of the child. It is always helpful to identify the family's concerns, priorities, and resources, and many teams have an assessment protocol for this process.

Teacher/Child-Care Provider Concerns. Given that assessments are typically time limited and may be context limited, it is vital to gather information from those who spend a good deal of time with the child and who see the child in varied environments.

Physical Features. Particular attention should be paid to oral-motor structure and function.

Intellectual Level. A psychological evaluation should be performed to establish the mental age of the child. The information is useful for profiling across skill areas and as a comparison at key transition periods: infant/toddler to preschool, and preschool to elementary school.

Articulation and Language Levels. Receptive versus expressive language, language sampling, or discourse analysis should be included because of processing issues raised previously. Pay particular attention to sequencing in storytelling, in following directions, and to pragmatics.

Audiologic Status. Every child who is at risk for communication disorders should have an audiological evaluation. Treatment for otitis media or sensorineural hearing loss may be indicated.

Socialization and Adaptation Skills. The Vineland Adaptive Behavior Scales (Sparrow, Balla, & Cicchetti, 1984) are recommended. The scales include four domains of behavior (Socialization, Communication, Motor Skills, and Daily Living Skills) and yield a score for each domain. The Socialization Scale, which encompasses interpersonal relationships, play and leisure time, and coping skills, is the most important of the scales. In addition, it is important to encourage caregivers to relate behaviors in the child that they perceive as problematic.

Alcohol History. The most important point to be made in this section is that professionals need not have an alcohol history in order to make a referral for suspected ARBD. Finding confirming information can be a problem for most professionals for the following reasons:

1. Asking about prenatal alcohol exposure makes most people uncomfortable. Most people would like to believe that this type of exposure does not happen. It is a rare professional who does not have negative attitudes about alcohol use in pregnant women, and gathering this information in a neutral fashion may be difficult.

2. Obtaining an alcohol history may be impossible because the child is in foster care or has been adopted and the birth history is unknown, or because the birth mother is not forthcoming.

3. Professionals fear that to ask a mother about alcohol use is an invasion of privacy or may violate privacy laws as well as increase professional liability.

The routine history-taking process affords professionals the easiest entry into the subject of alcohol intake during pregnancy. Information on maternal drinking history should be routinely asked in the workup of children of any age with developmental disabilities, attentional deficits, and/or conduct disorders (Streissguth et al., 1991). However, if information on maternal alcohol use can not be obtained by other service providers, it can be elicited by health care professionals when a referral is made.

Referral Process

After the team members have performed their assessment of the child and gathered pertinent information from the caregiver, they are ready to make the referral. The following are suggested steps for that process. First, inform your supervisor/administrator of the problem and your suspected diagnosis of ARBD. Then, call the closest genetics clinic and speak to the counselor about the procedure for referral to *rule out alcohol-related birth defects*. Ask the counselor what the parents should expect when they visit such as time involved, who should go along, and costs. Gather information from the classroom teacher and/or team regarding the possible diagnosis. Synthesize the information. Approach the mother or caregiver. It could occur at an Individualized Family Service Plan (IFSP) meeting, an Individualized Educational Plan Conference (IEPC), or as a private conversation. The conversation may be something like the following.

"Mrs. Smith, George seems to need help to pay attention and participate in his classroom at preschool and there are some things that I'm puzzled about. Have you ever had him evaluated by anyone other than here at the preschool?" Information on previous consultations should be entered into the child's record. You can then follow up by asking what was learned at those consultations. Did the evaluator have a reason or cause for the behaviors that you are seeing? Is the caregiver satisfied that everything is now known that could be known? Other questions should be asked, such as, "Is there anything in George's history or yours that might account for these concerns for his learning and paying attention?" The professional may want to start with prenatal and birth history to give a context for the discussion, for example, "Can you tell me about the time that you were pregnant with George?" and "Were there any factors that occurred during your pregnancy that may have had an impact on George?" Other questions focused on the health, medical care, and living circumstances of the mother during pregnancy may also lead to a discussion of alcohol use. Whether or not conclusive information is gained regarding alcohol use, the parent may be referred to a genetics clinic. For example, "There is a resource that could be very helpful to us here at the center/preschool that I would like you to consider. There is a team of specialists at the (hospital or other site of the genetics clinic) that specializes in diagnosing children's problems that probably started at or before birth. It's a genetics clinic. I have the phone number and the name of the person you should talk to. If you would like, I can call for an appointment for you."

The information you have about the procedures of the clinic should also be given at this time. The parent or caregiver should be reassured that even though a diagnosis might be troubling, it will enable professionals to better help the child. If available, a team member can offer to go along as an information source. Ask the caregiver to sign a release form giving permission to send copies of assessments and preschool information to the genetics clinic.

Synthesize the information and send a cover letter to the clinic explaining why the referral was made and providing pertinent information (Sparks, 1992).

Caregiver Reactions

Reactions to such a request are as varied as caregivers' personalities. It is possible that parents, particularly foster and adoptive parents, will welcome the opportunity to receive some help, especially if it means they can now obtain suitable programs for their child. It is also possible that caregivers will ignore your request out of fear or denial. If alcohol is an ongoing problem in the home, denial may be a fact of daily life. If you have planned collaboratively for this referral, and if you have the backing of team members and the administration, your united front may make the request more difficult to ignore.

Age-Specific Behaviors

There is considerable variability in the physical, academic, and behavioral characteristics of children with alcohol-related birth defect. In the following sections, common characteristics, derived from averaging across children with a wide spectrum of abilities, will be summarized with the caution that the individual child in one's caseload may vary from these patterns.

Infancy

At birth, babies with ARBD are often tremulous and irritable and have a weak sucking reflex and hypotonia. They also fail to tune out intrusive stimuli and involuntarily respond to noises and other environmental stimuli (lack of habituation). It is also usual for them to be readmitted to the hospital during the first few months of life for failure to thrive, pneumonia, and evaluation of heart defects, hip dysplasia, and developmental delay. Feeding difficulties are a concern to caretakers during this period. Sleep patterns may be erratic, with poor differentiation of sleep/wake cycles (Streissguth, 1990, 1997).

As the infants get older, they may be slow to master motor milestones, to start to say words, and to combine words. Adjusting to solid food is often difficult, and caregivers complain of poor appetites and disinterest in food (Streissguth, 1997). Common behaviors of infants and young children can be seen in Table 9-2.

Early Childhood

During this period, children with FAS are usually short and elf-like in manner and appearance. They flit from one thing to another, moving with "butterfly-like" movements. They seem alert, outgoing, excessively friendly, and

Table 9-2. Common Behaviors of Infancy and Early Childhood Linked to Alcohol-Related Birth Defects

Poor habituation
Sleep disturbances
Poor sleep/wake cycle
Poor sucking response
Failure to thrive
Distractibility/hyperactivity
Delays in walking/talking
Delays in toilet training
Difficulty following directions
Temper tantrums/disobedience
Prone to otitis media

Adapted from Streissguth (1990, 1997)

more interested in people than in objects. Their needs for bodily contact often seem insatiable; they like to touch, fondle, pat, and kiss. They are usually have a happy disposition but can be stubborn and unyielding in their demands.

Hyperactivity is most pronounced during these years. At home they may be "into everything," and their first preschool experience is often difficult because they "can't sit still a minute." They also are often fearless and do not respond well to verbal restrictions. They tend to wander away, go into the street, and need closer supervision than other children. Problems with coordination, fine motor control, and gross motor control become apparent as they try to draw and ride a tricycle (Streissguth, 1990; Streissguth et al., 1988).

Many caregivers find these children endearing during this period, and their slow development and poor performance are often excused on the basis of their small size. "He'll outgrow it" is a commonly expressed hope at this age, and developmental delays are often not taken seriously by the family. However, children with serious hyperactivity are usually diagnosed at this age. Alert preschool and Headstart teachers are often the first to recommend a diagnostic evaluation.

Coggins (1986) assessed social communicative behaviors in school-aged children and adolescents with ARBD. His survey of parents revealed the following characteristics about the children:

1. They were impulsive.

2. They had problems with concrete thinking, reasoning, and problem solving. Decisions were based on intuitive approaches to issues rather than made using inferential or logical judgments.

3. They had a restricted ability to learn from experience.

4. They possessed limited organizational skills.

5. They were talkative but not communicative; although loquacious, their talk was unrelated to the topic at hand.

6. They displayed poor social skills.

Interventions in Infancy and Early Childhood

Early diagnosis is desirable so that appropriate early interventions can prevent some disabilities and ameliorate others. However, according to Little, Snell, and Rosenfeld (1990), the prospect of general early identification of infants with FAS seems unlikely in light of a recent report from one of the largest obstetrical services in the United States documenting a 100 percent failure rate in diagnosing FAS at delivery. Once the diagnosis of FAS or FAE has been made, the team must undertake intervention with the birth or foster parents. Caregivers need to learn all they can about the signs, symptoms, medical, social, and behavioral consequences of alcohol-related disorders. This information is particularly important for birth mothers who are still drinking and at risk of having another affected child. Intervenors must be emphatic that mothers who are drinking must not breast-feed and that infants should not be given alcohol for colic or any other reason (Sparks, 1992).

Caregivers need to set realistic goals and expectations for their children and for themselves, particularly in the areas of social and academic functioning. Perhaps because of their verbal facility, children with alcohol-related disorders are often thought, on casual observation, to be brighter and more alert than test scores indicate, causing both caregivers and teachers to perceive them as lazy, stubborn, or unwilling to learn—a faulty perception. If caregivers are provided information early, frustration for them and for the child may be forestalled.

Caregivers should also be told about the child's need for consistent structure in the home environment and that the child may require much bodily contact. Ways of providing immediate reinforcement in discipline and setting reasonable goals should also be discussed before behavior becomes a problem. Some children have had abusive or neglectful home situations before they were placed with the present family; thus counseling may be needed to help the caregivers with symptoms that may occur as a result, such as withdrawal, inappropriate sexual activity, fears, and excessive demands on adults' time and attention (Streissguth et al., 1988).

Children with alcohol-related birth defects often have particular health needs, such as treatment for otitis media, eye problems, eating disorders, and dental needs. They should be seen for regular checkups by a physician who is aware of the diagnosis.

Preschool attendance is important to prepare the children for the school setting ahead. An extra year in a class for children with speech and language impairments or in a developmental kindergarten may also be helpful.

Use of Nontraditional Therapy Approaches

Speech and language therapy must encompass all forms of communication—the verbal, written, gestural, and behavioral skills that allow an individual to participate in a social environment. Professionals must teach children with ARBD to relate their needs to others in appropriate ways, whether verbally or through other communication systems. Professionals must think of communication skills in the context of social skills instruction: the two are inseparable and essential sets of skills needed to live and work in the community. Young children can learn to communicate their needs, interact with peers, and respond to others appropriately. This point cannot be overemphasized. Traditional speech therapy goals, such as using three new words in a sentence, are inappropriate. Functional goals, such as staying out of a stranger's car, are appropriate. The key concept is to focus on both present and future environments in which children will live and work, and to teach skills specific to those settings.

CASE STUDY: NATHAN

Let's go back to the meeting with Linda in her drug counselor's office. How, then, can Linda and her son Nathan be helped? First, Linda's good intentions as a mother should be confirmed. Generally, women do not begin drinking after they learn they are pregnant; they become pregnant while they are drinking. For the clinician, perhaps the hardest part of dealing with families where substance use is a factor is to be nonjudgmental. The most natural reaction is to be enraged that this child is affected by a condition that is 100 percent preventable. It cannot be overemphasized that, for the professional, dealing with one's own attitudes is far from easy.

From observing her and talking to her, it was obvious that Linda had done many good things with her son. He was attached to her and they clearly loved each other very much. When this love was pointed out, Linda's face relaxed a bit to nearly a smile. She was asked to tell more about her relationship with Nathan. After she described what her life had been like with Nathan, she was able to ask what her drinking had done to him. Only when she could ask for information was she ready to cope with that knowledge. There are no easy answers (for all the reasons discussed in the previous pages), but she at least could be encouraged that she had stopped drinking when she did and was becoming sober now.

After some discussion of her past and her feelings, Linda became more open and receptive, in contrast to the defensive posture she had assumed at the beginning of the meeting. She was asked what she thought her role with Nathan was now. She answered that she wanted to give him everything he wanted, including any toy that he saw on TV.

Linda could now understand that Nathan would probably need some special help, maybe for a long time, and that it was up to her to see that he got it.

She was told that he might learn differently from other children and might not easily remember what he learned from one day to the next. She was encouraged to start the process of getting him the special services that he needed by contacting the school district about an assessment. She was told that he would need an interdisciplinary assessment and then could possibly be enrolled in the area preschool, where he could receive intervention services. At this point, she looked alarmed and asked her counselor if she had to do anything that would interfere with her own recovery. Linda wanted to be sure that transporting Nathan to the assessment or, later, for intervention would not mean missing her own meetings. Her counselor assured her it would not and that the program would be supportive. The day-care teacher said that she would help Linda make the call to the school district.

Linda was assured that being a good mother meant doing what was the best thing for Nathan, and not necessarily what Nathan wanted her to do. It would not hurt their relationship if she told him no; in fact, he needed to learn what he could and could not do with other people. She was encouraged to begin attending the parenting classes and discussions held at the center. She acknowledged that she could use some help in getting Nathan to do what she wanted him to do. She left the meeting appearing resolved to enter Nathan in an early intervention program and to attend some of the parenting classes.

COCAINE EXPOSURE

Since the mid-1980s, when crack cocaine became readily available, a sense of alarm has swept the country concerning the effects of prenatal cocaine exposure on child development. Although there is no doubt that prenatal exposure can be detrimental, some damaging myths have been perpetuated.

The first myth is that all children exposed to cocaine will suffer adverse effects. In fact, most of the children exposed to prenatal drugs are not adversely affected. In most studies of cocaine use in pregnancy, less than half the neonates exposed to cocaine demonstrate effects of intrauterine cocaine exposure such as low birth weight, prematurity, intrauterine growth retardation, small head circumference, or neurobehavioral deficits (Chasnoff, Griffith, MacGregor, Dirkes, & Burns, 1989; Little, Snell, Klein, & Gilstrap, 1989).

The second myth is that "these children" require unprecedented resources. This prediction presumes that effective early intervention practices used for other high-risk preschoolers will not be adequate for children exposed to drugs and that all children affected by drug exposure will have to be served in special education programs (Rinkel, 1992). There is no doubt that many children exposed prenatally to drugs pose serious challenges to early intervention and school personnel. It is clear that prenatal exposure to cocaine constitutes a risk for development in many areas. However, the direct effects of the drug may not be the sole cause of a child's problems, nor are those effects irreversible. The important point is that there is no typical "cocaine-exposed" child. In fact, according to Kronstadt (1991), in many ways children prenatally exposed to drugs look much like other children who live in similarly chaotic homes or neighborhoods. Adverse effects may or may not be present and, if present, they may occur on a continuum of severity and may be capable of being ameliorated.

The third myth is the inevitability of negative outcomes. Early intervention works and is even more promising for children exposed to cocaine than it is for children prenatally exposed to alcohol (Sparks, 1992).

Passive Exposure

An emergency department of a large urban hospital recently found cocaine metabolite in the urine of more than 5 percent of the toddlers and children treated there for routine pediatric complaints (Randall, 1992). The most likely route of exposure is second-hand smoke inhaled when adult caregivers use free-base or crack cocaine. The physiological and behavioral effects of chronic environmental exposure to cocaine in children are not well established. Reported cases include transient neurological symptoms, such as drowsiness and unsteady gait, and seizures. Service providers who encounter such unexplained behaviors and suspect secondhand exposure should refer the child to a health professional.

Passive exposure may occur in breast-fed infants because cocaine is excreted in breast milk. Cocaine can be passed on to an infant in breast milk for 48 hours after the mother has used cocaine. Mothers who use cocaine must not breast-feed their infants. Infants may also be victims of intentional cocaine administration as a form of child abuse (Giacoia, 1990).

Risk versus Deficit

In this chapter, cocaine exposure will be considered a risk rather than the cause of any deficits the child may exhibit. There is a danger in professionals using a "deficit model" in thinking about children exposed to drugs. A deficit model assumes that the baby has experienced some neurochemical or other fundamental damage to the organism's capacities for self-organizing and self-adjustment. Symptoms indicative of drug exposure, such as small head circumference and problems with state control, can also be observed in full-term, otherwise healthy babies who have not been exposed to drugs. Yet any difficulty of the infant exposed to drugs is attributed to the single cause of drug exposure, and the complexities of the impact of drugs on parents and children are often deemed beyond understanding and preventive interventions—even beyond professional help. The deficit model can be used to rationalize giving up on infants exposed to drugs and their mothers (Weston, Ivins, Zuckerman, Jones, & Lopez, 1989).

A "risk model," on the other hand, recognizes that fetal exposure to drugs jeopardizes developmental processes but that the environment may contribute to positive developmental outcomes. Prospective studies of risk have repeatedly indicated that developmental outcomes are the product of both constitutional makeup and environment. The effects of the child on the environment and the environment on the child are consistent with Samaroff and Chandler's 1975 transactional model of development (Werner & Smith, 1982).

For example, it is well known that the most cogent risk factor for a newborn is low birth weight. Neonates prenatally exposed to cocaine are typically of low birth weight (Chouteau, Namerow, & Leppert, 1988; Little et al., 1989). In a recent, and particularly well done, study, McCormick, Brooks-Gunn, Workman-Daniels, Turner, and Peckham (1992) examined the range and cumulative nature of adverse health status at school age among children with lower birth weights. (Neonates exposed prenatally to cocaine were not identified as a separate group in this study.) They concluded that children born at very low birth weight experience higher rates of adverse health status at early school age across several individual dimensions of health. All low-birth-weight children in their study appeared to be at similar risk for "behavior problems" reported by their mothers, but lower IQ scores were concentrated among those whose birth weight was less than 1,000 grams. The authors also assessed the effect of environmental factors as reflected by maternal educational attainment. Children whose mothers had at least a high school education were found to have higher IQs at school age.

Excitable versus Depressed Behaviors

Lester et al. (1991) describe a consensus from the research that neurobehavioral patterns of infants exposed to cocaine can be divided into two extremes of behavior: excitable and depressed. The authors hypothesize that excitable behavior patterns are due to the direct, neurotoxic effects of cocaine, and the depressed behavior is due to the indirect effects of cocaine secondary to complications in the uterine environment, such as hypoxia and intrauterine growth retardation (IUGR).

Lester et al. (1991) describe excitable infants as easily aroused infants who show signs such as irritability, excessive and high-pitched crying, tremors, jitteriness, and hypertonicity. Depressed behavior refers to a decrease in functional activity. Infants who are depressed are underaroused, are difficult to wake, and have fleeting attention and low orientation and state control scores on the Neonatal Behavior Assessment Scale (Brazelton, 1984).

Some infants may show a mixed syndrome consisting of elements of both excitable and depressed behavior, for example, infants who have an initially high threshold for reactivity and appear depressed, but when stimulated become very reactive. Various combinations of excitable and depressed behavior may be observed in individual infants.

Within this conceptual framework, the manifestations of prenatal cocaine exposure will be addressed as they affect the child: physically and neurobehaviorally.

Physical Manifestations

Table 9-3 summarizes the physical manifestations observed in infants exposed prenatally to cocaine (Fulroth, Phillips, & Durand, 1989; Hadeed & Siegel, 1989; Howard, 1989). Head circumference is the most important manifestation for long-lasting effects. According to Chasnoff, Griffith, Freier, and Murray (1992), catch-up head growth may be an important biological marker in predicting long-term development in children exposed in utero to cocaine and other drugs.

In addition, some infants have congenital anomalies as a direct result of the decrease in blood supply to the fetus. These anomalies are disruptions, not malformations. That is, at any time during normal fetal development, interruptions in the blood supply can result in the death of cells. For example, cocaine taken during the time the fingers are developing can result in the constriction of vital blood vessels, causing an infarction: the cells in the fingers die and the fingers will fail to develop or drop off. Even more dangerous infarctions involve the infant's vascular system, namely, stroke and heart attack in utero (Chasnoff, 1992a). Infants born to women who use cocaine are also at risk of AIDS because of the higher incidence of AIDS in drug users.

Neurobehavioral Manifestations

According to Lester et al. (1991), no clear and consistent findings concerning neurobehavioral effects have been established. A number of studies note that infants have difficulty with state control (Anday, Cohen, Kelley, & Leitner, 1989; Chasnoff, Lewis, Griffith, & Wiley, 1989; Hume, O'Donnell, Stanger, Killam, & Gingras, 1989). Such infants are reported to: (a) be fussy and inconsolable, (b) lose state control when stimulated with touch or voice, and (c) look away when their gaze is engaged. Certainly such infants are dif-

---

Table 9-3. Physical Risks of Prenatal Cocaine Exposure

Small head circumference
Low birth weight from prematurity or intrauterine growth retardation
Intrauterine cerebral and cardiac infarctions —small strokes and heart attack
Congenital disruptions—cardiac, genitourinary, limb malformations
AIDS and other infections

Adapted from Fulroth, Phillips, & Durand (1989); Hadeed & Siegel, 1989; Howard (1989)

ficult to care for, putting bonding and attachment with a caregiver at risk. How these behaviors of infancy translate into long-term behaviors that interfere with language and with learning remains unclear, but it appears that prenatal drug exposure has predictable adverse effects on developmental processes that extend beyond the infancy period in many children, at least into toddlerhood. Those effects are summarized in Table 9-4 (see also Sparks, 1990).

Standardized Measures of Development

Chasnoff et al. (1992) used traditional methods of standardized test measurement. They have followed from birth a cohort of children exposed to drugs whose mothers sought recovery for themselves and intervention for their children. The mothers had prenatal care, good nutrition, and medical and developmental assessment and management, which reduced greatly the number of risk factors beyond drug exposure; thus, their study sample is a special group and not necessarily typical. Furthermore, their sample groups were exposed to polydrugs, that is, infants exposed to cocaine and other drugs plus alcohol were compared to a group exposed to other drugs plus alcohol without cocaine. The control group in this study had no drug exposure. The children were assessed at 3, 6, 12, 18, and 24 months. Development was measured by both the Mental Developmental Index (MDI) and the Psychomotor Developmental Index (PDI) of the Bayley Scales of Infant Development (Bayley, 1969). Head circumference was correlated with cocaine exposure at 12, 18, and 24 months, but not before 12 months. There were relatively few significant differences among the three groups on either the MDI or the PDI at 2 years of age. The authors speculate, however, that the Bayley Scales may not provide an accurate assessment of the problems of some children who were exposed to drugs. For example, infants exposed to drugs are reported to have difficulties with self-regulation (Chasnoff, 1992b). If the assessor reduces stimulation and focuses the child's attention during the testing procedure, the difficulty with self-regulation may not be apparent. It may be that test situations actually mask some of the self-regulatory difficulties experienced by children exposed to cocaine and other drugs. Chasnoff and colleagues speculate further that the manifestations of drug exposure may become evident later as these children must engage in increasingly complex thinking.

Table 9-4. Long-term Effects of Prenatal Cocaine Exposure

Reduced head circumference
Reduced self-regulation
Distractibility
Less representational play
Flat affect
Attachment problems

Observational Measures of Development

Another group of researchers (Howard, Beckwith, Rodning, & Kropenske, 1989; Rodning, Beckwith, & Howard, 1990) used observational methods in the belief that developmental and intelligence tests alone are inadequate in demonstrating the subtle deficits that would be most common in children exposed to drugs. They agree that children exposed to drugs can appear developmentally normal when externally structured and monitored by adults, as is the case in administering standardized tests. The capacities of children to meet daily challenges by actively engaging their environment, adapting their behaviors to the challenges in the environment, and initiating environmental changes to meet their own needs are salient dimensions of behavior that are not captured in the scoring of standardized developmental tests.

Rodning et al. (1990) compared 18-month-old toddlers exposed to drugs to a sample of high-risk, preterm toddlers. The observational setting was an unstructured free play situation that required self-organization, self-initiation, and follow-through without the assistance of the examiner to guide the task. The children exposed to drugs showed striking deficits in play and engaged in significantly less representational play than the high-risk, preterm children. Play for the majority of children exposed to drugs was characterized by scattering, batting, and picking up and putting down the toys rather than a sustained combining of toys, fantasy play, or curious exploration. Representational play events, such as combing one's hair, stirring a pot, or sitting a doll at a table were significantly less frequent and less varied in the group exposed to drugs than in the comparison group (Howard et al., 1989).

In addition, the majority of children exposed to drugs had insecure attachments characterized by disorganization rather than organized patterns of avoidance or ambivalence. The theme of disorganization was present in each of the developmental areas assessed—cognitive, social, and affective.

The highest percentage of insecure toddlers exposed to drugs was in the subgroup being raised by their biological mothers. In all but one case, these mothers continued to use drugs. The majority of toddlers exposed to drugs who were being reared by extended family members and foster mothers were rated as secure, and this percentage of security was not significantly different from the percentage of security in the preterm comparison group. The primacy of satisfying the addiction over the welfare of themselves and their children, the impairment from chronic drug use, and the consequent unavailability of mothers either on a high or coming down from a high suggest that the addicted mothers' abilities to be psychologically responsive was greatly impaired, despite their best intentions (Rodning et al., 1990).

Assessment

Professionals may use any normative or critierion-referenced test appropriate for the child's age and purpose for testing, for example, certifying eligibility for service or establishing intervention goals. Some measures of adaptability and coping are appropriate, such as the Vineland Adaptive Behavior Scales (Sparrow et al., 1984).

In addition to the usual assessment battery, emphasis must be given to qualities of the caregiver and to the quantity and quality of the interaction between the infant and caregiver. A number of observation instruments are available to guide the provider in assessing caregiver attributes. Typically, observations are recorded on a checklist while observing the caregiver in interaction with the infant or through direct caregiver interview. For many professionals, a standard part of the assessment includes videotaping the caregiver and child in a free play interaction.

Intervention with Infants

Infants exposed to drugs may range from very irritable to very passive, or they may have no problems with state control (Chasnoff et al., 1992). Irritable infants can reach a frantic-cry state very quickly, which should be avoided by quick caregiver response and soothing. Interaction should take place during quiet alert, not hyperalert, states. The infant may require swaddling and a pacifier to reach a quiet responsive state. The infant should guide the caregiver. His or her cues will indicate what he or she can tolerate and what he or she likes and dislikes. When infants are calm, they can be unwrapped to allow them to become used to controlling their own body movement. They can then be reswaddled, if and when they begin to lose control again, for example, if they begin to show fussy, diffuse movements (Lewis, Bennett, & Schmeder, 1989).

Some infants exposed to drugs show gastrointestinal difficulties throughout their first year of life, which tend to increase irritability and discomfort. The infants may also sleep for long periods of time and are at risk for inadequate nutrition unless wakened for feedings.

Caregivers will be affected by infant irritability, which may result in frustration and feelings of inadequacy in the mothering role and infant-caregiver attachment. If the caregiver is made aware of what to expect in the infant's behavior, negative judgments about the infant can be reduced.

Intervention with Toddlers and Preschool-Age Children

Three principles guide our intervention strategies for children exposed to cocaine, given the research to date:

1. Evaluate each child's threshold for self-regulation.

2. Work toward the child's understanding of his or her own threshold and help that child to take steps to regulate him- or herself. Regulation must begin from the outside—from those in the environment—and then be internalized.

3. Work with the caregiver as well as with the child to build confidence, attachment, and trust in both members of the dyad.

For these principles to work, we must look to the structure of the learning environment (e.g., in the home with the caregiver, in special services or in the classroom) and the individual child's interaction with that environment (e.g., setting and people).

When possible, use an Individual Family Service Plan (IFSP) format. The best planning comes from a team that includes the caregiver, so that the child is treated consistently at home and at school. Identify the family concerns and needs, keeping in mind what has been discussed about families where one or more members use drugs. The team should discuss all members' observations of the child's behavior and progress.

Preschool should be a place where children exposed to drugs can form attachments with adults and learn to trust. It is particularly important that the teachers and service providers are there consistently and turnover is kept to a minimum. Providing attachment is more important than any readiness or academic activities in the early years. These children need a teacher who realizes that they become sensitive and aware of the needs of others only by repeatedly having their own needs met.

Cole (1995) offered ways to help children establish acceptable methods of self-regulation in the classroom:

> Rules that are established must be kept to a minimum and stated clearly. However, children will not learn to cope with classroom expectation, recover from stressful circumstances, or become self-regulated simply by being told what to do and what not to do. Negotiations of acceptable behavior must be individualized and include dialogue, trial and error, and ongoing adaptations. Using headphones, pacing in the back of the room, going for a walk around the yard, or holding certain objects during transitions may work for one child, but not another, or may be possible in one setting, but not another. Initially, broader limits of acceptable behavior may need to be tolerated while getting to know the child. Help to organize the child's experience by reflecting back on what has occurred and what was said; be empathic, be authentic. (p. 134)

CASE STUDY: ROSE

Rose, a Caucasian toddler aged 2½, lives with her paternal grandmother, Martha; grandfather, Albert; and several other children in a small house in a rural area. Other children in the home are also grandchildren of Martha and Albert: Joe is 13, Velma is 6, and Jasper is 4. Sara, 5, is a foster child for whose care Martha and Albert are paid. Other family members are often present in the home. Madeline,14, another grandchild, spends most of her time in the home in the summer and acts as a primary caregiver for Rose. Rose's mother,

Margaret, visits the home about once per week. When she was pregnant with Rose, Margaret was known to use cocaine, alcohol, heroin, and methadone. She has not been in treatment and is still using a variety of substances. Rose's father, Bob, is Martha and Albert's son. He visits the children a few times per month. His substance history is unknown. He does not contribute to the children's care. His current girlfriend has just given birth to his seventh child. Martha and Albert have a chaotic home with many people living in a small space, but they provide stability and love for each of the children.

Rose receives weekly home visits from an early interventionist provided by her state's Department of Developmental Services. Rose initially qualified for service because of her risk status and a recognized developmental delay. With intervention, Rose's motor skills quickly progressed into the normal range. However, of greatest concern are Rose's aberrant behaviors. She is a fearless child who has a hard time understanding rules. She has to be watched constantly or she will run into the street, climb onto high places, or put inedible things, such as rocks and grass, in her mouth. Efforts to stop her with words are futile. On the other hand, she can be affectionate and make connections with others around her, especially with Martha and her aunt Madeline. Martha and Albert are understandably overwhelmed and in need of help with Rose's behavior. Rose's home visitor requested both a behavioral and a speech-language consultation from the home-visiting agency for the upcoming IFSP. In discussion with Martha and Albert, center-based placement seemed to be in Rose's best interest to give her structure in her environment and to give Martha needed respite from Rose and her constant care.

The purpose of the speech and language evaluation was to help determine eligibility and the appropriateness of another type of service, center-based early intervention, as well as to contribute to immediate solutions within the home-based intervention Rose now received. Both standardized testing (Preschool Language Scale–3, Zimmerman, Steiner, & Pond, 1992) and functional assessment were used: the former to establish eligibility under the state guidelines, and the latter for recommendations for the IFSP. Rose's scores on the PLS-3 were in the range of the 13th percentile. Her language skills were emerging, and home-based intervention was clearly making a difference in her responsiveness and communication. These scores made her ineligible for an infant-toddler program for children with special needs in her area. However, if Rose had low scores on another standardized test, she would qualify for center-based service. Since Rose's behaviors were the main concern, The Vineland Adaptive Behavior Scales, Interview Edition, Expanded Form (Sparrow et al., 1984) was also administered by the speech-language pathologist (SLP). The Daily Living Skills Domain, including subdomains of Personal, Domestic, and Community, were especially appropriate. The Community domain includes items on safety (demonstrates understanding that hot things are dangerous, for example) on which Rose had a score of zero. The results of this assessment instrument, along with the SLP's recommendation for center-based placement based on clinical judgment, were presented to the service coordinator.

The SLP also made recommendations to discuss with the family, home visitor, and service coordinator at the IFSP meeting. First and foremost were concerns for Rose's safety. She stressed that all persons in the family should use the same consistent hand signal and word for Stop! when Rose was in a dangerous situation. Second, she gave suggestions for increasing Rose's attention span and expressive and receptive language, remembering that all suggestions should be part of established household routines so as not to further burden Martha. After reviewing a typical day with the SLP, Martha identified bedtime as an optimal time to look at picture books and have conversations with Rose. Martha was also given the phone number of a "Grandparent's Warm Line," a support group for grandparents who are raising the children of their own children who use drugs.

Rose presented a problem that is common to children exposed prenatally to drugs: using standardized measures, they may not clearly qualify for special services designed for children who are developmentally delayed or who have clear disabilities. However, some of these children do need services. The professionals and family agreed that Rose's best placement would be in a small, center-based program with typically developing children who would be good models for her, where she could experience clear boundaries with immediate consequences for out-of-bounds behavior in order to establish methods of self-regulation.

It is unlikely that Rose will be placed in a center-based program until she is 3 years old and eligible for an early intervention preschool or Headstart class. Programs in her area for children with special needs from birth to age 3 are filled with children with more severe delays. She is clearly a child who may "fall between the cracks" of the system that is meant to serve her needs. Rose exhibits much potential and, with appropriate early intervention, can be expected to participate in regular education in the future. While waiting for a center-based placement, the SLP and early interventionist will work in tandem to support Martha and Albert in their efforts to help Rose further develop her communication and self-regulation skills.

SUMMARY

The fact of prenatal exposure to alcohol and cocaine does not necessarily mean that an infant will be adversely affected by that exposure. For children who are affected by alcohol-related birth defects, the maladaptive behaviors of the disorder continue throughout the life span, with the most important problems of communication involving discrepancies between language use and effectiveness. The most important problem for educational settings is poor attention; the most important problems of functioning in society are poor judgment and not understanding the consequences of behavior; and the most important problem in achievement is that it is lower than expected (Burgess & Streissguth, 1992).

Much more is known about alcohol-related disorders than is known about the consequences of prenatal cocaine exposure. It is important to remember that exposure poses a risk; a deficit may or may not be present. Early intervention works and is even more promising for children affected by cocaine than for those affected by alcohol. Some children who were exposed to drugs behave generally like children from the same environment who have had no prenatal exposure. Others, however, show deficits in representational play and caregiver attachments and suffer from general disorders across cognitive, social, and affective areas. In addition, a home where the main occupation is the procurement and use of drugs is not a nurturing environment for children. Thus, research studies that compare children who had prenatal exposure to drugs with children who were not exposed must control for the effects of the home environment.

The prognosis for children who were prenatally exposed to cocaine will not be known until the first cohort of affected children reaches young adulthood. The best intervention incorporates a collaborative IFSP format because the family, whether a foster family, adopted family, or family of origin, is central to success. Clearly, intervention calls for nontraditional and creative methods.

References

Abel, E. L., & Sokol, R. J. (1987). Incidence of fetal alcohol syndrome and economic impact of FAS-related anomalies. *Drug Alcohol Dependency, 19*, 51–70.

Anday, E. K., Cohen, M. E., Kelley, N. E., & Leitner, D. S. (1989). Effect of in utero cocaine exposure on startle and its modification. *Developmental Pharmacology and Therapeutics, 12*(3), 137–145.

Bayley, N. (1969). *Bayley Scales of Infant Development.* New York: Psychological Corporation.

Beck, J. (1984) Will drinking harm your unborn baby? *Detroit Free Press*, January 19.

Brazelton, T. B. (1984). *Neonatal behavior assessment scale* (2nd ed.). Philadelphia: Lippincott.

Burgess, D. M., & Streissguth, A. P. (1992). Fetal alcohol syndrome and fetal alcohol effects; Principles for educators. *Phi Delta Kappan, 74*, 24–30.

Burns, W. J., & Burns, K. A. (1988). Parenting dysfunction in chemically dependent women. In I. J. Chasnoff (Ed.), *Alcohol, drugs and parenting* (pp. 159–171). Boston: Kluwer Academic.

Chasnoff, I. J. (1992a, March). *Cocaine in pregnancy.* Paper presented at the New Perspectives on Substance-Exposed Infants Conference, Stanford University, Palo Alto, Calif.

Chasnoff, I. J. (1992b, May). *Drugs, alcohol, pregnancy and the child.* Paper presented at Drug Use in Pregnancy: Impact on Families and the Growing Child, National Association for Perinatal Addiction Research and Education (NAPARE) Conference, San Francisco.

Chasnoff, I. J., Griffith, D., Freier, C., & Murray, J. (1992). Cocaine/polydrug use in pregnancy: Two year follow-up. *Pediatrics, 51*(2), 284–289.

Chasnoff, I. J., Griffith, D. R., MacGregor, S., Dirkes, K., & Burns, K. A. (1989). Temporal patterns of cocaine use in pregnancy: Perinatal outcome. *Journal of the American Medical Association, 261*(12), 1741–1744.

Chasnoff, I. J., Lewis, D. E., Griffith, D. R., & Wiley, S. (1989.). Cocaine and pregnancy: Clinical and toxicological implications for the neonate. *Clinical Chemistry, 35*(7), 1276–1288.

Chouteau, M., Namerow, P. B., & Leppert, P. (1988). The effect of cocaine abuse on birth weight and gestational age. *Obstetrics and Gynecology, 72*(3), 351–354.

Clarren, S. K., & Astley, S. J. (1995, April). *A screening guide for fetal alcohol syndrome*. Paper presented at The Child with Special Needs Conference, San Francisco.

Clarren, S. K., & Smith, D. W. (1978). The fetal alcohol syndrome. *New England Journal of Medicine, 298*, 1063–1067.

Coggins, T. (1986). *Fetal alcohol syndrome*. Paper presented at the Annual Convention of the American Speech-Language and Hearing Association, New Orleans.

Cole, C. K. (1995). Classroom interventions for young children at risk. In G. H. Smith, C. D. Coles, M. D. Poulsen, & C. K. Cole (Eds.), *Children, families, and substance abuse*. Baltimore: Brookes.

Fulroth, R., Phillips, B., & Durand, J. J. (1989). Perinatal outcome of infants exposed to cocaine and/or heroin in utero. *American Journal of Diseases of Children, 143*(8), 905–1010.

Giacoia, G. P. (1990). Cocaine in the cradle: A hidden epidemic. *Southern Medical Journal, 83*(8), 947–951.

Giunta, C. T., & Streissguth, A. P. (1988, September). Patients with fetal alcohol syndrome and their caretakers. *The Journal of Contemporary Social Work, 69*(7), 453–459.

Hadeed, A. J., & Siegel, S. R. (1989). Maternal cocaine use during pregnancy: Effect on the newborn infant. *Pediatrics, 84*(2), 205–10.

Howard, J. (1989). Cocaine and its effects on the newborn. *Developmental Medicine and Child Neurology, 31*(2), 255–257.

Howard, J., Beckwith, L., Rodning, C., & Kropenske, V. (1989). The development of young children of substance-abusing parents: Insights from seven years of intervention and research. *Zero to Three, 2*(5), 8–12.

Hume, R. F., O'Donnell, K. J., Stanger, C. L., Killam, A. P., & Gingras, J. L. (1989). In utero cocaine exposure: Observations of fetal behavioral state may predict neonatal outcome. *American Journal of Obstetrics and Gynecology, 161*(3), 685–690.

Individuals with Disabilities Education Act Amendments of 1997, P. L. No. 105–117. (IDEA, 1997). U.S.C. Secs. 1400–1485.

Institute of Medicine (IOM), Stratton, K. R., Howe, C. J., & Battaglia, F. C. (Eds.). (1996). *Fetal alcohol syndrome: Diagnosis, epidemiology, prevention and treatment*. Washington: National Academy Press.

Jones, C. L., & Lopez, R. (1988). *Direct and indirect effects on infants of maternal drug abuse.* Washington, D.C.: Department of Health and Human Services National Institutes of Health.

Kronstadt, D. (1991). Complex developmental issues of prenatal drug exposure. *The Future of Children, Drug Exposed Infants, 1*(1), 36–49.

Lester, B., Corwin, M. J., Sepkoski, C., Seifer, R., Peucker, M., McLaughlin, S., & Golub, H. L. (1991). Neurobehavioral syndromes in cocaine-exposed newborn infants. *Child Development, 62,* 694–705.

Lewis, K. D., Bennett, B., & Schmeder, N. H. (1989). The care of infants menaced by cocaine abuse. *Maternal Child Nursing, 14*(5), 324–329.

Little, B. B., Snell, L. M., Klein, V. R., & Gilstrap, L. C. (1989). Cocaine abuse during pregnancy: Maternal and fetal implications. *Journal of Obstetrics and Gynecology, 73*(2), 157–160.

Little, B. B., Snell, L. M., & Rosenfeld, C. R. (1990). Failure to recognize fetal alcohol syndrome in newborn infants. *American Journal of Diseases of Children, 144,* 1142–1146.

Little, R. E., & Wendt, J. K. (1991). The effects of maternal drinking in the reproductive period: An epidemiologic review. *Journal of Substance Abuse, 3,* 187–204.

McBride, W. G. (1977). Thalidomide embryopathy. *Teratology, 16,* 79–82.

McCormick, M., Brooks-Gunn, J., Workman-Daniels, J., Turner, J., & Peckham, G. (1992). The health and developmental status of very low-birth-weight children at school age. *Journal of the American Medical Association, 276*(16), 2204–2208.

McKim, W. A. (1991). *Drugs and behavior: An introduction to behavioral pharmacology* (2nd ed.). Englewood Cliffs, N.J.: Prentice-Hall.

Randall, T. (1992). Infants, children test positive for cocaine after exposure to second-hand crack smoke. *Journal of the American Medical Association, 267*(8), 1044–1045.

Riley, E. P., & Vorhees, C. V. (1986). *Handbook of behavioral teratology.* New York: Plenum Press.

Rinkel, P. (1992). *Myths and stereotypes about long term effects of prenatal alcohol and other drug exposure (PADE)* (Perinatal Addiction Research and Education Update, 1–3). Chicago: National Association for Perinatal Addiction Research and Education.

Rodning, C., Beckwith, L., & Howard, J. (1990, March). *Characteristics of attachment organization and play organization in prenatally drug-exposed toddlers.* Paper presented at the Workshop on Children and Parental Illicit Drug Use: Research, Clinical and Policy Issues. National Research Council, Institute of Medicine, Washington.

Rosett, H. L. (1979). Clinical pharmacology and the fetal alcohol syndrome. In E. Majchrowitz & E. P. Noble (Eds.), *Biochemistry and pharmacology of ethanol* (Vol. 2, pp. 485–510). New York: Plenum.

Samaroff, A., & Chandler, M. J. (1975). Reproductive risk and the continuum of caretaking casualty. In F. D. Horowitz, M. Hetherinton, S.

Scarr-Salapatek, & G. Siegel (Eds.), *Review of child development research* (Vol. 4, pp. 187–244). Chicago: University of Chicago Press.

Schafer, W. (1991). President's Column. The infant crier. *Michigan Association for Infant Mental Health, 55,* 1–2.

Sparks, S. (1990). *A synthesis review of behaviors displayed by neonates with antenatal cocaine exposure.* Unpublished manuscript.

Sparks, S. (1992). *Children of prenatal substance abuse.* San Diego: Singular Press.

Sparrow, S. S., Balla, D. A., & Cicchetti, D. V. (1984). *Vineland Adaptive Behavior Scales.* Circle Pines, Minn.: American Guidance Service.

Streissguth, A. P. (1990, May). *Fetal alcohol syndrome and fetal alcohol effect.* Paper presented at the National Council on Alcoholism of Michigan Workshop, Lansing.

Streissguth, A. P. (1997). *Fetal alcohol syndrome: A guide for families and communities.* Baltimore: Brookes.

Streissguth, A. P., LeDue, R. A., & Randels, S. P. (1988). A manual on adolescents and adults with fetal alcohol syndrome with special references to American Indians (2nd ed.). Albuquerque, N.M.: Indian Health Service.

Streissguth, A. P., Aase, J. M., Clarren, S. K., Randels, S. P., LaDue, R. A., & Smith, D. F. (1991). Fetal alcohol syndrome in adolescents and adults. *Journal of the American Medical Association, 265,* 1961–1967.

Streissguth, A. P., Sampson, P. D., & Barr, H. M. (1989). Neurobehavioral dose-response effects of prenatal alcohol exposure in humans from infancy to adulthood. *Annals of the New York Academy of Sciences, 562,* 145–158.

Vorhees, C. V., & Butcher, R. E. (1982). Behavioral teratogenicity. In K. Snell (Ed.), *Developmental toxicology* (pp. 247–298). New York: Wiley.

Werner, E., & Smith, R. (1982). *Vulnerable but invincible.* New York: McGraw-Hill.

Weston, D. R., Ivins, B., Zuckerman, B., Jones, C., & Lopez, R. (1989). Drug exposed babies: Research and clinical issues. *Zero to Three, 9*(5) 1–7.

Wilson, J. G. (1977). A new area of concern in teratology. *Teratology, 16,* 227–228.

Zimmerman, I., Steiner, V., & Pond, R. (1992). Preschool Language Scale–3. San Antonio, Tex.: Psychological Corporation.

Human Immunodeficiency Virus (HIV) Infection in Young Children

Genine Sander Scott
M.A., CCC-SLP
Speech-Language Pathologist
Chapel Hill, North Carolina
and
Thomas L. Layton, Ph.D., CCC-SLP
Professor
Communication Sciences and Disorders
North Carolina Central University
Durham

Key Terms

acquired immunodeficiency syndrome (AIDS)
antiretroviral
Candida esophagitis
candidiasis
cryptococcus
cytomegalovirus
diplegia
dysarthria
dysphagia

encephalopathy
HIV seropositive
human immunodeficiency virus (HIV)
hyperreflexia
hypogammaglobulinemia
immunocompromised
lymphadenopathy
microencephaly
odynophagia

opportunistic infections or diseases
otitis media
ototoxicity
perinatal
polymerase

pseudobulbar palsy
seroreverted
transcriptase
trunkal hypertonia
virion

Overview

The first cases of pediatric **acquired immunodeficiency syndrome (AIDS)** were reported in 1982, or about one year after reports of the first adult cases (Rogers, 1988, p. 324). Since then, and up to December 1996, there have been 7,629 reported cases of AIDS in children in the United States (Centers for Disease Control [CDC], 1996). Alarmingly, this figure represents only a portion of the number of **human immunodeficiency virus (HIV)** infected children who will eventually develop AIDS (Ammann, 1994; Wolters, 1992). This is especially true since women comprise 20 percent of all adults reported with AIDS (CDC, 1996), and the heterosexual transmission of the disease has begun to increase. Therefore, the proportion of children infected with HIV will assuredly increase too.

In children, AIDS is a multisystemic disease. Whereas its manifestations are numerous, the most frequent findings in the pediatric population are neurodevelopmental abnormalities (Rubinstein, 1989). A review of the literature reveals that the nervous system of the **immunocompromised** child (one whose immunologic mechanism is deficient) can be damaged in a variety of ways (Belman et al., 1988; Civitello, 1991-92; Diamond, 1989; Diamond & Cohen, 1992; Krikorian & Wrobel, 1991). For instance, the virus can invade the brain directly, producing HIV **encephalopathy** (any brain disorder), or it can affect the development of the maturing nervous system, resulting in **microencephaly** (abnormally small brain) and atrophy. In addition, HIV infection can lead to **cryptococcus** (yeast-like fungus) and **cytomegalovirus** (the group of herpes viruses), opportunistic infections of the central nervous system. **Opportunistic infections** or diseases are ailments that occur secondary to a compromised immune system.

Research has indicated that HIV-related neuropathologies produce cognitive, behavioral, and motor deficits (Nozyce et al., 1994). For the early intervention professional, these deficits translate into possible feeding or **dysphagia** (swallowing) issues, articulation disorders, **dysarthria** (disturbances of speech due to paralysis, incoordination, or spasticity of oral musculature secondary to progressive encephalopathy), and/or inadequate respiratory support for speech (Eddy & Whittle-Seiden, 1991; Pressman, 1992). The early interventionist also should be aware of HIV-related otopathologies, especially recurrent **otitis media**, which may occur in 45 percent of the pediatric group (Falloon, Eddy, Wiener, & Pizzo, 1989). Furthermore, the early interventionist should note oral/pharyngeal manifestations, such as **candidiasis** (yeast infection), presenting as hoarseness or **odynophagia** (painful swallowing) and the effect of the disease on language function. This chapter targets the identification, communicative assessment, and treatment of the child who is immunosuppressed.

ETIOLOGY

Human immunodeficiency virus (HIV) causes a progressive disease that moves along a continuum of increasing severity. Acquired immunodeficiency syndrome (AIDS) marks a point somewhere late on that continuum, or the point where an HIV-infected individual contracts any of a list of opportunistic infections, neoplasms, or other symptoms indicative of severe immunodeficiency (CDC, 1987a). In both the pediatric and adult population, the HIV disease varies from asymptomatic to symptomatic infection and inevitably leads to fatal immunosuppression.

Although it is not a major cause of infant mortality, HIV ranks among the 10 leading causes of death for children 1 to 4 years of age (Gayle, Selik, & Chu, 1990). Moreover, approximately 1 percent (7,629/581,429) of all CDC-reported AIDS cases (CDC, 1996) were under 13 years of age; 81 percent of these children were under the age of 5 years (CDC, 1990).

The number of minority children infected with HIV greatly surpasses the number of infected European-American children. In 1996, more than half of all children with HIV in the United States were African American (58 percent, or 4,409 African American children out of the 7,629 children in the United States reported with HIV infection; see Goodwin, 1996, p. 1418). Hispanic American children comprised 1,770 (23 percent), whereas their European American counterparts made up 1,369 (18 percent) of all infected children in the United States. Perhaps minorities, especially African Americans, may be over-represented in this population due to a combination of factors, including poverty and denial that certain behaviors may increase risk of infection (Washington, 1996). Furthermore, injection drug use, prevalent in some African-American, as well as urban, communities, has led to high rates of HIV transmission (Washington, 1996).

HIV: The Virion

HIV belongs to a group of viruses (i.e., a **virion**) known as lentiviruses ("lenti" meaning "slow"). The median period from the time an adult acquires HIV infection to the diagnosis of AIDS is about 8–10 years (Berkelman, Heyward, Stehr-Green, & Curran, 1989). However, HIV infection progresses more rapidly in children (Ammann, 1994; Frederick, Mascola, Eller, O'Neil, & Byers, 1994; Nair, 1992; Oxtoby, 1991; Rogers, 1988). Although the longest reported time from pediatric HIV infection to AIDS diagnosis is 9 years (Rogers, 1988), the typical period is 8 to 17 months (Ammann, 1994), with the median period being 8 months for children with high-risk mothers and 19 months for children receiving transfusions (Rogers, 1988). According to Maldonado and Petru (1994), these data underestimate the incubation period of perinatal HIV infection because they represent pediatric AIDS cases which were diagnosed and reported early in the HIV epidemic. They report that 20 percent of infants with perinatally acquired HIV infection will develop CDC-defined AIDS in the first year of life, followed by 8 percent of such infants per year thereafter. Regardless of the length of asymptomatic infection, once HIV has progressed to AIDS, death usually follows within 2 years (Fox, 1991).

Pediatric HIV infection and its manifestations result from the indirect effect of HIV on the immune system and the direct effect of HIV infection in specific organ systems. It is important that all professionals become familiar with the way HIV invades the human body to better understand the virus's presenting clinical manifestations and their implications on the assessment and treatment of the immunocompromised child.

Outside a host cell, HIV exists as an organized, multilayered particle known as a virion (Fox, 1991; Young, 1994). Figure 10-1 displays the life cycle of the HIV virion through its many stages of development. The virion consists of a center of ribonucleic acid (RNA) and reverse **transcriptase** (a genetic transfer) enclosed by an inner core of proteins, which in turn is surrounded by a knobby-shaped sticky envelope of glycoproteins (gp120 and gp41), which bind and anchor the virus into the host-cell receptor. HIV targets predominantly those cells having a special "receptor" protein (known as CD4); these include white blood cells (macrophages) and T-helper cells (T-4 lymphocytes). After docking onto and merging with the surface of the host cell, the virion transforms the host cell into an "HIV factory." This process begins as RNA and proteins flow into the host cell's cytoplasm. The reverse transcriptase creates a dioxyribonucleic acid (DNA) copy of the viral RNA genome (stage I copy). The DNA copy is then copied, creating a DNA double helix, or provirus (stage II). This provirus enters the nucleus of the host cell and becomes spliced into the host cell's DNA, where it remains for the life of the cell. Although it may exist as an unproductive, "silent" infection, the provirus may be productive, generating more viral RNA. The viral RNA passes out of the host cell nucleus, migrates into the cell cytoplasm, and causes the cell cytoplasm to manufacture the components of the virus. The new virions bud through the host cell membrane, acquiring a lipid bilayer coating as they leave. The body's tissue fluids carry the newly manufactured virions throughout the body to infect more cells. Therefore, by primarily attacking the T-helper cells, the virus causes a depletion of these cells and a reversal of the normal T4 to T8 lymphocyte ratio, yielding more suppressor than helper lymphocytes. This change decreases host defenses to both infection and neoplastic transformation. For more information regarding the cellular invasion of HIV in the human body, refer to Young (1994).

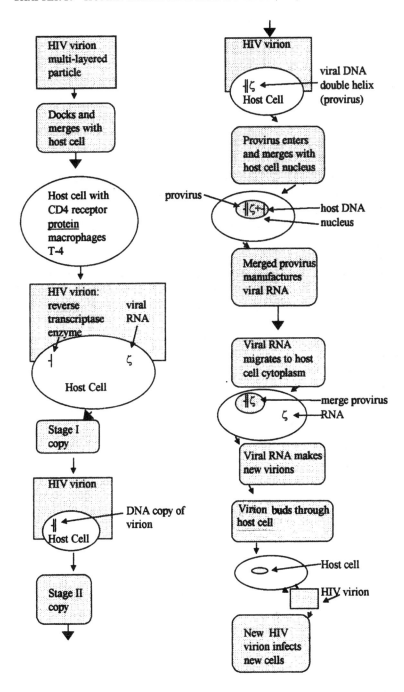

Figure 10-1.   Life cycle of HIV and other lentiviruses. Adapted from Fox, C. (1991). *AIDS and HIV diseases.* Carolina Biology Readers, Research Issue #20, Carolina Biological Supply Company, Burlington, N.C.

Acquisition of HIV

Children acquire HIV in essentially three ways (Simonds & Rogers, 1992). First, they may acquire it parenterally, by shared contaminated needles or other sharp objects, accidental blood exposure, transfusion of blood or other blood products, and tissue or organ transplantation. The second means is sexual transmission, by contact with infected semen, genital secretions, or blood. The third and primary way children acquire HIV is by **perinatal** transmission: through exposure to their infected mothers via maternal-fetal or maternal-infant contacts (Ammann, 1994; Ginzburg, Trainor, & Reis, 1990; Oxtoby, 1991; Rogers, 1988; Simonds & Rogers, 1992). Oxtoby (1991) asserts that perinatal transmission accounts for 80 percent of all pediatric HIV cases in the United States.

Perinatal transmission of HIV can occur: (1) in utero from the mother to the fetus, (2) at the time of delivery by contact with infected blood or vaginal secretions, and (3) through breastfeeding. Increased rates of transmission have been associated with preterm delivery, low maternal anti-gp120 antibody, low maternal CD4 counts, elevated maternal p24 antigen titers, elevated maternal viral levels, maternal injection drug use, lack of prenatal care, and poor clinical condition of the mother (Blanche et al., 1994). Only 25–40 percent of all children born to women infected with HIV, however, actually acquire the disease (Ginzburg et al., 1990; Oxtoby, 1991; Simonds & Rogers, 1992).

DIAGNOSIS

Diagnosis of perinatal HIV infection can be problematic, due to the passively transferred maternal antibodies that can persist in the infant's blood up to 15 months of age (Maldonado & Petru, 1994). Therefore, a baby is usually **HIV seropositive** (showing presence of HIV) after birth because the presence of the HIV antibody is detected with the most common tests, namely, the enzyme-linked immunosorbent assay (ELISA) and the Western blot. To detect true HIV infection as soon as possible in infants born to HIV-infected mothers, investigators have turned to other, more direct measures, such as immune complex dissociation (ICD) p24 antigen, **polymerase** (any enzyme catalyzing a polymerization) chain reaction (PCR), and HIV culture testing. PCR and HIV culture are generally regarded to be sufficiently sensitive and specific to detect the infection in children by the age of 6 months (Maldonado & Petru, 1994). In fact, Maldonado and Petru consider HIV culture the "gold standard" for diagnosis of perinatal infection.

Because virtually all children born to HIV-infected mothers are positive at birth (CDC, 1994c), HIV culture and p24 antigen assay testing should be performed every month for the first 3 months, then every 2 to 3 months until the child is 18 months of age. While some children will be confirmed HIV-positive at that time, others born to infected mothers may serorevert. That is, they may lose their maternally acquired antibodies, thereby changing their status from HIV-positive to HIV-negative (Lepage et al., 1992). Although **seroreverted** children rarely again become seropositive, Lepage et al. (1992) emphasize that seroreversion in children born to seropositive mothers does not, per se, guarantee that the child is uninfected by HIV.

Opportunistic Diseases

The immunocompromised child is subject to a myriad of opportunistic diseases. The most common HIV-related clinical manifestations in this population include: (1) nonspecific symptoms, such as failure to thrive, recurrent fever, anorexia, and generalized **lymphadenopathy** (disease process affecting the lymph nodes); (2) organ system–related diseases (e.g., progressive encephalopathy, peripheral neuropathy, and lymphocytic interstitial pneumonia); (3) infectious complications, examples of which are tuberculosis, ***Candida* esophagitis** (yeast infection of the oral cavity), and cytomegalovirus; and (4) malignancies, especially lymphomas of the non-Hodgkin's type (Hoyt & Oleske, 1992; Maldonado & Petru, 1994). Children with perinatal HIV infection are especially prone to B-cell dysfunction (B-cells are part of the immune system). This dysfunction may eventually yield B-cell depletion, **hypogammaglobulinemia** (decreased quantity of immunoglobulins and increased susceptibility to infection), and recurrent bacterial infections. Yet, the most prevalent of the CDC-defined indicator diseases in children is *Pneumocystis carinii* pneumonia (PCP), at 32 percent (CDC, 1992, 1993a). Table 10-1 lists frequencies of CDC-defined AIDS indicator diseases. As infected children live longer due to **antiretroviral therapy** (drug treatment to combat opportunistic infections), and as prophylactic therapy prevents some of the more common opportunistic infections, new clinical and pathologic disease processes may be observed (Hoyt & Oleske, 1992).

Table 10-1.   Frequency of CDC-defined AIDS Indicator Disease in Reported Pediatric CDC-defined Cases, 1991 and 1992.*

Indicator Disease	Frequency
Pneumocystis carinii pneumonia (PCP)	32%
Lymphoid interstitial pneumonitis (LIP)	21%
Recurrent bacterial infections	15%
HIV encephalopathy	15%
HIV wasting syndrome	14%
Candida esophagitis	12%
Kaposi's sarcoma	rare in children

*(CDC, January 1992; CDC, January 1993a).

According to Lee and Safrin (1994, p. 4.6), "the potential for drug interactions and adverse reactions is great in patients with HIV disease." The authors explain that this is due not only to the multiple drugs prescribed to combat the opportunistic infections associated with HIV, but also to the higher incidence of adverse reactions to commonly used drugs among infected patients. Reactions may range from nausea, vomiting, diarrhea or rash—as with trimethoprim-sulfamethoxazole, the treatment of choice for *Pneumocystis carinii* pneumonia (Coleman, 1994; Peiperl, 1993)—to bone marrow toxicity and myelosuppression—as with flucytosine, which is commonly prescribed for cryptococcosis (Coleman, 1994; Peiperl, 1993).

In addition to medications for opportunistic infections, the child with HIV may be receiving antiretroviral therapy. Jenkins (1994) explains that antiretroviral therapy is provided when a child is enrolled in clinical trials, which administer experimental treatments and monitor for disease progression. AZT (zidovudine, azidothymidine), dideoxylinosine (didanosine, ddI), and dideoxycytidine (zalcitabine, ddC) comprise most of the drugs used in these pediatric clinical trials. However, AZT is currently the only licensed antiretroviral drug for treating HIV infections in infants and children (Jenkins, 1994). Jenkins notes considerable hematologic toxicity in AZT-treated children, although pharmacokinetic studies of continuous intravenous AZT have reported improvement in neurodevelopmental scores, motor function, intellectual function, and weight gain.

Recently, reports of **ototoxicity** (a toxic effect on the ear) associated with certain medications have appeared in the otolaryngologic literature. Examples of reported treatments include eflornithine and trimethoprim sulfamethoxazole (Sahai & Berry, 1989), acyclovir, amphotericin B, azidothymidine (AZT), furosemide, pentamidine and aminoglycoside antibiotics (Kohan, Hammerschlag, & Holliday, 1990; Sooy, 1987; Tami & Lee, 1994). The astute professional working with the immunocompromised child should be familiar with antiretroviral therapies, as well as the more commonly prescribed medications and their side effects, particularly noting those that may be ototoxic. A detailed discussion of these drugs goes beyond the scope of this chapter; see Coleman (1994), Jenkins (1994), Lee and Safrin (1994), or Peiperl (1993) for further information on this topic.

Definition of Pediatric HIV

The case definition of pediatric HIV infection has evolved over the years to accommodate the diverse range of clinical presentations. The 1987 CDC classification system is often referred to in articles regarding children infected with HIV. The system has been simplified to three primary classes. The letter "P" denotes the pediatric classification system, distinguishing it from the CDC's adult HIV classification scheme. Thus, the class P-0, or indeterminate infection, applies to those children less than 15 months old in whom the HIV infection has not been determined. Class P-1 designates children under the age of 13 years whose HIV infection has been confirmed but who are asymptomatic or present without clinical symptoms. Finally, pediatric patients who are symptomatic, that is, presenting with the full or partial spectrum of clinical symptoms of HIV, are classified as class P-2 (CDC, 1987b).

Prompted by additional knowledge about the progression of HIV disease among children, the Centers for Disease Control revised the above definition in 1994 (see Table 10-2). In the new system, the prefix "E" denotes perinatally exposed children, whereas "SR" designates perinatally exposed, but seroreverted, individuals. The class "N" applies to those children under age 13 years with confirmed HIV infection, but who are asymptomatic. Pediatric patients who are both infected and symptomatic are categorized according to severity of symptoms. Thus, "A" indicates "mild," "B" "moderate," and "C" "severe symptomatic" infection. The reader is referred to the CDC's (1994c) revised classification system for specific information regarding category definitions and/or clinical symptoms presenting in the pediatric population.

NEUROPATHOLOGY OF HIV INFECTION IN CHILDREN

Neurologic abnormalities occur frequently in children with HIV infection (Belman et al., 1985, 1986; Brouwers, Belman, & Epstein, 1991; Civitello, 1991-92; Diamond et al., 1990; Kozlowski, 1992; Wiley, Belman, Dickson, Rubenstein, & Nelson, 1990). Essentially, the collective research of these works illustrates that

Table 10-2. Pediatric Human Immunodeficiency Virus (HIV) Classification

		Clinical Categories		
Immunologic categories	N: No sign/ symptoms	A: Mild signs/ symptoms	B:[†] Moderate signs/ symptoms	C:[†] Severe signs/ symptoms
1. No evidence of suppression	N1	A1	B1	C1
2. Evidence of moderate suppression	N2	A2	B2	C2
3. Severe suppression	N3	A3	B3	C3

Note: Children whose HIV infection status is not confirmed are classified by using the above grid with a letter E (for perinatally exposed) placed before the appropriate classification code (e.g., EN2).
[†]Both Category C and lymphoid interstitial pneumonitis in Category B are reportable to state and local health departments as acquired immunodeficiency syndrome.
Source: CDC, 1994c, p. 2.

the nervous system of the immunocompromised child can be damaged in a variety of ways. These include direct invasion of the mature brain (producing HIV encephalopathy) or the developing brain and nervous system (resulting in atrophy and microencephaly). Furthermore, HIV encephalopathy may frequently produce the following features, occurring in either a static or a progressive course, at varying rates of deterioration: pyramidal tract signs, weakness, ataxia, and rarely, seizures and extrapyramidal signs, such as tremor or athetosis (Diamond & Cohen, 1992; Falloon et al., 1989; Schmitt, Seeger, Kreuz, Enenkel, & Jacobi, 1991). As previously stated, HIV may also lead to opportunistic infections of the central nervous system. Civitello (1991–92) suggests that most of the CNS impairment seen in children is secondary to direct HIV infection of the brain.

HIV-related neuropathologies produce cognitive, behavioral and motor deficits (Mellins, Levenson, Zawadzki, Kairam, & Weston, 1994). In fact, developmental delay has been observed in 90 percent of children with HIV infection (Williams, 1987). Behavioral abnormalities, manifested as disruptions in attention and concentration, accompanied by hyperactivity may also occur (Armstrong, Sejdel, & Swales, 1993; Klindworth, Dokecki, Baumeister, & Kupstas, 1989). Schmitt et al. (1991), for example, found autistic behavior combined with deterioration in play and loss of language skills in their study of 75 children infected with, or exposed to, HIV. In addition, they observed aggression, anxiety, and some depression.

Deficits in fine and gross motor skills are common (Armstrong et al., 1993), and include **pseudobulbar palsy** (paralysis of bulbar nerves), **trunkal hypertonia** (extreme tension in trunk), spastic **diplegia** (paralysis on both sides of body) or quadriplegia, **hyperreflexia** (exaggeration of deep tendon reflexes), pyramidal signs, myoclonus (contractions or spasms of muscles), and focal or more generalized seizures (Harris, 1992). Thus, a child with HIV may exhibit low axial tone, interfering with competence in attaining righting skills against gravity and posturing of the lower extremities and preventing weight bearing and transitions from one position to another.

The cumulative effects of the above cognitive, behavioral, and motor difficulties may translate into oral/pharyngeal/laryngeal manifestations related to the HIV infection (Eddy & Whittle-Seiden, 1991; Pressman, 1992).

ORAL MANIFESTATIONS OF HIV INFECTION IN CHILDREN

Among the reported opportunistic infections is candidiasis (i.e., thrush or an oral infection), which is the most common oral condition in individuals with AIDS (Tami & Lee, 1994), occurring in more than half of infected patients with CD4 counts under 200 (Peiperl, 1993). Moreover, when presenting in the esophagus, it is the second most common AIDS-defining opportunistic pathogen in the United States, after PCP (Farizio et al., 1992).

Essentially, candidiasis is a yeast infection of the mouth and esophagus, characterized by white plaque-like lesions, reddened mucous membranes, hoarseness and some discomfort in chewing and swallowing (Peiperl, 1993; Tami & Lee, 1994; Thomas, 1993). Even when oral candidiasis has been treated and cleared, it often persists in the trachea (Pressman, 1992) as well as the esophagus (Tavitian, Raufman, & Rosenthal, 1986), affecting up to 12 percent of infected children (CDC, 1992, 1993a).

Another oral manifestation associated with HIV is salivary gland disease. This includes xerostomia, or dryness of the mouth, diffuse glandular swelling, or benign lymphoepithelial cysts (Tami & Lee, 1994). Parotid enlargement due to lymphocytic infiltration is also reported and may occur in up to 30 percent of infected children (Williams, 1987). While not reporting forms of salivary gland disease, Pressman (1992) has noted both herpes gingivostomatitis (inflammation of the gingiva and oral mucous membranes) and cytomegalovirus esophagitis (a group of herpes viruses) in her investigation.

The presence of oral pathogens, or oral diseases, in the child with HIV has many implications for the professional. In her study of 96 children, Pressman (1992; see also Tables 10-3 & 10-4) reported voice disorders in approximately 13 percent of the children, with 67 percent of those children presenting with hoarseness. She also found equal representation (17%) of denasal, hoarse vocal quality, and hypernasal vocal quality. Although citing progressive encephalopathy as the origin of the weak, hypernasal voices, Pressman generally associated hoarseness with candidiasis, stating that a hoarse voice may be a marker for this infection. However, Pressman carefully notes that one cannot assume candidiasis is always the source of hoarseness. In fact, one should consider vocal cord nodules and/or granulomas as possible etiologies as well.

In addition to voice disorders, Pressman (1992) reported that about 21 percent of the children in her study evidenced dysphagia. Her examinations revealed problems in the oral preparatory, oral, and pharyngeal phases of swallowing. Specific complaints of the children's caregivers included coughing on food or liquid, failure to thrive, slow feeding, and gagging on solids or chewables. Pressman adds that, in many cases, gagging resulted from hypersensitivity secondary to oral defensiveness, relating to lack of experience with a variety of foods. Etiologies for dysphagia consisted of encephalopathy, neuromuscular discoordination, and odynophagia (painful swallowing) related to candida esophagitis, herpes gingivostomatitis, and CMV esophagitis.

OTOLOGIC DISEASES ASSOCIATED WITH PEDIATRIC AIDS

In recent years, the otolaryngologic literature has documented a myriad of AIDS-related otologic manifestations. These are often a result of bacterial, fungal and viral pathogens that invade the immunocompromised patient, the ototoxic medications used to treat them, cutaneous and oral lesions, or neuropathy of the eighth cranial nerve (Falloon et al., 1989; Williams, 1987). Many AIDS-related otologic diseases have different prevalence rates in pediatric than in adult AIDS populations (Sculerati & Borkowsky, 1990). A review of the literature suggests that children with HIV frequently experience bacterial infections of the ear, otitis externa and various forms of otitis media (Chanock & McIntosh, 1989; Church, 1987; Johnson et al., 1989; Pahwa et al., 1986; Pinkert et al., 1993; Principi et al., 1991; Sculerati & Borkowsky, 1990; Smith & Canalis, 1989). The appearance, however, of other otopathologies in the pediatric population are rare.

As with noninfected children, **otitis media** (OM, inflammation of the middle ear) commonly presents in children with AIDS, in part due to eustachian tube dysfunction typical in this age group, as well as to depressed cell-mediated immunity, which markedly increases their susceptibility (Kohan, Rothstein, & Cohen, 1988) and antibody dysfunction. Currently, there is no evidence that HIV-infected patients have a higher incidence of complications of otitis media than the general public (Morris & Prasad, 1990; Tami & Lee, 1994). However, research indicates that children diagnosed as P-2 infected with HIV (i.e., those children who were both HIV-positive and symptomatic), in addition to those children with lower T4 cell counts, are at greater risk (47 percent vs. 18 percent) of recurrent acute otitis media (AOM) than children diagnosed P-1 who were HIV-positive and asymptomatic (Barnett, Klein, Pelton, & Luginbuhl, 1992; Principi et al., 1991). A review of the literature documents acute OM, recurrent OM, or OM with effusion (fluid) in the pediatric HIV population. In addition, an 80 percent incidence of serous OM has been reported (Smith & Canalis, 1989). Regardless of the form of infection, children with OM typically experience a 21 to 30 dB hearing loss (Bess & Humes, 1990).

Acute otitis media (AOM) typically causes recurrent ear pain and fever, and, in the infected population, usually results from *Streptococcus pneumoniae* or *Haemophilus influenzae*. Also found in infected children are recurrent otitis media (ROM), occurring in 45 percent (Falloon et al., 1989) and serous otitis media. Serous otitis media (SOM) is presumably due to poor eustachian tube function; however, nasopharyngeal tumors, allergies, viral infections or adenoidal hypertrophy from the HIV virus may be contributing causes (Sooy, 1987). Furthermore, children with AIDS may experience otitis media with effusion (OME), in which relatively asymptomatic effusion takes place without signs of inflammation.

Otitis media responds well to oral antimicrobial therapy such as ampicillin, amoxicillin, erythromycin, or ciprofloxacin. However, failure of response may require tympanocentesis and a fluid culture, with the antibiotics changed according to culture results (Morris & Prasad, 1990). In cases of recurrent otitis media, or in infections that have responded poorly to antimicrobial therapy, myringotomy and tympanometry tubes or surgical drainage may be necessary (Poole, Postma, & Cohen, 1984).

A hearing loss of any kind has far-reaching consequences in the pediatric AIDS population. A hearing impairment in this population, coupled with the developmental delay frequently seen in pediatric AIDS patients (Williams, 1987), could interfere with language learning and dramatically inhibit communication. Thus, the need for hearing evaluation in this population cannot be overemphasized.

LANGUAGE FUNCTION IN CHILDREN INFECTED WITH HIV

The initial research investigating neurological AIDS-related manifestations only peripherally documented developmental delays in language within the pediatric population. Later research generalized results to a discussion of linguistic function, at times in a cursory manner (Cohen et al., 1991; Diamond et al., 1987; Epstein et al., 1986; Msellati et al., 1993). Only a handful of studies have specifically tested language dysfunction in children infected with HIV (Belman et al., 1988; Condini et al., 1991; Havens, Whitaker, Feldman, Alvardo, & Erhardt, 1993; McCardle et al., 1991; Pressman 1992; Ultman et al., 1985; Wolters, 1992; Wolters, Brouwers, Moss, & Pizzo, 1995). However, not all of these studies reported in detail the results of their language testing (Belman et al., 1988; Ultmann et al., 1985). Tables 10-3 and 10-4 summarize five investigations that more closely examine language function within the pediatric HIV population.

Of the five studies, all used some method of standardized testing to measure receptive and expressive language. Pressman (1992), for example, administered the Preschool Language Scale (Zimmerman & Dodson, 1979), as well as the Birth to Three Developmental Scale (Bangs, 1979), Early Learning Accomplishment Profile (ELAP), (Glover, Preminger, & Sanford, 1978); Hawaii Early Learning Profile (HELP), (Furuno et al., 1984); Peabody Picture Vocabulary Test (PPVT), (Dunn, 1959); and Expressive One-Word Picture Vocabulary Test (EOWPVT), (Gardner, 1979). For children 3 years of age and above, Pressman (1992) noted that vocabulary tests were emphasized because she found these tests very sensitive to change in neurological status. Pressman also found that over 69 percent of her 96 subjects showed moderate to profound deficits in receptive and expressive language. Pressman looked at a wide range of factors that influenced communication, from articulation disorders to vocal quality and dysphagia. However, she did not provide a detailed discussion of her test results. Pressman reported that many factors could have contributed to the high incidence of language delay and developmental abnormalities exhibited by her subjects. These factors included prenatal, medical, environmental, and psychological factors associated with HIV, as well as living in the inner city. Another factor possibly influencing the results was that those subjects over 3 years of age were assessed only by vocabulary testing, which reveals merely one level of language function (Pressman, 1992).

The Havens et al. (1993) study provided more details on language functioning on the Receptive One-Word Picture Vocabulary Tests (Gardner, 1985) and Expressive One-Word Picture Vocabulary Test (Gardner, 1990). Havens and colleagues matched children who were HIV-positive for age, sex, and race

Table 10-3. Summary of Five Studies that Reported Language Dysfunction in Children Infected with HIV: Part 1

Source	Pop. Size	Age/Grouping	Family	Medication	Speech Devel. Task/Tools	Naming Task/Tools	Comprehension Task/Tools
Condini et al. (1991)	36 Matched: 18 infected 18 non-infected	18–30 months	Implied with mothers	Not on Mx during study	DQ=Brunet-Lezine Scale	- Drawn objects (hand, spoon) - Model objects (car, bus) -Verb indicating drawn action	-Selects 7 drawn objects -Selects 12 model objects -9 action verbs (Child given 3 drawings showing 3 objects. Child had to indicate object needed to perform a certain action.)
Havens et al. (1993)	60 26 HIV+ 14 seroreverted 20 controls (born to substance using mother)	5 to 12 years (X = 7:4 years) Matched: age, sex, race; all children were exposed to drug use in utero	All were in foster care	Not Specified			
McCardle et al. (1991)	27 8 HIV+ via blood 19 perinatally exposed [7 infected 12 uninfected (seroreverted)]	Not Given	Not Given	3/7 infected (class P-2) received AZT			

(continues)

Table 10-3. (continued)

Source	Pop. Size	Age/Grouping	Family	Medication	Speech Devel. Task/Tools	Naming Task/Tools	Comprehension Task/Tools
Pressman (1992)	96	4 months to 17:3 years	Many in single parent homes	Not Specified	Test instrument not specified, but 27% reported to be deficient in articulation		
Wolters (1992) Dissertation Wolters et al. (1995)	36 27 infected mother to child; 9 infected by transfusions; 21 with HIV-related enceph-alophathy; 15 nonenceph-alophathic 20 uninfected siblings	1 to 10 years (X = 5:5 years)	Not Specified	Not on Mx at time of testing			

Table 10-4. Breakdown of Five Studies That Reported Language Dysfunction in Children Infected with HIV: Part 2

Source	Memory	Vocal Quality	Cog Function	Lang Develop	Receptive Lang	Express Lang	Visual Processing	Conclusions
Condini et al. (1991)			3/15 HIV+ showed cognitive deficits	20 minute language sample to obtain MLU				-Children who were HIV-infected but not ill had delayed language production (lower MLU's) compared to children who were non-infected born to mothers who were HIV-infected. -Delay more evident at beginning of language devel. (year 2) than later for HIV-inf. Children. (Groups were similar during year 3). -Language is strong area for children with HIV-infection, but data indicate language is impaired.
Havens et al. (1993)	Stanford-Binet (Fourth Ed): Short Term Memory		Stanford-Binet (Fourth Ed): Verbal Reason Quant Reason Composite		Gardner One-Word Picture Vocabulary Test of Receptive Language	Gardner One-Word Picture Vocabulary Test of Expressive Language	Stanford-Binet (Fourth Ed): Abstract Visual Reasoning	-Psychiatric disorder tests -All groups had low-average language - Children with HIV+ were deficient cognitively in short-term memory -Behavior problems due to in-utero drug exposure -Genetic factors and background more important influence on cognitive and language function than HIV

(continues)

Table 10-4. continued

Source	Memory	Vocal Quality	Cog Function	Lang Develop	Receptive Lang	Express Lang	Visual Processing	Conclusions
McCardle et al. (1991)			3/15 HIV+ showed cognitive deficits	Test Instrument not specified. However, 12/15 children who were HIV+ reported to have language deficits		5/7 perinatal had language deficits 6 of these 7 had an expressive deficit		- No definite pattern of language deficit for child infected w/HIV via blood products -Language ability, especially expressive, seems vulnerable to HIV -25% seroreverters showed language deficits, albeit w/ no specific pattern
Pressman (1992)		12.5% voice disordered 17% denasal 67% hoarse 17% weak hypernasal		-Birth-3 Scale -Early Learning Accomp Profile -HELP	-Pre-School Language Scale -PPVT -Expressive One-Word Vocabulary Test	-Pre-School Language Scale		-69%+ showed moderate-to-profound deficits in receptive/expressive language -Hoarseness due to candidiasis -Many factors such as prenatal, environmental and psychological factors associated with HIV may have contributed to the high incidence of language delay exhibited by subjects
Wolters (1992) Dissertation Wolters et al. (1995)					-Reynell Developmental Language Scale -Clinical Eval of Language Functions-Revised	-Reynell Developmental Language Scale -Clinical Eval of Language Functions-Revised		-Children w/AIDS exhibit lower expressive language than receptive language -Children with enceph perform poorer than children who were nonenceph on receptive and expressive language

with children who had no history of HIV. Nearly all of the children were born to substance-using mothers, and all of the children were in foster care. Havens et al. found that, although the receptive and expressive scores fell in the low average range across the board, there was no difference between children who were HIV-positive, seroreverted, and the control children (see Table 10-3 and 10-4). Havens and associates concluded that genetic factors and/or background, such as prenatal drug exposure, were possibly more important influences of cognitive and language function than HIV infection itself.

In another study that controlled for developmentally influential factors, McCardle et al. (1991) examined 27 children, 8 of whom had acquired HIV via blood products and 19 of whom were exposed to HIV perinatally (7 infected, 12 uninfected, or seroreverted). Neurodevelopmental skills, especially language, were targeted, although the authors failed to specify the manner of skill assessment. Their study's population, all participants in the U.S. Military Pediatric HIV program, had fewer background risk factors that might have influenced cognitive and/or linguistic performance. Although specific risk factors were not detailed, the authors described their subjects as a "more stable, healthy population with less maternal IV drug abuse" (p. 187). McCardle et al. found that 12 of the 15 infected children manifested some form of language deficit. However, no definite pattern of language deficit emerged for the 8 children who acquired HIV via blood products. Still, linguistic ability, especially expressive language, appeared particularly vulnerable to HIV, with 71 percent (5/7) of the children exposed perinatally exhibiting language deficits and 86 percent (6/7) demonstrating expressive difficulties. In addition, 25 percent (4/12) of the children who were seroreverted (i.e., perinatally exposed, uninfected) had language impairments, albeit with no specific pattern regarding receptive versus expressive language. McCardle et al. concluded that language ability, especially expressive language, seemed vulnerable to HIV. McCardle et al. (1991) purported that children who were seroreverters were at neurodevelopmental risk and should be monitored for neurodevelopmental and linguistic progress.

Two of the five studies reported in Tables 10-3 and 10-4 were quite thorough in their investigation of language development in children infected with HIV. In the first, Wolters (1992; Wolters et al., 1995) examined receptive and expressive language in 36 children with AIDS (21 encephalopathic, 15 nonencephalopathic), ages 1 to 12 years (with a mean age of 5; 5). Wolters used the Reynell Developmental Language Scales (Reynell & Huntley, 1985) and the Clinical Evaluation of Language Functions–Revised (Semel, Wiig, & Secord, 1987) as her diagnostic instruments. Her results indicated that the children with AIDS exhibited lower expressive language scores than they did receptive language. In addition, she found that the children with encephalopathy performed poorer than the children without encephalopathy, on both receptive and expressive language functions. From these results, Wolters concluded that HIV affects the language abilities of children with AIDS, particularly their expressive language skills. Also, Wolters noted that advanced HIV disease in the CNS yields significantly more impairments in expressive and receptive language.

Despite Wolters's (1992) thoroughness, she did not match subjects by age or employ a control group. Also, family status was not reported, which could have altered her overall results. Further, 27 of her children acquired the virus vertically (i.e., from mother to child), whereas 9 became infected by transfusion. Since Jason, Stehr-Green, and Hohman (1988) reported that children with hemophilia who acquire HIV infection via transfusion differ from infants with perinatally acquired HIV infection, this difference could have influenced the results. Not only do children with hemophilia and HIV suffer more often from different opportunistic infections than their perinatally acquired counterparts, but they also have a premorbid history of normal language acquisition. Infants infected from birth or within the first 2 years generally lack this period of normalcy (Jason et al., 1988).

Finally, Condini et al. (1991) matched 18 children infected with HIV with 18 children who were non-infected but exposed, ages 18 to 30 months. After employing the Brunet-Lezine Scale (Brunet & Lezine, 1967) to determine the children's developmental quotient, the children were asked to name drawn and model objects, as well as drawings depicting action verbs. Comprehension skills were examined with similar measures. Condini and his associates also obtained a 20-minute spontaneous language sample from each child to determine mean length of utterance (MLU).

Condini et al.'s results were supportive of those of Pressman (1992), Havens et al. (1993), and Wolters (1992). They found children infected with HIV with no opportunistic diseases exhibited significantly lower MLUs compared to noninfected children born to mothers infected with HIV. This delay in language production was more apparent at the beginning of language development (during the 2nd year of life) than in later years. That is, despite a slow start in language development, the infected children reached comparable language levels with the noninfected children by approximately 3 years of age. Condini et al.'s (1991) investigation supported the conclusion that HIV infection appears to impair the beginning rather than the later development of language in children who are HIV-infected, but not ill.

As a whole these five studies are of interest; however, most evidence some methodological weakness. First, the researchers often used subjects whose age span differed dramatically (Havens et al., 1993; Wolters, 1992; Wolters et al., 1995). The Pressman (1992) study had the largest age range, spanning nearly 17 years (from 4 months to 17 years, 3 months). This, of course, is problematic because language abilities and measures to evaluate language of a 4-month-old significantly differ from those used with a 17-year-old. Older children have acquired many more language and concepts skills than younger children. Therefore, it is difficult to cite any thing more than gross generalizations of overall language abilities, and comparisons of specific skills cannot and should not be made.

Furthermore, two of the studies did not specify family status, which may be an important variable for language and overall development (McCardle et al., 1991; Wolters, 1992). Often the environment of the child infected with HIV is unstable, depending on the caregiver-child relationship (Wiener & Septimus, 1991). Thus, an important variable may be whether the child infected with HIV lives with his/her biological parents, a guardian, or a foster family. Even if a child who is infected is with his/her biological parents, the language-learning environment may be adversely affected due to the health of a mother, father, or siblings who are infected with HIV.

Finally, two of the five investigations did not specify whether the children took medication during the study (Havens et al., 1993; Pressman, 1992). This information is critical to the interpretation of the studies because medication can resolve many of the HIV-related opportunistic infections, thereby positively affecting language development and/or test performance. It can also cause negative side-effects, affecting testing (Pizzo & Wilfert, 1991). Clearly, it may be important for researchers to note whether the subjects took medication during the trial and to list the name of the medication in order to identify possible drug-related effects.

ASSESSMENT

Given the number of developmental difficulties that these children display, as well as the complexity of medical, social, and educational issues involved with this population, a multidisciplinary (several different professions assessing the child) approach to both assessment and intervention is critical (Cohen & Diamond, 1992). Of course, the nature of the infection, in addition to the variety of opportunistic pathogens that manifest within the immunocompromised child, makes medical management a necessity. Thus, general medical assessment is needed initially to determine the status of the mother's health and/or infection during pregnancy, the amount of prenatal care, and the course of the neonate after delivery. In addition, pediatric medical assessment should establish baselines and follow-up regarding nutrition, weight gain, growth history, and recurrent illnesses.

In addition to general medical assessment, assessment by a number of medical specialists may be involved. For instance, immunologists and infectious disease specialists may diagnose and treat opportunistic infections. Other specialists (e.g., pulmonary disease experts and otolaryngologists) may be called upon as consultants along the course of the child's disease to treat these infections, as well. The child infected with HIV may also experience failure to thrive and feeding difficulties due to dysphagia. A nutritional assessment can be done to evaluate the child's diet, feeding techniques, and schedule (Cohen & Diamond, 1992).

Diamond and Cohen (1992) also noted that developmental delay may be the first manifestation of HIV symptomatology, as well as of neurological dysfunction in children congenitally infected with HIV. Certainly, with the risk of the development of neuropathologies, a neurodevelopmental assessment is warranted (Cohen & Diamond, 1992). The neurological examination should determine presence of physical characteristics associated with congenital HIV or other syndromes, type and degree of neurological dysfunction, if any, and developmental and behavioral status.

Psychological testing can determine the level of cognitive functioning. The clinician should also evaluate behavior and, when appropriate, make recommendations about management strategies. The cognitive profile of each child will vary depending on age and stage of disease progression, but poor performance may generally be expected due to encephalopathy, as well as environmental factors and possible language deficits (Cohen & Diamond, 1992). Motor impairment may also negatively affect the results of cognitive assessments designed to test visual-motor coordination, drawing, or block building (e.g., the McCarthy Scales of Children's Abilities; McCarthy, 1972).

Living with HIV means living with the stresses that often accompany the infection. For example, the child with HIV may experience painful medical treatments, occasional hospitalizations that may disrupt the child's routine, and side effects of antiretroviral therapy or medications used for opportunistic infections. The child may exhibit HIV-related psychiatric symptoms and/or dementia that may require special services as well as special attention of parents and caregivers. Parents of the children may themselves be chronically ill, or drug- or substance-dependent, thereby rendering them less capable of providing adequate or consistent child care. The child may be in a foster home or a series of homes. In addition, the family and the immunocompromised child must face the social stigma associated with HIV infection (Klindworth et al., 1989). All of these "stressors," while independently already difficult to handle, may occur simultaneously. Social service assessment can facilitate coping strategies for the family/caregivers. Cohen and Diamond (1992) emphasize that, under all circumstances, the needs of the family/caregivers must be carefully considered and plans must be formulated to deal with their concerns.

Educational assessment can help to determine the child's educational needs and the specific special educational interventions that might be necessary (Cohen & Diamond, 1992). This is true not only for preschoolers, but also for school-age children, who, because of developmental deficits, may require special education and/or early intervention services.

Due to the many motoric difficulties, especially oral-motor complications, services provided by an occupational and physical therapist seem warranted. The occupational therapist can assist in daily living activities as well as the swallowing and feeding needs of the child. A physical therapist can help with large muscle coordination and fine motor activities.

In addition to the previously listed types of assessment, speech, language, and hearing evaluations are essential. Because the child with HIV may experience a variety of otopathologies, especially otitis media, audiologic evaluation is warranted. Moreover, because the development of expressive language skills in infants and children infected with HIV may be an early indicator of HIV-associated CNS disease, Wolters et al. (1995) noted the clinical importance for comprehensive speech and language testing. These authors also recommend speech and language services throughout the course of the disease to provide evaluation, and rehabilitation therapy, as well as alternative communication systems to prevent, improve, and compensate for the language and speech deficits observed in the pediatric population.

A full battery of speech and language instruments is recommended to evaluate and obtain a complete picture of the speech and language abilities of the child with HIV. To begin with, an oral mechanism examination is needed to grossly evaluate cranial nerve function necessary for producing and sequencing sounds. Acoustic measures, such as fundamental frequency and pitch perturbation (jitter), can assess the perceptual qualities of pitch and voice quality, while an s/z ratio may be taken to estimate function of the vocal folds. A subjective rating of voice quality (e.g., hoarseness or degree of nasality) may also prove useful.

The clinician should administer standardized and nonstandardized tests which target both receptive and expressive language skills. Two reported instruments in the literature for older children include the Reynell Developmental Language Scale–Revised (Reynell & Huntley, 1985) and the Clinical Evaluation of Language Fundamentals–Revised (Semel et al., 1987). For younger children, the Early Language Milestone Scale (ELMS), (Walker, Gugenheim, Downs, & Northern, 1989); MacArthur Communicative Development Inventories (Fenson et al., 1993); and Communication and Symbolic Behavior Scales (Wetherby & Prizant, 1990) are currently used instruments, along with play-based assessment (Linder, 1990). To obtain a naturalistic, spontaneous language sample, the focus should extend beyond the free play situation and include personal and elicited narratives (Lund & Duchan, 1988). Furthermore, because vocabulary tests are sensitive to changes in neurological status (Pressman, 1992), assessment should include receptive and expressive vocabulary evaluation, for example, the Peabody Picture Vocabulary Test–Revised (Dunn & Dunn, 1981) and the Expressive One-Word Picture Vocabulary Test (Gardner, 1979). Articulation testing is also recommended. The Goldman-Fristoe Test of Articulation (Goldman & Fristoe, 1986) is a commonly used test; however, we feel that the additional information such as that obtained on the Khan-Lewis Phonological Analysis (Khan & Lewis, 1986), especially related to phonological processes, is also important in assessment.

Due to the frequency of dysphagia in this population, the speech-language pathologist may also be involved with swallow assessments. In her work with children infected with HIV, Pressman (1992) employed the Modified Barium Swallow Study (MBSS). However, the acutely symptomatic child may either be on contact isolation precautions or may be too ill to sustain movement or exposure to radiation. In such cases, Fiberoptic Endoscopic Examination of Swallowing (FEES) may be used at the patient's bedside. As usual, the professional performing the Modified Barium Swallow Study or FEES should carefully follow standard precautions as set by the medical facility or hospital. Examples of standard precautions include, but are not limited to, wearing gloves with contact or possible contact with blood and/or bodily fluids and hand washing after contact with every patient.

Regardless of the roles of the professionals who may be involved with the child who has HIV, Cohen and Diamond (1992) call for a team process and collaborative information sharing in order to provide the best care to the family and the child.

The following two cases are of girls who were born to mothers who are HIV-positive. The first girl, Lydia, unfortunately, was infected with the virus; Olivia, fortunately, was not infected. The two cases are presented here to demonstrate possible communication problems and other related difficulties associated with the virus.

CASE STUDY: LYDIA

Lydia, an African-American girl aged 5;2, with perinatally acquired AIDS, was seen by two speech-language pathologists during a 4-month course of treatment at a university hospital. Lydia was the youngest of her siblings, of which there were three. Because her parents had both died from complications of AIDS, Lydia lived with her maternal aunt. Each of the siblings lived with various relatives in another state.

According to medical report, Lydia was born following a 35-week pregnancy to a mother who was HIV-positive. Records also indicated that Lydia experienced withdrawals secondary to prenatal exposure to drugs, which her mother had apparently used throughout her pregnancy with Lydia. Thus, Lydia was exposed prenatally to HIV as well as to drugs.

A series of tests confirmed Lydia's HIV-positive status. By age 7 months, she had already become symptomatic, developing respiratory distress, oral thrush (candidiasis), and failure to thrive. In fact, Lydia's weight, both at birth and at 7 months, fell at the 5th percentile.

By 1 year of age, Lydia received AZT, which failed to retard the progression of AIDS. She then was placed on a protocol where she received ddC salvagen. This medication was soon discontinued because Lydia demonstrated progressive central nervous system disease, characterized by a regression of motor and language milestones. A chart report at this time revealed that Lydia stopped walking and exhibited decreased language, though no specific examples of the loss were given.

As Lydia grew older, her disease continued to progress, and she experienced bouts of candidal esophagitis, chronic sinusitis, HIV encephalopathy and spastic diplegia. Records show calcification of the basal ganglia present since she was aged 4;2. When Lydia was not in the hospital, her aunt placed her in an area preschool program.

At the time of her last hospitalization, Lydia was aged 5;2 and had a low CD4 count of 40 (CD4 counts, however, are more variable in children and may not be as good an indicator of infection status in children as in adults.) As is common with later stages of the virus, Lydia was plagued by numerous medical complications, such as HIV encephalopathy. Her diagnosis also included pulmonary disease; therefore, she was treated with a bronchoscopy, intubated, and placed on a conventional ventilator. She required a series of chest tubes for pressure regulation, as well as a Bivona trach to reduce air leakage. After 3 months of hospitalization, Lydia's respiratory status stabilized. She was weaned from the ventilator and later decannulated.

Lydia also experienced many electrolyte abnormalities, especially hypokalemia (extreme potassium depletion of the blood), which was exacerbated by persistent diarrhea. After 2½ months of hospitalization, Lydia's liver function became impaired, possibly secondary to potentially hepatotoxic medications. Thus, ddI and AZT (used to combat the AIDS virus), in addition to fluconazole (for oral thrush), were discontinued.

Notes from the infectious disease specialist following her case revealed that, over the course of her hospital stay, Lydia had multiple infections. These included Pneumocystis carinii pneumonia (PCP), *tracheal flu, oral thrush, fungal duodenitis (inflammation of first part of small intestine) and tracheal,* Methicillin-resistant Staphylococcus aureus (MSRA). *The tracheal MRSA, which is spread by touching an infected person or things with which an infected person has come in contact, placed Lydia on contact isolation. Thus, Lydia was placed in a private room, and masks, gowns and gloves were required when entering the room and working with the child. All infections were managed with pharmacotherapy. Morphine helped relieve the child's pain from her deteriorating condition, numerous procedures, and multiple infections.*

A pediatric neurologist addressed Lydia's spastic diplegia. A physical therapist worked with her daily to maintain range of motion and strength, and orthopedic specialists fitted short leg and stretching casts to counter Lydia's severe equinous contractures, which reduced proper foot position, making it difficult to bear weight.

Lydia had already been hospitalized for over 2 months when the speech-language pathologists were called in to evaluate, and possibly augment, the child's communication skills. An initial cursory evaluation at bedside revealed Lydia to be weak and somnolent, demonstrating intermittent periods of alertness. In subsequent sessions Lydia communicated her immediate needs via gestures and head nods as well as verbally. Vocal function was weak and breathy. She phonated in short bursts of speech, in part due to her reduced respiratory capacity secondary to PCP. Air leakage around the tracheostomy tube as Lydia attempted to phonate also contributed to her impaired vocal quality. Lydia was not referred for an audiological evaluation in view of her deteriorating condition. Her interaction with the therapist at the time of the examination suggested that her hearing was within functional limits.

Because of the severity of Lydia's condition, nonstandardized, informal assessment instruments were the best method to evaluate the child. Informal assessment revealed that Lydia could point to body parts on command and could understand and execute simple, one-step directions on herself and on another (e.g., she fed herself and then a baby doll at the examiner's request). From this assessment, it appeared that, while Lydia demonstrated functional communicative intent, her comprehension ability was somewhat impaired, likely due to HIV encephalopathy.

To augment her existing communication abilities, a variety of assistive devices were tried. A digital voice output device was used initially, but Lydia showed little interest in the pictures and appeared to be too weak to push the buttons that activated the electronic voice. Next, a small Cooper-Rand electrolarynx in the shape of a child's toy was tried to circumvent the problem of picture identification. The electrolarynx consists of a plastic tube to be placed in the oral cavity and a tone generator. Speech is created when words are mouthed around the plastic tube while the tone generator is activated. Although Lydia seemed extremely interested in this device, she was too weak to push the tone generator button and demonstrated a sucking reflex whenever the flexible tube was placed in her mouth.

The therapist then introduced a Passy-Muir valve. Because Lydia experienced air leakage around the site of her trach, which produced breathy, effortful phonation, it was believed the Passy-Muir would reduce the air leak and, consequently, facilitate more efficient speech. The valve was gradually left on for increasingly longer periods of time. Lydia successfully used the Passy-Muir valve to produce speech, but she also relied upon gestures and head nods for communication. With the stabilization of her respiratory status, Lydia was decannulated, eliminating the need for the Passy-Muir valve. Without the trach to interfere, Lydia could phonate independently. Although the speech-language pathologist initially noted a weak vocal quality, Lydia's voice was noticeably stronger at the time of the last visit.

During her 4-month period of hospitalization, Lydia was followed by a number of professionals to treat and relieve the infections and symptoms secondary to the AIDS virus. Speech-language pathologists, respiratory therapists, infectious disease, gastroenterology and cardiovascular specialists, nutritionists, social workers and physical therapists, in addition to physicians from Ear, Nose, and Throat (ENT), Radiology, Pediatric Psychology, Orthopedics, and Pediatric Neurology, completed the team. Upon discharge, Lydia's case manager, an infectious disease specialist, recommended a nasogastral tube to maintain gastrointestinal status, continued parenteral nutrition in 24-hour periods, liberal administration of medications for pain management, and follow-up by hospice. The prognosis for the child was poor.

Lydia died at her aunt's home 2 weeks after discharge, due to complications of AIDS. She was aged 5;6.

CASE STUDY: OLIVIA

When seen at a university speech and hearing clinic for a complete speech, language, and hearing evaluation, Olivia was a delightful African-American girl aged 3;8, who lived in the same household with her mother, stepfather, and five older siblings. The mother described her pregnancy with Olivia as being "normal," "nine months," and "free of complications." However, Olivia's mother had been diagnosed HIV-positive, causing Olivia to be perinatally exposed to HIV. Although Olivia initially tested positive for carrying HIV antibodies at birth, by 18 months of age she was tested and found to be uninfected with the virus. She was thereby classified as seroreverted according to the 1994 (CDC, 1994c) revised definition of HIV infection in children. Olivia's mother also reported that her daughter experienced withdrawals and the "shakes" secondary to exposure to crack cocaine, which the mother had used up to 2 days prior to Olivia's birth. Moreover, the mother reportedly received zidovudine (AZT) as part of a clinical trial in an attempt to reduce the risk of transmission of HIV to the baby. Thus, Olivia was exposed in utero not only to HIV, but also to crack cocaine and AZT, as well.

According to parental report, Olivia seemed to be within normal limits for reaching her language and motor developmental milestones. The mother noted that Olivia babbled at 9 months, said her first word at 12 months, rolled over at 3 to 4 months, sat up at 5 months, crawled at 7 months, and walked at 12 months.

When Olivia was aged 3;8, a one-time diagnostic protocol was administered that included standard and nonstandardized measures of oral-motor function, voice, hearing, cognitive, and language testing. An assessment of oral-motor skills using the Robbins and Klee (1987) diagnostic protocol revealed that Olivia's vocal tract structures and their relationships were within normal limits but her performance on the tasks to test oral-motor function was scattered. For instance, Olivia accomplished single tasks well (e.g., sucking through a straw); yet when she was asked to rapidly coordinate several movements during diadochokinetic tasks, her performance was impaired. Her vocal function (i.e., fundamental frequency and s/z ratio) fell within normal limits for her age and gender, and a perceptual rating indicated her voice was within normal limits. Audiologic evaluation revealed a mild hearing loss, most likely due to fluid present in the middle ear, as implied by her tympanograms. However, the conductive hearing loss had little apparent effect on Olivia's test taking abilities, because she interacted well with the examiner and followed directions with ease.

Olivia's findings in cognitive ability, as determined on the Perceptual-Performance Scales of the McCarthy Scales of Children's Abilities (McCarthy, 1972), were approximately at, or slightly above, age level. Results were the following: (1) Block Building, 4;0 to 4;6, (2) Draw-A-Design, 3;6, (3) Draw-A-Child, 4;0 to 4;6, and (4) Conceptual Grouping, 4;6. Olivia's scores on the Tapping Sequence, a measure of short-term auditory memory, visual-motor coordination, and attention, placed her below the 2;6-to-3;0 level, suggesting that Olivia had deficits in these areas. Nevertheless, overall performance on the McCarthy Scales suggested that Olivia was cognitively at or above age level. Thus, based upon these test results, it appears that perinatal exposure to HIV and other drugs had had no affect on Olivia's cognitive abilities.

The Goldman-Fristoe Test of Articulation (Goldman & Fristoe, 1986) and the Khan-Lewis Phonological Analysis (Khan & Lewis, 1986) were used to assess Olivia's articulation skills and phonological processes. On the Goldman-Fristoe Test, Olivia obtained a composite score of 19, or 3;10, placing her slightly above chronological age for articulation. However, the type of errors she demonstrated would suggest that many were not developmental and could be problematic for her in the future. Two phonological processes that were nondevelopmental included glottal replacements (e.g., /vaeʔum/ for "vacuum") and backing to velars (/kɪfɪki/ for "Christmas tree"). Olivia also presented several developmental phonological processes, including: (1) final consonant deletions (e.g., /hau/ for "house"), (2) stridency deletion (e.g., /mae:/ for "matches"), (3) cluster simplification (e.g., /tov/ for "stove"), (4) velar fronting (e.g., /tar/ for "car"), (5) consonant harmony (e.g., /fm/ for "thumb"), (6) syllable reduction (e.g., /fon/ for "telephone"), and (7) final devoicing (e.g., /bɛ/ for "bed"). Taken together, most of these processes were expected for a child of her age; however, it is of interest to point out that two of Olivia's siblings manifested the same phonological-processing errors (Scott, 1995). Thus, despite the developmental nature of her errors, there appears to be a strong familial association. This draws into question whether Olivia's pattern of phonology can be attributed to a developmental, cultural, or familial pattern. Olivia and her two siblings did exhibit some dialectal features typical of African-American English vernacular speakers, such as absence of the -s suffix marking in third-person singular, deletion of the copula, cluster reduction, and cluster simplification (Scott, 1995). However, because the youngsters held common developmental, as well as nondevelopmental processes, and because they were siblings, it could be argued that familial differences may be a cofactor in Olivia's articulation performance. Furthermore, the mother reported speech problems as being prevalent in her family, which lends additional support to the existence of a familial relation.

The standardized tests indicated that Olivia scored at the 1st percentile in receptive vocabulary on the Peabody Picture Vocabulary Test–Revised (Dunn & Dunn, 1981), with an age equivalent of 2;3, and at the 1st percentile in expressive vocabulary on the Expressive One-Word Picture Vocabulary Test–Revised (Gardner, 1990), with an age equivalent of 2;11. Thus, on both receptive and expressive vocabulary, she performed below her age-level of 3;8. However, she performed at age level in the areas of general language comprehension on the Reynell Developmental Scales–Revised (Reynell & Huntley, 1985), with Verbal Comprehension at the 55th percentile, age equivalent of 3;11; and, in overall expressive language, also on the Reynell Scales, her Expressive Language was at the 71st percentile, with an age equivalent of 3;11 to 4;0. Thus, *in spite of Olivia's poor performance in vocabulary, her language abilities appeared to be age appropriate, or commensurate to her cognitive skills, as measured on the McCarthy (McCarthy, 1972).*

A 20-minute, 100-utterance spontaneous language sample was obtained. This consisted of free play interaction, as suggested by Lund and Duchan (1988), between Olivia and the senior author. The language sample was audiotaped and later entered and analyzed with SALT I (Systematic Analysis of Language Transcripts), (Miller & Chapman, 1993).

Several measures were obtained from the language sample, and most indicated age appropriate development. That is, Olivia's mean length of utterance (MLU), a general index of grammatical development, was 3.31, placing her at an age equivalent of 3;3. Her Type-Token Ratio (TTR), a general semantic measure of language, was .38, or only slightly below a TTR of .45 to .50 for children of her age (Templin, 1957). The number of mazes (i.e., false starts and/or reformulations within an utterance) that Olivia produced totaled 10, a number well within expectations for her age level (Miller, 1981). This suggests that Olivia was essentially fluent in her language sample and had no word-finding problems.

In addition to the SALT I analysis, a Developmental Sentence Score (DSS), (Lee, 1974), and Black English Sentence Score (BESS), (Nelson, 1993), were also obtained. Olivia scored age 2;6 on the DSS and below age 3;0 on the BESS. Her performance was not age appropriate on either measure.

Taken together, the language sample and the standardized test results suggest that Olivia's cognitive and language performance were, for the most part, developmentally age appropriate. Therefore, neither exposure to HIV nor to its at-risk behaviors (e.g., parental intravenous drug use during pregnancy) had much effect on her expressive and receptive language. This finding is somewhat unexpected, considering what has been reported in the literature regarding children who have been exposed to HIV and other drugs. On the other hand, while pregnant with Olivia, her mother received AZT as part of a clinical trial; this antiretroviral therapy may have prevented the detrimental effects experienced by many children who are perinatally exposed and/or seroreverted. Certainly, Olivia had mildly depressed receptive and expressive vocabulary scores, which may have been the result of the HIV exposure, but her overall cognitive and language skills appeared to be age appropriate. Nevertheless, as McCardle et al. (1991) suggested, Olivia, as a child who was seroreverted and HIV exposed, should be followed for possible later neurodevelopmental and linguistic problems.

SUMMARY

It has been estimated that 25 to 40 percent of all children born to women infected with HIV actually acquire the disease (Ginzburg et al., 1990; Oxtoby, 1991; Simonds & Rogers, 1992). Although previous research has compared language function in these children, the information was cursory and only peripherally documented developmental delays. This chapter has discussed the communication deficits experienced by children who were perinatally exposed to HIV or HIV-at-risk behaviors. However, the reader is reminded that in performing and discussing studies of the communication skills of children with HIV, it is quite difficult to ascertain what factors influence the deficits these children may, or may not, exhibit. In addition to the HIV, factors like poor prenatal care, poor postnatal care, prematurity, and drug exposure, as well as sociocultural factors (e.g., foster care, poverty), all may affect the communication abilities of these children. Therefore, it is probably more correct to discuss the abilities and/or deficits of these children with a constellation of factors related to the HIV, than to attribute such deficits directly to the virus itself.

Furthermore, the reader is cautioned not to view children who were perinatally exposed to this disease as "exposed." Nor should the reader look at the child with HIV as a representation of a disease surrounded by a multiplicity of potential problems. Rather, each child must be viewed with hope as an individual who may blossom through team effort.

In his chapter entitled, "Growing Up with AIDS—Preschool and School Years: Community Concern" (1989), William H. Ginsburg aptly observes:

> Pediatric AIDS cannot be ignored. Society has the responsibility to take care of each of its members, and perhaps its greatest responsibility is to the young, regardless of how short their lives may be. The fact that a child will die does not reduce his or her worth or our responsibility. With education, thought, planning, and adequate funding, each child will be able to develop to his or her full capacity. Great strides will be made to integrate the irrational fears surrounding a very real condition into the rational realm of the mind of society. (pp. 42–43)

Indeed, the responsibility belongs to each professional, family member, or other person who encounters the child during this period.

References

Ammann, A. J. (1994). Overview of pediatric HIV disease. In P. T. Cohen, M. A. Sande, & P. A. Volberding (Eds.), *The AIDS knowledge base: A textbook on HIV disease from the University of California, San Francisco, and the San Francisco General Hospital* (pp. 8.1-1–8.1-7). Boston: Little, Brown.

Armstrong, F. D., Sejdel, J. F., & Swales, T. P. (1993). Pediatric HIV infection: A neuropsychological and educational challenge. *Journal of Learning Disabilities, 26*(2), 92–103.

Bangs, T. E. (1979). *Birth to Three Developmental Scale*. Allen, Tex.: DLM Teaching Resources.

Barnett, E. D., Klein, J. O., Pelton, S. I., & Luginbuhl, L. M. (1992). Otitis media in children born to human immunodeficiency virus–infected mothers. *Pediatric Infectious Diseases Journal, 11*(5), 360–364.

Belman, A. L., Diamond, G., Dickson, D., Horoupian, D., Llena, J., Lantos, G., & Rubinstein, A. (1988). Pediatric acquired immunodeficiency syndrome: Neurologic syndromes. *American Journal of Diseases in Children, 142,* 29–35.

Belman, A. L., Lantos, G., Horoupian, D., Novick, B. E., Ultmann, M. H., Dickson, D. W., & Rubinstein, A. (1986). AIDS: Calcification of the basal ganglia in infants and children. *Neurology, 36,* 1192–1199.

Belman, A. L., Ultmann, M. H., Horoupian, D., Novick, B., Spiro, A. J., Rubinstein, A., Kurtzberg, D., & Cone-Wesson, B. (1985). Neurological complications in infants and children with acquired immune deficiency syndrome. *Annals of Neurology, 18,* 560–566.

Berkelman, R., Heyward, W., Stehr-Green, J., & Curran, J. (1989). Epidemiology of human immunodeficiency virus infection and acquired immunodeficiency syndrome. *American Journal of Medicine, 86,* 761–770.

Bess, F. H., & Humes, L. E. (1990). *Audiology: The fundamentals.* Baltimore: Williams & Wilkins.

Blanche, S., Mayaux, M. J., Rouzioux, C., Teglas, J. P., Firtion, G., Monpoux, F., Ciraru-Vigneron, N., Meier, F., Tricoire, J., Courpotin, C., Vilmer, E., Griscelli, C., & Delfraissy, J. F. (1994). Relation of the course of HIV infection in children to the severity of the disease in the mothers at delivery. *New England Journal of Medicine, 330,* 308–312.

Brouwers, P., Belman, A. L., & Epstein, L. G. (1991). Central nervous system involvement: Manifestations and evaluation. In P. A. Pizzo, & C. M. Wilfert (Eds.), *Pediatric AIDS: The challenge of HIV infection in infants, children, and adolescents* (pp. 318–335). Baltimore: Williams, & Wilkins.

Brunet, O., & Lezine, I. (1967). *Scala di Sviluppo Psicomotorio della Prima Infanzia.* Firenze, Italy: OS.

Centers for Disease Control. (1987a). Classification system for human immunodeficiency virus (HIV) infection in children under 13 years of age. *Morbidity and Mortality Weekly Report, 36*(15), 225–230, 235–236.

CDC. (1987b). Revision of the CDC surveillance case definition for acquired immunodeficiency syndrome. *Morbidity and Mortality Weekly Report, 26,* 3S–15S.

CDC. (1990, November). HIV/AIDS surveillance report. *Morbidity and Mortality Weekly Report, 9.*

CDC. (1992, January). *HIV/AIDS Surveillance Report,* 1–22.

CDC. (1993a, January). *HIV/AIDS Surveillance Report,* 1–22.

CDC. (1993b). *Morbidity and Mortality Weekly Report, 42*(51–52), 997.

CDC. (1994a, September 9). AIDS among racial/ethnic minorities—United States, 1993. *Morbidity and Mortality Weekly Report, 43*(35), p. 644.

CDC. (1994b). Update: Impact of the expanded AIDS surveillance case definition for adolescents and adults on case reporting—United States, 1993. *Morbidity and Mortality Weekly Report, 43*(9), 167.

CDC. (1994c, September 30). 1994 revised classification system for human immunodeficiency virus infection in children less than 13 years of age. *Morbidity and Mortality Weekly Report, 43*(RR-12), 1–11.

CDC. (1996, December). *HIV/AIDS Surveillance Report,* 1–34.

Chanock, S. J., & McIntosh, K. (1989). Pediatric infection with the human immunodeficiency virus: Issues for the otorhinolaryngologist. *Otolaryngology Clinics of North America, 22,* 537–560.

Church, J. A. (1987). Human immunodeficiency virus (HIV) infection at Children's Hospital of Los Angeles: Recurrent otitis media of chronic sinusitis as the presenting process in pediatric AIDS. *Immunology Allergy Practice, 9,* 25–31.

Civitello, L. A. (1991–92). Neurologic complications of HIV infection in children. *Pediatric Neurosurgery, 17,* 104–112.

Cohen, S. E., & Diamond, G. W. (1992). Developmental assessment of children with HIV infections. In A. C. Crocker, H. J. Cohen, & T. A. Kastno (Eds.), *HIV infection and developmental disabilities: A resource for service providers* (pp. 53–61). Baltimore: Brookes.

Cohen, S. E., Mundy, T., Karassik, B., Lieb, L., Ludwig, D. D., & Ward, J. (1991). Neuropsychological functioning in human immunodeficiency virus type 1 seropositive children infected through neonatal blood transfusion. *Pediatrics, 88*(1), 58–68.

Coleman, R. (1994). HIV-related drug information. In P. T. Cohen, M. A. Sande, & P. A. Volberding (Eds.), *The AIDS knowledge base: A textbook on HIV disease from the University of California, San Francisco, and the San Francisco General Hospital* (pp. 4.7-1–4.7-12). Boston: Little, Brown.

Condini, A., Axia, G., Cattelan, C., D'Urso, M. R., Laverda, A. M., Viero, F., & Zacchello, F. (1991). Development of language in 18–30-month-old HIV-1–infected but not ill children. *AIDS, 5,* 735–739.

Diamond, G. W. (1989). Developmental problems in children with HIV infection. *Mental Retardation, 27*(4), 213–217.

Diamond, G. W., & Cohen, H. J. (1992). Developmental disabilities in children with HIV infection. In A. C. Crocker, H. J. Cohen, & T. A. Kastner (Eds.), *HIV infection and developmental disabilities: A resource for service providers* (pp. 33–42). Baltimore: Brookes.

Diamond, G. W., Gurdin, P., Wiznia, A. A., Belman, A. L., Rubinstein, A., & Cohen, H. J. (1990). Effects of congenital HIV infection on neurodevelopmental status of babies in foster care. *Developmental Medicine and Child Neurology, 32,* 999–1005.

Diamond, G. W., Kaufman, J., Belman, A. L., Cohen, L., Cohen, H. J., & Rubinstein, A. (1987). Characterization of cognitive functioning in a subgroup of children with congenital HIV infection. *Archives of Clinical Neuropsychology, 2,* 245–256.

Dunn, L. M. (1959). *Peabody Picture Vocabulary Test.* Circle Pines, Minn.: American Guidance Service.

Dunn, L. M. (1981). *Peabody Language Development Kits–Revised: Level I.* Circle Pines, Minn.: American Guidance Service.

Dunn, L. M., & Dunn, L. M. (1981). *Peabody Picture Vocabulary Test–Revised.* Circle Pines, Minn.: American Guidance Service.

Eddy, J., & Whittle-Seiden, S. (1991). Nursing issues in the care of HIV-infected children. In P. A. Pizzo & C. M. Wilfert (Eds.), *Pediatric AIDS: The challenge of HIV infection in infants, children, and adolescents* (pp. 561–568). Baltimore: Williams & Wilkins.

Epstein, L. G., Sharer, L. R., Oleske, J. M., Connor, E. M., Goudsmit, J., Bagdon, L., Robert-Guroff, M., & Koenigsberger, M. R. (1986). Neurologic manifestations of human immunodeficiency virus infection in children. *Pediatrics, 78*(4), 678–687.

Falloon, J., Eddy, J., Wiener, L., & Pizzo, P. A. (1989). Human immunodeficiency virus infection in children. *The Journal of Pediatrics, 114*(1), 1–30.

Farizio, K., Buehler, J., Chamberland, M., Whyte, B., Froelicher, E., Hopkins, S., Reed, C., Mokotoff, E., Cohn, D., Troxler, S., Phelps, A., & Berkelman, R. (1992). Spectrum of disease in persons with human immunodeficiency virus infection in the United States. *Journal of the American Medical Association, 267,* 1798–1805.

Fenson, L., Dale, P., Reznick, J., Thal, D., Bates, E., Hartung, J., Pethick, S., & Reilly, J. (1993). *MacArthur Communicative Development Inventories.* San Diego: Singular Publishing Group.

Fox, C. H. (1991). AIDS and HIV diseases. In J. J. Head (Ed.), *Carolina biology readers,* Research Issue No. 20 (pp. 1–16). Burlington, N.C.: Carolina Biological Supply Company.

Frederick, T., Mascola, L., Eller, A., O'Neil, L., & Byers, B. (1994). Progression of human immunodeficiency virus disease among infants and children infected perinatally with human immunodeficiency virus; or through neonatal blood transfusion. *Pediatric Infectious Disease Journal, 13,* 1091–1097.

Furuno, S., Inatsuka, T., O'Reilly, K., Hosaka, C., Zeisloft, B., & Allman, T. (1984). *Hawaii Early Learning Profile (HELP).* Palo Alto, Calif.: VORT.

Gardner, M. F. (1979). *Expressive One-Word Picture Vocabulary Test.* Novato, Calif.: Academic Therapy Publications.

Gardner, M. F. (1985). *Receptive One-Word Picture Vocabulary Test.* Novato, Calif.: Academic Therapy Publications.

Gardner, M. F. (1990). *Expressive One-Word Picture Vocabulary Test–Revised.* Novato, Calif.: Academic Therapy Publications

Gayle, J. A., Selik, R. M., & Chu, S. Y. (1990, July). Surveillance for AIDS and HIV infection among Black and Hispanic children and women of childbearing age, 1981–1989. *MMWR CDC Surveillance Summaries, 39*(SS–3), 23–30.

Ginsburg, W. H. (1989). Growing up with AIDS—Preschool and school years: Community concerns. In H. Adam (Ed.), *Pediatric AIDS: Report of the twentieth Ross roundtable on critical approaches to common pediatric problems* (pp. 40–45). Columbus, Ohio: Ross Laboratories.

Ginzburg, H. M., Trainor, J., & Reis, E. (1990). A review of epidemiologic trends in HIV infection of women and children. *Pediatric AIDS and HIV Infection: Fetus to Adolescent, 1*(1), 11–15.

Glover, M. E., Preminger, J. L., & Sanford, A. R. (1978). *Early Learning Accomplishment Profile (ELAP)*. Winston-Salem, N.C.: Kaplan.

Goldman, R., & Fristoe, M. (1986). *Goldman-Fristoe Test of Articulation*. Circle Pines, Minn.: American Guidance Service.

Goodwin, S. (1996). *AIDS reference guide: A source book for planners and decision makers*. Washington D.C.: Atlantic Information Services.

Harris, M. H. (1992). Habilitative and rehabilitative needs of children with HIV infection. In A. C. Crocker, H. J. Cohen, & T. A. Kastner (Eds.), *HIV infection and developmental disabilities: A resource for service providers* (pp. 85–94). Baltimore: Brookes.

Havens, J., Whitaker, A., Feldman, J., Alvardo, L., & Erhardt, A. (1993). A controlled study of cognitive and language function in school-aged HIV-infected children. *Annual New York Academy of Science, 693*, 249–251.

Hoyt, L. G., & Oleske, J. M. (1992). The clinical spectrum of HIV infection in infants and children: An overview. In R. Yogev & E. Connor (Eds.), *Management of HIV infection in infants and children* (pp. 227–245). St. Louis: Mosby Year Book.

Jason, J. M., Stehr-Green, J., & Hohman, R. C. (1988). Human immunodeficiency virus in hemophiliac children. *Pediatrics, 82*, 565–570.

Jenkins, M. (1994). Treatment of pediatric HIV disease. In P. T. Cohen, M. A. Sande, & P. A. Volberding (Eds.), *The AIDS knowledge base: A textbook on HIV disease from the University of California, San Francisco, and the San Francisco General Hospital* (pp. 8.3-1–8.3-17). Boston: Little, Brown.

Johnson, J. P., Nair, P., Hines, S. E., Seiden, S. W., Alger, L., Revie, D. R., O'Neil, K. M., & Hebel, R. (1989). Natural history and serologic diagnosis of infants born to human immunodeficiency virus infected women. *American Journal of Diseases in Children, 143*, 1147–1153.

Khan, M. L., & Lewis, N. P. (1986). *Khan-Lewis Phonological Analysis*. Circle Pines, Minn.: American Guidance Service.

Klindworth, L. M., Dokecki, P. R., Baumeister, A. A., & Kupstas, F. D. (1989). Perspectives: Pediatric AIDS, developmental disabilities, and education: A review. *AIDS Education and Prevention, 1*(4), 291–302.

Kohan, D., Hammerschlag, P. E., & Holliday, R. A. (1990). Otologic disease in AIDS patients: CT correlation. *Laryngoscope, 100*, 1326–1330.

Kohan, D., Rothstein, S. G., & Cohen, N. L. (1988). Otologic disease in patients with acquired immunodeficiency syndrome. *Annals of Otology, Rhinology and Laryngology, 97*, 636–640.

Kozlowski, P. B. (1992). Neuropathology of HIV infection in children. In A. C. Crocker, H. J. Cohen, & T. A. Kastner (Eds.), *HIV infection and developmental disabilities: A resource for service providers* (pp. 25–31). Baltimore: Brookes.

Krikorian, R., & Wrobel, A. J. (1991). Cognitive impairment in HIV infection. *AIDS, 5*(12), 1501–1507.

Lee, B. L., & Safrin S. (1994). Drug interactions and toxicities in patients with HIV disease. In P. T. Cohen, M. A. Sande, & P. A. Volberding (Eds.), *The AIDS knowledge base: A textbook on HIV disease from the University of California, San Francisco, and the San Francisco General Hospital* (pp. 4.6-1–4.6-18). Boston: Little, Brown.

Lee, L. L. (1974). *Developmental Sentence Analysis: A Grammatical Assessment Procedure for Speech and Language Clinicians*. Evanston, Ill.: Northwestern University Press.

Lepage, P., Van de Perre, P., Simonon, A., Msellati, P., Hitimana, D-G., & Dabis, F. (1992). Transient seroreversion in children born to human immunodeficiency virus 1-infected mothers. *The Pediatric Infectious Disease Journal, 11*(10), 892–894.

Linder, T. (1990). *Transdisciplinary play-based assessment*. Baltimore: Brookes.

Lund, N., & Duchan, J. (1988). *Assessing children's language in naturalistic contexts*. Englewood Cliffs, N.J.: Prentice-Hall.

Maldonado, Y. A., & Petru, A. (1994). Diagnosis of pediatric HIV disease. In P. T. Cohen, M. A. Sande, & P. A. Volberding (Eds.), *The AIDS knowledge base: A textbook on HIV disease from the University of California, San Francisco, and the San Francisco General Hospital* (pp. 8.2-1–8.2-10). Boston: Little, Brown.

Maternal factors involved in mother-to-child transmission of HIV-1. (Report of a Consensus Workshop, Sienna, Italy, January 17–18, 1992). (1992). *Journal of Acquired Immune Deficiency Syndrome, 5*, 1019–1029.

McCardle, P., Nannis, E., Smith, R., & Fischer, G. (1991, June 16–21). Patterns of perinatal HIV-related language deficit. *International Conference of AIDS, 7*(2).

McCarthy, D. (1972). *McCarthy Scales of Children's Abilities*. New York: Psychological Corporation.

Mellins, C., Levenson, R., Zawadzki, R., Kairam, R., & Weston, M. (1994). Effects of pediatric HIV infection and prenatal drug exposure on mental and psychomotor development. *Journal of Pediatric Psychology, 19*, 617–627.

Miller, J. (1981). *Assessing language production in children: Experimental procedures*. Baltimore: University Park Press.

Miller, J., & Chapman, R. (1993). *Systematic Analysis of Language Transcripts (SALT I): Version 3.0*. University of Wisconsin–Madison, Language Analysis Laboratory, Waisman Center.

Morris, M. S., & Prasad, S. (1990). Otologic disease in the acquired immunodeficiency syndrome. *Ear, Nose and Throat Journal, 69*, 451–453.

Msellati, P., Lepage, P., Hitimana, D-G., Van Goethem, C., Van de Perre, P., & Dabis, F. (1993). Neurodevelopmental testing of children born to human immunodeficiency virus type 1 seropositive and seronegative mothers: A prospective cohort study in Kigali, Rwanda. *Pediatrics, 92*(6), 843–848.

Nair, P. (1992). Early identification of HIV infection in children. *Pediatric AIDS and HIV Infection: Fetus to Adolescent, 3*(1), 40–44.

National Center for Health Statistics. (1989). Annual summary of births, marriages, divorces, and deaths: United States, 1988. *Monthly Vital Statistics Report, 37*(13). Hyattsville, Md.: Public Health Service.

Nelson, N. W. (1993). *Childhood language disorders in context: Infancy through adolescence.* New York: Macmillan.

Nozyce, M., Hittelman, J., Muenz, L., Durako, S., Fischer, M., & Willoughby, A. (1994). Effect of perinatally acquired human immunodeficiency virus infection on neurodevelopment in children during the first two years of life. *Pediatrics, 94*, 883–91.

Oxtoby, M. J. (1991). Perinatally acquired HIV infection. In P. A. Pizzo & C. M. Wilfert (Eds.), *Pediatric AIDS: The challenge of HIV infection in infants, children, and adolescents* (pp. 3–21). Baltimore: Williams & Wilkins.

Pahwa, S., Kaplan, M., & Fikrig, S., Pahwa, R., Sarngadharan, M. G., Popovic, M., & Gallo, R. (1986). Spectrum of human T-cell lymphotropic virus type III infection in children: Recognition of symptomatic, asymptomatic and seronegative patients. *Journal of the American Medical Association, 255*, 2299–2305.

Peiperl, L. (1993). *Manual of HIV/AIDS therapy.* Fountain Valley, Calif.: Current Clinical Strategies Publishing International.

Pinkert, H., Harper, M. B., Cooper, T., & Fleisher, G. R. (1993). HIV-infected children in the pediatric emergency department. *Pediatric Emergency Care, 9*(5), 265–269.

Pizzo, P. A., & Wilfert, C. (1991). Treatment considerations for children with HIV infection. In P. A. Pizzo, & C. M. Wilfert (Eds.), *Pediatric AIDS: The challenge of HIV infection in infants, children, and adolescents* (pp. 478–494). Baltimore: Williams & Wilkins.

Poole, M. D, Postma, D., & Cohen, M. S. (1984). Pyogenic otorhinologic infections in acquired immune deficiency syndrome. *Archives of Otolaryngology, 110*, 130–131.

Pressman, H. (1992). Communication disorders and dysphagia in pediatric AIDS. *Asha, 34*, 45–47.

Principi, N., Marchisio, P., Tornaghi, R., Onorato, J., Massirioni, E., & Picco, P. (1991). Acute otitis media in human immunodeficiency virus-infected children. *Pediatrics, 88*(3), 566–571.

Reynell, J., & Huntley, M. (1985). *Reynell Developmental Language Scales–Revised.* Windsor, U.K.: NFER-Nelson.

Robbins, J., & Klee, T. (1987). Clinical assessment of oropharyngeal motor development in young children. *Journal of Speech and Hearing Disorders, 52*, 271–277.

Rogers, M. G. (1988). Pediatric HIV infection: Epidemiology, etiopathogenesis and transmission. *Pediatric Annals, 17*(5), 325–331.

Rubinstein, A. (1989). Background, epidemiology, and impact of HIV infection in children. *Mental Retardation, 27*(4), 209–211.

Sahai, J., & Berry, A. J. (1989). Eflornithine for the treatment of *Pneumocystis carinii* pneumonia in patients with the acquired immunodeficiency syndrome: A preliminary review. *Pharmacotherapy, 9*(1), 29–33.

Schmitt, B., Seeger, J., Kreuz, W., Enenkel, S., & Jacobi, G. (1991). Central nervous system involvement of children with HIV infection. *Developmental Medicine and Child Neurology, 33*, 535–540.

Scott, G. S. (1995). *Communication skills in three siblings perinatally-exposed to HIV or HIV at-risk behaviors.* M. S. thesis, University of North Carolina, Chapel Hill.

Sculerati, N., & Borkowsky, W. (1990). Pediatric human immunodeficiency virus infection: an otolaryngologist's perspective. *The Journal of Otolaryngology, 19*(3), 182–188.

Semel, E., Wiig, E., & Secord, W. (1987). *Clinical Evaluation of Language Fundamentals–Revised.* San Antonio, Tex.: Psychological Corporation.

Sicklick, M. J., & Rubinstein, A. (1992). Types of HIV infection and the course of the disease. In A. C. Crocker, H. J. Cohen, & T. A. Kastner (Eds.), *HIV infection and developmental disabilities: A resource for service providers* (pp. 15–23). Baltimore: Brookes.

Simonds, R. J., & Rogers, M. F. (1992). Epidemiology of HIV in children and other populations. In A. C. Crocker, H. J. Cohen, & T. A. Kastner (Eds.), *HIV infection and developmental disabilities: A resource for service providers* (pp. 3–13). Baltimore: Brookes.

Smith, M. E., & Canalis, R. F. (1989). Otologic manifestations of AIDS: The otosyphilis connection. *Laryngoscope, 99*, 365–372.

Sooy, C. D. (1987). The impact of AIDS on otolaryngology—Head and neck surgery. *Advances in Otolaryngology—Head and Neck Surgery, 1*, 1–28.

Sparks, S. N. (1993). *Children of prenatal substance abuse.* San Diego: Singular Publishing Group.

Tami, T. A., & Lee, K. C. (1994). Otolaryngologic manifestations of HIV disease. In P. T. Cohen, M. A. Sande, & P. A. Volberding (Eds.), *The AIDS knowledge base: A textbook on HIV disease from the University of California, San Francisco, and the San Francisco General Hospital* (pp. 5.29-1 – 5.29-25). Boston: Little, Brown.

Tavitian, A., Raufman, J. P., & Rosenthal, L. E. (1986). Oral candidiasis as a marker for esophageal candidiasis in the acquired immunodeficiency syndrome. *Annals of Internal Medicine, 104*, 54–55.

Templin, M. (1957). *Certain language skills in children: Their development and interrelationships.* (Institute of Child Welfare, Monograph No. 26). Minneapolis: University of Minnesota Press.

Thomas, C. L. (1993). *Taber's cyclopedic medical dictionary: Edition 17.* Philadelphia: Davis.

Ultmann, M. H., Belman, A. L., Ruff, H. A., Novick, B. E., Cone-Wesson, B., Cohen, H. J., & Rubinstein, A. (1985). Developmental abnormalities in infants and children with acquired immunodeficiency syndrome (AIDS) and AIDS-related complex. *Developmental Medicine and Child Neurology, 27,* 563–571.

Walker, D., Gugenheim, S., Downs, M., & Northern, J. (1989). Early Language Milestone Scale and language screening of young children. *Pediatrics, 83,* 284–288.

Washington, H. (1996, spring/summer). HIV among African Americans. *Harvard AIDS Review.* Available: www.hsph.harvard.edu/Organizations/hai/publications/har_ss96_afam.

Wetherby, A., & Prizant, B. (1990). *Communication and symbolic behavior scales.* Chicago: Riverside.

Wiener, L., & Septimus, A. (1991). Psychosocial consideration and support for the child and family. In P. A. Pizzo, & C. M. Wilfert (Eds.), *Pediatric AIDS: The challenge of HIV infection in infants, children, and adolescents* (pp. 577–594). Baltimore: Williams & Wilkins.

Wiley, C. A., Belman, A. L., Dickson, D. W., Rubinstein, A., & Nelson, J. A. (1990). Human immunodeficiency virus within the brains of children with AIDS. *Clinical Neuropathology, 9*(1), 1–6.

Williams, M. A. (1987). Head and neck findings in pediatric acquired immune deficiency syndrome. *Laryngoscope, 99,* 365–372.

Wolters, P. L. (1992). *The receptive and expressive language functioning of children with acquired immune deficiency syndrome.* Unpublished doctoral dissertation, University of North Carolina, Chapel Hill.

Wolters, P. L., Brouwers, P., Moss, H. A., & Pizzo, P. A. (1995). Differential receptive and expressive language functioning of children with symptomatic HIV disease and relation to CT scan brain abnormalities. *Pediatrics, 95*(1), 112–119.

Young, J. A. T. (1994). The replication cycle of HIV-1. In P. T. Cohen, M. A. Sande, & P. A. Volberding (Eds.), *The AIDS knowledge base: A textbook on HIV disease from the University of California, San Francisco, and the San Francisco General Hospital* (pp. 3.1-1–3.1-12). Boston: Little, Brown.

Zimmerman, I. L., & Dodson, S. (1979). *Preschool Language Scale–Revised.* Columbus, Ohio: Merrill.

Deafness and Hearing Impairment in Young Children

Laura W. Kretschmer, Ed.D., CCC-A
Professor, University of Cincinnati
Ohio
and
Richard R. Kretschmer, Jr., Ed.D.
Professor, University of Cincinnati
Ohio

Key Terms

air conduction	mixed type hearing loss
Auditory Brainstem Response	otoacoustic emissions (OAEs)
bone conduction	personal FM systems
conductive hearing loss	pure tone
Cued Speech	pure-tone averages (PTAs)
deictics	sensorineural hearing loss

Overview

In the last decade, hearing impairment has become the most common disability of school-age children in regular education (Ross, Brackett, & Maxon, 1991). There is reason to believe that the same is true for infants and preschool children who are otherwise typically developing, as well as those who have mental retardation and/or multiple disabilities (Fritsch & Sommer, 1991; Strome, 1981). If hearing impairment should no longer be labeled a low incidence disability, and if it occurs frequently among young children with multiple developmental disabilities, then it is important that its effects be recognized and appreciated by anyone who interacts with infants, toddlers, or preschool-age children.

By way of review, Figure 11-1 is offered to remind the reader of the components of the peripheral human auditory system. As noted, any hearing disorder that affects Part 1 (the external ear) or Part 2 (the middle ear) and results in a loss of hearing sensitivity is termed a **conductive hearing loss**. Conductive hearing loss can be of any degree up to moderately severe and can occur in one or both ears, but it is also generally amenable to medical/surgical treatment. Causes of conductive hearing loss include chronic otitis media, impacted wax in the external canal, and congenital anomalies of the external and/or middle ear. Any diseases, injuries, drugs or genetic syndromes that affect Part 3 (inner ear and Cranial Nerve VIII), the portion that receives sensory information and conducts it to the central nervous system, might result in a **sensorineural hearing loss**. Sensorineural hearing losses can be of any degree from marginal to profound in one or both ears. This type of loss typically cannot be improved by medical or surgical intervention, but it can be managed by use of amplification and habilitation. A combination of conductive and sensorineural pathologies results in a so-called **mixed type hearing loss**. Mixed hearing loss might be caused by both middle and inner ear developmental anomalies occurring in the same child. Young children with sen-

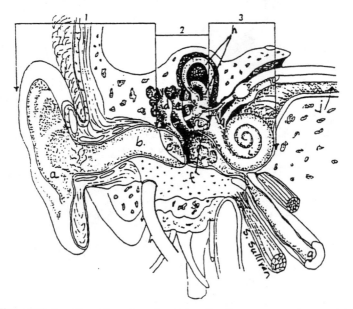

Figure 11-1.　Frontal section of peripheral auditory system, Showing (1) external ear (a. pinna, b. external auditory canal); (2) middle ear (c. eardrum or tympanic membrane, d. malleus, e. incus, f. stapes, g. eustachian or auditory tube connecting middle ear to nasopharynx); (3) inner ear (h. balance system, i. cochlea, j. auditory nerve fibers of Cranial Nerve VIII).

sorineural hearing loss are just as susceptible to acquiring middle ear disorders as are children with normal hearing.

The hearing levels of children (and adults) are described most commonly in terms of both the type, as defined above, and the degree of loss, with the latter using **pure-tone averages (PTAs)**. Table 11-1 contains a list of descriptive terms and their equivalent pure-tone average ranges. PTAs are used widely to define children's hearing status, whether in audiological reports or in legislation establishing eligibility for educational services. While it is useful to be familiar with the general implications of these terms, it should be stressed that they represent only one aspect of a child's auditory and communication potential. The type of hearing loss, the age of identification of that loss and the quality of subsequent management, including use of hearing aids, are all equally important factors in understanding auditory potential. For purposes of our discussion, we will use the terms from Table 11-1 to describe children's hearing status. Deafness, a term often used in the medical literature to refer to any degree of hearing loss, in this chapter will describe the hearing status of children with profound and/or total hearing loss in both ears. The terms *hearing impairment* and *hard of hearing* will be used to describe any child whose hearing sensitivity in both ears is not within the normal range (0–15 dB HL). In contemporary American society, the term *Deaf* (capital *D*) has assumed political and cultural implications. That is, many in the adult community of persons who, regardless of hearing levels, use American Sign Language (ASL) prefer to be identified as members of the Deaf Community, sharing both language and Deaf Culture. This issue is of interest to our discussion because parents of infants and children who are newly

Table 11-1.	Classification of Hearing Impairment by Pure-Tone Average in the Better Ear
Normal Limits	0-15 dB HL (for young children)
Minimal Hearing Loss	16-30 dB HL; Unilateral permanent hearing loss 35 dB or >, PTA of 35 dB or > in the better ear for two or more frequencies 2, 3, 4, 6, 8 K Hz;
Mild Hearing Loss	31-40 dB HL
Moderate Hearing Loss	41-55 dB HL
Moderately Severe Hearing Loss	56-70 dB HL
Severe Hearing Loss	71-90 dB HL
Profound Hearing Loss	91+ dB HL

Pure-Tone Average is defined as the average of the air conduction thresholds at 500, 1000, and 2000 Hz expressed as a whole number and calculated separately for each ear, except as noted for minimal hearing loss.

identified with deafness are called on to decide the mode of communication they will use with their child. If sign language is chosen, then the particular form must also be selected from several choices, including ASL. Selection of ASL does not automatically place the child in Deaf Culture, but it carries implications for language learning and future social interactions for a family when the child's parents are not deaf. For background on the concerns of the Deaf Community and information about Deaf Culture, the reader is referred to popular literature such as Anders (1995), Padden and Humphries (1988), Padden and Ramsay (1993), Paul and Quigley (1994), Reagan (1990), and Solomon (1994). A further discussion of these issues follows in the section on social characteristics of children who are deaf.

ETIOLOGY

Several professional societies have cooperated to develop a list of risk factors or etiologies that place any newborn, infant, or young child at risk for hearing loss. Table 11-2 shows the most recent risk factors suggested by the Joint Committee on Infant Hearing, a group that includes the American Speech-Language-Hearing Association and other groups concerned about early identification of hearing loss (Joint Committee on Infant Hearing, 1994). The factors listed here may cause mild to profound hearing loss in one or both ears, or place the newborn, infant or young child at risk for later acquisition of, as noted in Table 11-2, a significant conductive, sensorineural, or mixed hearing loss. The reader should note that a portion of the conditions referenced in Table 11-2, even if screened for in the newborn, require monitoring and routine follow-up through the preschool years.

Maternal infections and genetic factors figure prominently in this listing for newborns. It is estimated that 30 to 50 percent of congenital hearing loss for which no other factors can be identified is caused by autosomal recessive deafness (Downs & Pike, 1991). Autosomal recessive deafness is a condition in which the infant inherits sensorineural hearing loss of mild to profound degree, most commonly bilateral in extent, with both congenital onset or onset and progression in early to middle childhood, and not associated with other disabilities or stigmata. As with any congenital disability, hearing impairment may be a complication of prematurity and the problems associated with management of low and very low birthweight infants. For example, premature infants with insufficient lung development experience both respiratory compromise and the risk of lung and systemic infections. Administration of drugs that are highly toxic to the inner ear, and lead to severe or profound bilateral hearing impairment, may be part of the life-saving measures employed.

Risk factors for infants and toddlers include acquired diseases such as bacterial meningitis and common childhood viral infections. Contemporary immunization programs, if fully implemented, could significantly reduce the complication of hearing loss in such diseases. Indeed, in the United States,

Table 11-2. Indicators Associated with Sensorineural and/or Conductive Hearing Loss in Neonates and Young Children

A. For use with neonates (birth through 28 days) when universal hearing screening is not available.
   1. Family history of hereditary childhood sensorineural hearing loss.
   2. In utero infections such as cytomegalovirus, herpes, rubella, syphilis, toxoplasmosis.
   3. Craniofacial anomalies, including malformations of the pinna and ear canal.
   4. Birth weight less than 1,500 grams (3.3 lbs).
   5. Hyperbilirubinemia at a serum level requiring exchange transfusion. (levels are set by hospital)
   6. Ototoxic medications, including but not limited to aminoglycoside antibiotics used repeatedly or with loop diuretics.
   7. Bacterial meningitis
   8. Apgar scores of 0–4 at 1 minute and 0–6 at 5 minutes.
   9. Mechanical ventilation lasting 5 days or longer.
   10. Stigmata or other findings associated with a syndrome known to include a sensorineural and/or conductive hearing loss

B. For use with infants (29 days through 2 years) when certain health conditions develop that require rescreening.
   1. Parent/caregiver concern regarding hearing, speech, language, and/or developmental delay.
   2. Bacterial meningitis or other infections associated with sensorineural hearing loss.
   3. Head trauma associated with loss of consciousness or skull fracture.
   4. Stigmata or other findings associated with a syndrome or association known to include a sensorineural and/or conductive hearing loss.
   5. Ototoxic medications including but not limited to chemotherapy agents, aminoglycoside antibiotics used in multiple courses or in combination with loop diuretics.
   6. Recurrent or persistent otitis media with effusion for at least 3 months

C. For use with infants (29 days through 3 years) who require periodic monitoring of hearing. Some newborns and infants may pass initial hearing screening but require periodic monitoring of hearing to detect delayed-onset sensorineural and/or conductive hearing loss. Infants with these indicators require hearing evaluation at least every six months until age 3, and at appropriate intervals thereafter.

Indicators associated with delayed-onset sensorineural hearing loss include:
   1. Family history of hereditary childhood hearing loss.
   2. In utero infections such as cytomegalovirus, herpes, rubella, syphilis, or toxoplasmosis.
   3. Neurofibromatosis Type II and neurodegenerative disorders.

Indicators associated with conductive hearing loss include:
   1. Recurrent or persistent otitis media with effusion.
   2. Anatomic deformities and other disorders that affect eustachian tube function.
   3. Neurodegenerative disorders.

Reprinted by permission from the Joint Committee on Infant Hearing. (1994). 1994 position statement. *Asha, 36,* 38–41. American Speech-Language-Hearing Association. Washington, D.C.

we have made some progress in immunization. More than one bacterial meningitis vaccine has been developed that can be used with infants as young as 2 months of age. If current trends continue in the reduction of the number of cases of *Haemophilus influenzae* bacterial meningitis, a decrease of as much as one-third in the number of cases of severe bilateral hearing loss in children under 5 years of age might be expected annually in this country (Stein & Boyer, 1994). Australia already reports a substantial reduction in the number of children with severe and profound hearing loss due to the elimination of rubella and problems of Rh incompatibility (Upfold, 1988). Due to space limitations, only a few of the risk factors listed in Table 11-2 can be considered in this chapter. Readers are referred to a variety of excellent texts such as Hayes and Northern (1996) or Shprintzen (1997) for detailed discussions on the range of syndromes and conditions associated with hearing impairment in young children.

Otitis Media Epidemic?

Otitis media (OM) is listed in Table 11-2 as a risk factor beginning after the first month of life. The contemporary data on the prevalence and the incidence of middle ear disorder suggests that families and professionals are faced with an epidemic of OM, especially the variation of fluid accumulation in the middle ear, without other problems, so-called otitis media with effusion (OME). In a substantial number of cases, OME is associated with mild bilateral conductive hearing loss that some link to the delayed onset of speech and language in infants, toddlers, and young children. In the mid-1990s, treatment and research on middle ear infections was a $4 billion drain on the health care system, with $2 billion of that spent on medical and surgical intervention (Ince, 1994). This fact, combined with a range of opinion in the medical community about management of middle ear disease, led to a 1994 Department of Health and Human Services (HHS) consensus conference of Otitis Media (Stool et al., 1994). Appendix 11-1 summarizes the recommendations of this national conference with regard to medical management of this disease. While the issues of medical costs to the family and ill health for the child are critical, the concern of speech and hearing and other early intervention professionals is about the presence of the mild (to moderate) bilateral conductive hearing loss that frequently accompanies OME. The natural history of a middle ear disorder from development of fluid to return to a typically functioning air-filled middle ear is about 3 months. If the disorder does not start from an upper respiratory infection, with an earache, the condition of OME is not a painful one for the child. Thus its presence, and the mild hearing loss frequently associated with it, is not easily recognized by parents, day care workers or other adults around the child. Diagnosis of OME is best done by a physician through visual or otoscopic examination of the external canal and the eardrum and through use of immittance measurement screening. The reader is referred to Appendix 11-2 for a complete description of hearing screening procedures for infants and young children. If hearing loss accompanies the disorder, leading to a minimum of 3 months of lost auditory experience and, likely, 6 months to a year before detection and resolution, then OME with hearing loss must be considered a critical factor in altering the speech and language acquisition opportunities of the young child (Flexer, 1994; Northern & Downs, 1994). Children with limited access to health care, especially Native Americans, infants, toddlers, and young children in day care, children in environmentally polluted city or rural environments (often all these factors affect the same children), children with Down syndrome, those with allergies and with congenital head and neck anomalies, are all at risk for chronic OM or OME. The HHS consensus conference mentioned previously (Stool et al., 1994) recommends that professionals simply expect OME in any infant, toddler, or young child and act accordingly with regard to routine screening and management. The authors concur strongly with this recommendation.

The question of long-term effects of OME on speech and language acquisition including discourse abilities, attention, and subsequent school learning continues to be debated. There have been literally dozens of studies, in the United States and around the world, on the prevalence, incidence, and long-term effects, or lack thereof, on speech production, auditory perception, language comprehension and performance, cognitive abilities, and social-emotional status of children. The studies have been retrospective/cross-sectional, prospective and longitudinal, examining children of various ages, socio-economic and educational backgrounds with a range of statistical/epidemiological and qualitative research approaches. A researcher such as Paradise (1981), who has long been critical of studies of the effects of OM or OME, contends that the definitive study has yet to be done on the question of associations between OM occurring at common levels of frequency during the first few years of life and long-lasting developmental problems in speech, language, cognitive, or social-emotional development (Paradise, 1997). The very comprehensive text edited by Roberts, Wallace, and Henderson (1997) includes a chapter by Paradise as well as detailed reports on studies from the late 1960s to the present. While the statistical relationship between a history of OM and various developmental problems is equivocal, a number of studies have identified definite long-term effects on language, auditory, and learning abilities in children with a substantial early history of OM (Gravel & Wallace, 1995; Gravel, Wallace, & Abraham, 1991; Nozza, 1994; Nozza, Rossman, Bond, & Miller, 1990; Paden, Novack, & Beiter, 1987; Reichman & Healey, 1983). This evidence, along with the authors' own experience, convinces us that history of early co-occurrence of OME and hearing loss in young children who have delayed onset of language and speech should be sufficient cause to initiate medical management, parental counseling, and intervention with the child and family. While the effects of such problems in infancy and early childhood may be reversible, children who do not have this problem attended to until school age are at particular risk for school failure. Because these children are frequently children of color or those from restricted economic circumstances who reside in inner cities or in rural poverty, who attend day care and have less access to health care, they are already at risk for school failure and do not need any additional burdens (Bauer, Kretschmer, Kretschmer, & Hess, 1993).

Wernersbach (1996, 1997) reports the intriguing finding that altered middle ear status as measured by tympanometric changes, and presumably feelings of illness that accompany such middle ear alterations, had a noticeable effect on the teacher's interaction style with three preschool children who were observed over a 6-month period. These alterations included increased focus on physical management and a sharp decline in the richness and scaffolding of the teacher's talk. In addition, Vernon-Faegans, Menlove, and Volling (1996) found that children who suffered from chronic otitis media in the first 3 years of life played alone more often and had fewer verbal interactions, either positive or negative, with their playmates. Combined, these results suggest that the effects of otitis media may well affect the ability of young children to establish meaningful relationships with others, either because of changes in the child him- or herself or in the child's communication partners, who may be attempting to adapt their patterns of communication to the child's lack of responsiveness. Such observations suggest that research should examine a variety of factors in the environment, in addition to the child, in order to understand the full effects of OM. Appendix 11-1 provides some basic management suggestions for clinicians, teachers, and parents who interact with children with OM and its associated hearing loss. The text edited by Roberts et al. (1997) should also be consulted for a range of resources and suggestions for families and professionals.

CASE STUDY: EVAN

Evan was a reserved 20-month-old boy. As his parents' first child and the first grandchild, he was showered with attention and surrounded by talk. Although generally healthy, he was treated several times in the first 2 years of life for ear infections and upper respiratory illnesses through the health maintenance organization (HMO) to which his parents belong. Because his parents both work, he has been in day care with Mrs. Brown, who keeps him and her own two children in her home, where she is observed to be a very communicative caregiver. At 20 months he was not combining words and had a spoken vocabulary of about 10 clear words, including: hi, bye, no, boo-boo (bear), bee(big), daddy, and mama. His mother noted that he had always been quiet (i.e., not much vocalization as an infant), although he cried appropriately. He liked to watch videos and play with large toys. He would imitate a variety of words when prompted by his parents and grandparents, all of whom believed that direct imitation is an important process in language acquisition. He seemed to hear most of what was said to him except when he was engrossed in a task or playing in another room. At Evan's most recent medical checkup, the HMO pediatrician noted that he appeared to have fluid in both middle ears and referred him to the approved otologist. Evan was scheduled for placement of pressure equalization tubes in both tympanic membranes. Because his adenoids were found to be unusually large and clearly were obstructing his breathing, they were also removed. A presurgical hearing evaluation at the hospital audiology clinic showed a 40 dB bilateral conductive hearing loss. Post-surgical hearing evaluation showed pure tone sensitivity well within normal limits bilaterally. Within 3 weeks of the surgery, Evan acquired 30 new words, started to combine the ones he had, and was seen to sway to music and to talk to his bear. His parents (and grandparents) were astonished by the explosion in his speech and language acquisition since they assumed that boys were always slow to talk.

DIAGNOSIS

The identification of hearing loss at birth or in early infancy has been a goal of the audiology profession for more than 30 years. The Joint Committee on Infant Hearing (1982) has recommended since 1982 that intervention for children with significant hearing loss be initiated by 6 months of age. The average age of identification in this country, however, is still about 18 months of age, with a further delay of 4 months to 1 year in initiation of intervention, depending on the quality of advice of the initial evaluator (Mace, Wallace, Whan, & Stelmachowicz, 1991). The advice of family physicians and pediatricians, who are the initial contact for two-thirds of families who suspect a hearing loss in their child, continues to be a barrier to early identification (Coplan, 1987; Kurtzer-White & Luterman 1997; Smith, 1998). Clearly, a critical component of early identification must be improved education for both physicians and the public.

The problem of finding an inexpensive, reliable, and accurate procedure for rapidly screening the hearing of every infant born has been a daunting one. Because of efforts by speech, hearing, educational and medical professionals concerned about identifying children who are deaf or hard of hearing at the earliest possible age, in 1997 some 34 states reported some activity relative to hearing screening of newborns, and 19 of those states have addressed the screening of newborns through legislation (Penn & Abbott, 1997). These programs typically employ a high-risk registry with factors such as those shown in Table 11-2, along with some hearing screening procedure such as observing infant response to calibrated signals, or automated procedures such as **Auditory Brainstem Response (ABR)** tests to measure the adequacy of inner ear and auditory nervous system function. The idea of a federally mandated early identification program has been put forward for many years. At a national conference in 1993, attention was drawn to the availability of an efficient and relatively inexpensive instrumental procedure involving the measurement of **otoacoustic emissions (OAEs)**, which could be used as the basis for a universal screening program (National Institutes of Health, 1993). This procedure, which involves non-invasive measurement of preneural cochlear echoes, has been used successfully in several European countries as a universal hearing screening procedure. It appears to meet the requirements for an inexpensive, rapid, and reliable procedure, and as such it is being researched in this country. Appendix 11-2 contains an explanation of ABR and OAE testing as implemented in the state of Rhode Island for universal screening (Mauk & White, 1995). Other procedures for hearing screening of children 0–5 years are also explained in Appendix 11-2.

In addition to concerns about procedures for screening, there is some controversy about the advisability of trying to identify infants with hearing loss before 6 to 12 months of age (Bess & Paradise, 1994). The concerns include (a) whether sufficient rehabilitation services are available to assist all the infants and their families who would be identified regardless of location; (b) whether accurate identification can be achieved without excessive numbers of false positive results; (c) whether such early identification makes an appreciable difference to the infant's subsequent communication and social development; (d) the efficacy of fitting amplification devices in the earliest months of life; and (e) the general expense of adding another screening test to those presently required and paid for by the health care system. That is, what is the cost-benefit equation in view of the fact that as many as 50 percent of children identified with hearing loss apparently are born with normal hearing or are not identified by the current risk factor screening (Elssman, Matkin, & Sabo, 1987; Mauk, White, Mortensen, & Behrens, 1991)?

The first of these concerns is the only one the authors would concede to be a problem. Although pediatric diagnostic and habilitation professionals are available in large metropolitan areas, many families must travel long distances to obtain quality diagnostic and follow-up services. Concern about the lack of research to prove the positive effects of early identification and assistance on the acquisition of communication and the development of social maturity in children with significant hearing loss is misplaced, since there are hundreds, even thousands, of children and families who have had the benefit of early diagnosis and management who will attest to its efficacy. (See Mauk and White, 1995, for a detailed discussion of the rationale for and benefits of early intervention, as well as Yoshinaga-Itano, 1995a.) Hearing aids have been routinely fitted on infants younger than 6 months of age for more than 30 years. Finally, hearing loss is so much more common than problems such as phenylketonuria (PKU), which is routinely screened for, and the consequences of lack of early identification are so serious that, to the authors' way of thinking, a financial argument is not justified. A substantial portion of pediatric audiologists have long advocated for universal screening, most notably, Marion Downs (1993, 1994). The reader is referred to other contemporary sources such as Gravel, Diefendorf, and Matkin (1994); Mauk and White (1995); Northern and Hayes (1994); Spivak (1998); White, Behrens and Strickland (1995); and Yoshinaga-Itano (1995b) for further support for this procedure.

Clearly, universal hearing screening would not solve the whole identification problem. As noted, only about 50 percent of children with congenital onset of hearing loss have identifiable risk factors in their history, or hearing loss at birth. Still, universal infant hearing-screening procedures, as well as the hearing screening of all toddlers and preschool children by audiologists, pediatricians, health clinics, day-care, and preschool programs, is advocated if early identification is to be improved.

HEARING ASSESSMENT IN INFANTS AND YOUNG CHILDREN

The competent diagnosis of hearing loss in infants and young children requires estimates of hearing sensitivity that are both *ear specific* and *frequency specific* before amplification fitting is finalized and before all management decisions can be made. Pure-tone audiometric testing estimates best hearing sensitivity for **pure-tone** signals from 250 through 8000 Hertz (Hz), including sensitivity for signals presented through the **air conduction** pathway as well as through the **bone conduction** pathway for each ear, and can and should be obtained on any infant, toddler, or young child suspected of having a hearing loss (Figure 11-1). These data, which will indicate type (conductive, sensorineural, or mixed), degree (mild to total), configuration of the loss (poorer sensitivity in the high frequencies, poorer in the low frequencies, etc.), and number (unilateral, bilateral) of ears involved, can be obtained on otherwise typically developing children younger than 6 months of age through the use of electrophysiologic testing such as ABR, and after 6 months of age through the use of ABR as well as play-type procedures such as Visual Reinforcement Audiometry (Gravel, 1994; Hall, 1992). Because such testing requires tester experience and ability as well as appropriate equipment, the diagnosis of hearing loss in very young children is best accomplished in a setting where there is a team of experts, including a pediatric otologist, a pediatric audiologist, and habilitation specialists, who may be audiologists, speech-language pathologists, or teachers of the deaf and hard-of-hearing. Further, these experts should have the perspective that once hearing loss is identified and quantified and medical/surgical management is initiated, the focus should be on family-centered assessment and intervention.

As noted, identification audiometry or hearing screening should continue routinely in all programs for infants, toddlers, and young children, particularly those with special needs or with early language impairment. Even with typically developing children, it has been shown that in regular education programs as many as 40 percent of preschool and kindergarten students do not pass a hearing screening at 15 dB HL (lower limits of normal for a child as shown in Table 11-1) on any given day (Flexer, 1989), nor do 75 percent of children in classes for children with learning disabilities (Ray, Sarff, & Glassford, 1984).

Hearing screening for young children should include, at a minimum, the use of limited frequency pure-tone audiometry, screening for middle ear disorders using immittance measures, and visual inspection of head, neck, external ears and tympanic membranes. (See Appendix 11-2 for more specific guidelines).

PHYSICAL, SOCIAL, AND COGNITIVE CHARACTERISTICS

Deafness or hearing impairment affects the physical, social, and cognitive characteristics of children. Early onset hearing loss is typically an invisible condition, since physical damage is to internal auditory structures such as the middle or inner ears. The infant or toddler is unable to report on its presence except by behavior such as lack of response to the auditory environment and/or delayed onset of vocalization and spoken language. Even those indicators may be unreliable due to the wide variation in the degree and extent of hearing impairment. The child with a unilateral hearing loss might show problems primarily in sound localization or in listening in noisy environments. The child with a fluctuating mild hearing loss due to OME may show inconsistent behavior, only a mild delay in language onset, or attention problems only in specific communication situations. As a consequence, the authors will offer only general cautions or points about physical, social, and cognitive characteristics in the sections that follow.

Physical Characteristics

There are no specific physical characteristics that are routinely associated with childhood deafness or hearing loss. Hearing loss can occur in children with severe head and neck anomalies such as cleft palate, or a range of syndromes (sequences or associations) with life-threatening features, or in infants who are otherwise developing typically in all respects. However, the frequency with which syndromes or associations of physical characteristics include hearing impairment as a feature makes it incumbent on persons working with all young children with special needs to be sure that hearing status is clearly established in every child. This is particularly true for those infants and children whose syndromes involve defects in major organs or systems, particularly the heart, the limbs, or the integumentary (skin/pigment) system. A detailed description of common syndromes that include hearing impairment can be found in resources such as Fritsch and Sommer (1991), Northern and Downs (1994), or Shprintzen (1997).

The association of hearing loss with visual disorders needs to be stressed as a physical issue. The prevalence of visual disorders in the population of persons who are deaf or hearing impaired is about twice that of the typical population (60% vs. 30%), (Johnson, 1991; Silberman, 1981). Unfortunately, a large proportion of these visual disorders are not detected early, either because they are progressive in nature, with onset in adolescence or young adulthood in persons with congenital severe to profound hearing loss, or because vision is thought to be too difficult to assess in young children with limited communication. Routine vision screening is as important in infants, toddlers, and children with deafness or hearing impairment as a routine test of hearing status.

Social and Cognitive Characteristics

The population of children who are deaf or hearing impaired is so varied that it is not possible to attribute any social characteristics to the group as a whole. It is, unfortunately, true that references to *the deaf* or to *the Deaf Community* continue to be used as if this population were monolithic in nature. Congenital severe or profound bilateral hearing loss, which is not identified early, generally results in language/communication delays in young children. These delays in language acquisition, rather than the deafness itself, account for the social/emotional immaturity which is often observed in interpersonal and family relationships and subsequent learning in the child who is deaf (Schum, 1991).

There is no persuasive evidence that children who are deaf or hearing impaired have differences in cognitive ability when compared to the typical population, assuming that the cause of the deafness does not also effect neurological development. The fact that many more children with short gestation periods, low birth weight, and multiple system impairments are surviving to enter educational programs does suggest that the cognitively intact child with simple genetic hearing loss may constitute a smaller percentage of those with childhood deafness than was the case even 10 years ago. Thus, it may be that more of today's young children who are deaf or hearing impaired will have learning and developmental problems than previously. However, one of the simplest explanations for some early speech, language, or discourse acquisition difficulties as well as social interaction problems is still an undetected and unmanaged peripheral hearing loss. So-called minimal hearing losses, particularly those of a fluctuating nature, can be particularly pernicious in this respect and, in the authors' view, offer a clear explanation for some communication development problems.

The issue of defining social and/or cognitive characteristics in children with deafness brings us once again to the topic of Deaf Culture versus the condition of deafness. The Deaf Culture movement in this country is frequently marked as entering public consciousness with the strike by students at Gallaudet University in Washington, D.C., against the appointment, in 1988, of a president who was not deaf. The subsequent appointment to the post of a faculty member who was deaf and the activism of segments of the adult deaf sign language community have worked to redefine deafness, not as a handicap or disability but as a variation on the human theme. This effort has struck a chord in many professionals who are not deaf but who interact with children and/or adults who are deaf and their families. The results of this movement have included the development of Deaf Studies programs in many universities, the promotion of American Sign Language as the *natural* language of persons who are deaf, as well as a variety of debates in educational settings and public forums between members of the Deaf Community and parents and educators of children who are deaf or hearing impaired (Barringer, 1993). Because in this country only about 10 percent of children who are deaf have parents who are themselves deaf, only children whose deaf parents also use sign language could reasonably be said to have ASL as a natural language. The remaining 90 percent-plus of children who are deaf or hearing impaired are born into an environment where some spoken language is the norm. Since the vast majority of these students have mild to severe hearing loss, they will learn and use spoken language for their educational and social interactions. The reader is warned that preferred mode of communication arguments have a long and bitter history in this country, a history that often leaves a child and his or her parents in the middle, dealing with the emotional effects of the diagnosis of hearing impairment and all the myths that this evokes, as well as the urgent need to establish communication with the child. This discussion is not offered to force the reader to take a position on this issue. Rather, it is mentioned as a warning that working with parents and other professionals in the area of deafness presents many challenges related to differences in beliefs and values.

EFFECTS OF DEAFNESS AND HEARING IMPAIRMENT ON COMMUNICATION ABILITIES

This section will include some brief comments on the diagnostic value of infant vocalization, as well as some information on the development of interpersonal communication. This section also addresses issues related to interactions between parents and their children who are hearing impaired, followed by sections on the acquisition of language forms and functions and of literacy. The issues in this section are not tied to either the communication mode in which parent-child interactions take place, or the mode through which the child acquires comprehension and expression of language/communication. In other words, for interpersonal communication, it is not critical whether interactions occur in spoken or signed mode. It is critical, however, that those interactions are abundant, comprehensible, contextually rich, and authentic.

Infant Vocalization

To understand the effects of significant (70 dB or greater PTA) bilateral hearing loss on preverbal infant vocalization, a grand synthetic model of infant

Table 11-3. Preverbal Vocalizations in the Grand Synthetic Model of Infant Vocal Development from Birth to 1:0 Year of Age

A. The PHONATION STAGE (Quasivowels with normal phonation) 0-2 months
This stage manifests initial vocal control abilities that will be brought to bear in speech, especially phonation and attempts to form the oral cavity for resonance.

B. The PRIMITIVE ARTICULATION STAGE (Gooing and protosyllables with glottals) 1-4 months of age
This stage shows initiation of back of the mouth plus phonation vocalization.

C. The EXPANSION OR EXPLORATORY STAGE (Fully vocalic sounds, lip trills, squeals, yells, growls, whispers, marginal babbling) 3-8 months of age
This stage reflects the infant's exploration of vocal pitch, intensity and lip control, and the initiation of vocal timing control as the infant may produce syllables with an elongated nucleus or shaky vocal transitions.

D. The CANONICAL STAGE (well-formed syllables with appropriate timing and repetition of elements, e.g., bah-bah-bah) 5-10 months of age
If a baby does not enter the CANONICAL stage before 11 months of age and is healthy otherwise, there is reason for concern about hearing status.

E. The INTEGRATIVE STAGE (Babbling and speaking together) 9-18 months of age
This stage has also been referred to as the jargon stage, which reflects the infant's mastery of vocal control and her advancement toward first real words.

Adapted from Oller, Delgado, Lynch & Steffens (1990, November). Transcription and categorization of child speech and infant sounds. Short Course presentation at the American Speech-Language-Hearing Association National Convention, Seattle, Washington.

vocal development, as suggested by Oller, Delgado, Lynch, & Steffens (1990), is offered as background (Table 11-3). As can be seen, the *canonical,* or so-called babbling, stage of infant vocalization is achieved by typically developing infants with normal hearing, and even, presumably, by those with moderate bilateral hearing loss, before 11 months of age. Oller and Eilers (Eilers & Oller, 1994; Oller & Eilers, 1988) have established clearly that the *absence* of babbling or absence of reduplicated syllables in the vocalizations of infants who are 11 months of age and older should trigger an alarm, in parents, physicians, audiologists, or any persons who work with families and young children, to the possibility of severe bilateral hearing loss. An immediate referral for a complete audiological evaluation and medical examination is indicated.

Interpersonal Communication

Models of language acquisition emphasize at least three basic components of this process. First, infants and toddlers must be exposed to and actively engaged in meaningful communication with adults or older children who model the language to be learned. Such interactions are, by definition, bidirectional in nature (Van Kleeck, 1985). That is, to have an interaction, infants must react to, and modify, their efforts according to the adult reaction, and *just as important,* the adults must react to the infant's communicative attempts and modify their efforts as well. Together they construct a social relationship that is both emotionally satisfying and communicatively productive. Thus, research directed toward the study of adult-child interactions must consider both the interactive nature of this process and the communication behaviors of individual partners. Second, infants must have an opportunity to act on the input they are receiving, to determine the semantic and syntactic regularities of the language system so that they can learn how these regularities can be used in ongoing conversation exchanges (Musselman & Kircaali-Iftar, 1996). Children typically learn about language as they are engaged in conversation. In conversation, children learn how to formulate linguistic rules and simultaneously how to use these rules in communication. Research on language acquisition should include descriptions of the acquisition of linguistic rules and their use in discourse. Third, it has been traditionally thought that children learn interpersonal communication first and then master print, if it exists in their culture. However, studies on early literacy acquisition now support the simultaneous acquisition of print and interpersonal communication when a rich print environment is available to the child from the moment of birth (Baghban, 1984; Cochran-Smith, 1984; Dyson, 1989; Heath, 1983; Koppenhaver, Coleman, Kalman, & Yoder, 1992; Taylor, 1983; Taylor & Dorsey-Gaines, 1988; Wells, 1986).

Studies examining language and communication development in children who are deaf or hearing impaired have tended to address the nature of the language learning environment and the acquisition of the linguistic/communication rules of the language used in that environment. It seems reasonable to examine these two bodies of research to identify any underlying themes that might assist the reader in understanding the effects of deafness and hearing impairment on language acquisition.

Parent-Child Interaction.   A number of studies have examined the nature of the communication interactions between mothers with normal hearing and their children who are deaf (Cheskin, 1981; Connard & Kantor, 1988; Cross, Johnson-Morris, & Nienhuys, 1980; Greenberg, 1980; Kenworthy, 1986; Mac-Turk, Meadow-Orlans, Koester, & Spencer, 1993; Musselman & Churchill, 1991, 1992, 1993; Musselman, Lindsay, & Wilson, 1988; Nienhuys, Cross, & Horsborough, 1984; Power, Wood, Wood, & MacDougall, 1990; Spencer & Gutfreund, 1990; Swisher, 1992; White, 1984), between mothers and their children when both are deaf (de Villiers, Bibeau, Ramos, & Gatty, 1993; Erting, Prezioso, & O'Grady Hynes, 1990; Harris, Clibbens, Chasin, & Tibbitts, 1989; Lartz & Lestina, 1995; Lartz & McCollum, 1990; Snitzer Reilly, McIntire, & Bellugi, 1990b) and, in some cases, have compared the mother-child communication interactions of these two groups (Jamieson, 1994; Meadow,

Greenberg, Erting, & Carmichael, 1981; Prendergast & McCollum, 1996; Spencer, 1996; Spencer & Meadow-Orlans, 1996). Studies of mothers with normal hearing and their infants with hearing loss have involved English-speaking mothers as well as mothers who speak Brazilian Portuguese (da Cunha Pereira & De Lemos, 1990) or Italian (Volterra, Beronesi, & Massoni, 1990). Most of these studies require the mothers to interact with their children in a laboratory setting, using a specific task such as solving a problem or playing with toys, while being videotaped. The results have been interpreted as showing that the conversational exchanges between mothers and infants when both are deaf are freer and less structured than those between mothers who have normal hearing and their infants with hearing loss. Mothers who have normal hearing are typically described as more controlling and directive of the conversation and less responsive to their children's communication attempts. However, it should be noted that there are subgroups of mothers with normal hearing who have infants who are deaf, rendering statistical comparisons among these dyads difficult to interpret (Prendergast, 1992; Robinshaw & Evans, 1995). Indeed, when comparing the interactions of both mothers and children with normal hearing with those of mothers whose children had mild to moderate hearing impairments, Tanksley (1993) reported no significant differences. When it is understood that many of the studies employing mothers with normal hearing use laboratory rather than naturalistic settings, and show only the smallest, most artificial slice of parent-child interaction, it makes sense that any conclusions are likely to stereotype or to incompletely describe the communication styles of mothers who hear.

Even so, what does distinguish the communication interactions of mothers who are deaf from those who are not? Several important features emerge. First, during the initial months of a child's development, mothers who are deaf engage in substantial affective contact with their children, through either physical touch or facial expressions (Erting et al., 1990; Snitzer et al., 1990b). Second, they support their own communication efforts with contextual cues such as attention getting pointing, exaggerated communication, nonlinguistic gestures, and/or holding objects while talking about them (de Villiers et al., 1993; Harris et al., 1989; Prendergast, 1992). Third, they scaffold their communication by embedding it in context that allows the child to enter into the interaction as well (Erting et al., 1990; Jamieson, 1994; Lartz & Lestina, 1995). The importance of these efforts by mothers who are deaf cannot be overly stressed. Masataka (1996) found that, like infants with normal hearing, who responded better to audiotaped speech directed toward infants than toward adults, infants who were deaf showed greater attention and affective responsiveness to videotaped infant-directed signing than to adult-directed signing. In general, most parents who have normal hearing do not easily adopt such strategies when their children are identified as having a severe hearing loss, in spite of the fact that both deaf and hearing infants seem to engage in comparable types and rates of adult-eliciting behaviors (Smith-Gray & Koester, 1995).

The research focusing on mother-child interactions where both partners are deaf seems to suggest the absence of a directive approach, which stands in contrast to research on hearing mother–deaf child interactions. However, using a social interaction model, Caissie and Cole (1993) have argued that while mothers with normal hearing do use directives, they do so in specific but facilitating ways. Moreover, these directives are used with both children who have normal hearing or children who are deaf. Namely, they observed that directives were used with children who exhibited less advanced language abilities, regardless of hearing status. It is their contention that directives may act as a facilitator of conversational turntaking by providing a frame for communication events. Interestingly, a similar argument was advanced by Mahoney and Neville-Smith (1996) for children with developmental delays, by Thiemann-Stagge (1993) for children with cerebral palsy who use communication devices, by Tucker (1995) for children with severe to profound multiple handicaps, and by Seery, Kretschmer, and Elgas (in press) for children with autism. Based on this perspective, it would seem that, even though some mothers of children with special needs may be highly directive, their use of such strategies is likely to be an attempt to cope with the unusual communication demands of a child exhibiting language acquisition problems. These directive communication interactions should be considered part of the social reality constructed between parents and their child with special needs as they struggle to establish a meaningful, loving relationship. Moreover, as children who are deaf or hearing impaired become more mature in their ability to use a variety of symbol systems communicatively, changes in interactional patterns also occur. Thus, the early directive styles of these mothers may be a function of their child's ability to communicate rather than a pattern fixed by hearing status (Nohara, MacKay, & Trehub, 1995).

A further thought about why parents may exhibit a directive approach to interaction comes from Musselman and Churchill (1992), who suggested that one of the reasons for breakdowns in communication interaction between children who have hearing loss and their parents may be the parents' conception of the purpose of such interactions. Parents who have no experience with deafness may be more concerned with the form aspects of communication, rather than the content or purpose of the communication act. In the authors' experience, parents are often counseled to behave in this manner. The introduction of hearing aids and/or sign language to persons not familiar with either may inhibit the type and length of interactions as well. Further, the psychological distancing effects of a diagnosis of deafness may serve to undermine parents' confidence in their ability to communicate with their children, thus having a further effect on their communication styles (Brown, Maxwell, & Browning, 1990; Greenberg, Calderon, & Kusche, 1984; Howell, 1984; Swisher, 1984, 1992).

The point regarding parent experience was made dramatically in Paterson's 1990 study of a French-Canadian father interacting in spoken French with his daughter, who was the second child with a hearing loss born into the family.

The father-child interactions were observed in the first 3 weeks after the introduction of a hearing aid, but prior to professional intervention and counseling. Paterson observed that the parent-child interactions were quite conversational in nature, leading her to suggest, among other things, that careful attention to the interactional strengths of the family should precede any recommendations that professionals make about changes needed in the parents' communication interaction style.

As noted, laboratory situations can constrain or narrowly focus the interactions between mother and child. What happens when research strategies are adopted that focus on more naturalistic interactions over a long period of time? Plapinger and Kretschmer (1991) reported a longitudinal (13 months' duration) intensive study of one mother who had normal hearing and her preschool age daughter who was deaf that involved observing and videotaping communication interactions in the home. Two types of interactions were identified, namely, conversational and teaching. The teaching interactions showed the mother to be controlling, inflexible, and directed toward the perfection of language forms, while the conversational interactions were closer to those described for mothers who were deaf or hearing mothers with typically developing children.

In a study of naturalistic communication in community settings such as shopping malls, Brown et al. (1990) found that "In contrast to behavior of hearing mothers in laboratory settings, who (especially those who do not sign) have tended to be inflexible, controlling, didactic, intrusive, and disapproving . . . these (hearing) parents were approving, flexible, and unintrusive most of the time" (p. 58).

It would seem unrealistic to expect that parents would interact with their children, deaf or not, in the same way throughout the day. Unlike parents who are deaf and through their own life experience are likely to be more comfortable with communicating in various modes, parents with normal hearing often are counseled, or decide on their own, to adopt the attitude that they are teachers (or therapists) and must meld this role into their primary job of parenting. Indeed, most of the parents in the Brown et al. (1990) study did exactly that, expecting in most situations to need to interpret for and protect their children with hearing loss. Such attitudes cannot help but have an effect on parents' interactions with their children, especially if they are coached in this view by the professionals around them who are, properly, concerned about establishing and developing mature communication in the child with a hearing loss.

Despite the quantity of research on parents who have children who are deaf, there is a dearth of information on parent-child interactions in families where the child is hard-of-hearing. In one of the few longitudinal studies available, Uzuner (1993) examined the interactions between Adam, a 4-year-old child with a moderate bilateral hearing loss, and his mother while she read to him and to one or both of his siblings, who had normal hearing. At the time of the study, Adam spoke in multiword utterances and was beginning to use complexities such as coordination, relativization, and complementation. He was receiving intensive speech and language therapy to promote his language development. Analysis of the interactions indicated that when initially observed, his mother employed a teacher's style with Adam. Adam was observed to be able to participate fully in the book reading interactions, often using aided hearing alone. It can be deduced from this family's contacts with speech and hearing professionals and from his mother's own reports that Adam's mother had accepted the viewpoint that she must "teach" her child both language and content during her interactions with him. Adam showed that he could participate and understand as well as his siblings in book reading without didactic structure. As a consequence, his mother gradually returned to her natural style, which was a very good one for encouraging talk about the stories she was reading.

Besides interaction with parents, many toddlers and preschool-age children who are deaf or hearing impaired are enrolled in formal parent-infant and preschool educational programs. For some children, their only systematic exposure to interpersonal communication (sign or spoken language) occurs in this setting. Even though these environments are specifically designated for very young children, it is the authors' observation that there is often too much emphasis on school-related experiences in ways that are similar to traditional classrooms for older children who are deaf. This means a highly didactic and controlling environment, where constant testing of the child's knowledge is the norm, and teachers who are instructed to be highly controlling and directive (Bishop & Gregory, 1985; Burns-Hoffman, 1992; Fox, 1980; Wood & Wood, 1987; Wood, Wood, Griffiths, & Howarth, 1986). Preschool-age children who are deaf or hard-of-hearing can learn to express complex language in school settings if they are provided with interactional opportunities. For example, Burns-Hoffman (1992) reported on school interactions that involved personal narratives where her subject, who was hard-of-hearing, showed high verbal output, especially when the teacher supported such efforts. Thus, as is true with parents, teachers also fall along a continuum from those who are highly interactive and communicative to those who tightly control communication. It seems likely that the most progress in communication development will occur when every environment supports rich interactions with the child (Beattie & Kysela, 1995).

Acquisition of Language Forms and Functions

The issue of the acquisition of the rule systems underlying the semantic, syntactic, and discourse components of the primary languages to which children who are deaf or hearing impaired are being exposed will be considered next. To begin this section, a few comments on the factors affecting language acquisition in children who are deaf or hearing impaired are in order. The age of onset and the age of identification of the hearing loss, the extent of family support, and the availability of professional services will all affect the acquisition, development, and complexity of language in children who are deaf or have moderate to severe hearing impairment. Children with hearing loss are not a monolithic group, since some children are identified well before the 1st year of age and, with appropriate intervention and comprehensible interactive language input, will approximate typical language development milestones in terms of age and sequence. Other children may not be identified until ages 3 or 4, have only limited language experiences outside of school, and struggle their whole lives to achieve adequate interpersonal communication abilities in any mode. Still other children may be identified late but, with appropriate interactive communication experiences, will develop interpersonal abilities in one or more modes that are very like those of persons who are not hearing impaired.

If amplified hearing is of benefit to a particular child, the age at which the hearing aid starts being worn full time, works consistently, and is used in communication can also be a critical factor in shaping the language acquisition process. With the ideal circumstances of early identification and accommodation, it is generally agreed that, if the gestural language of children who are deaf or hard-of-hearing is included, a full range of communication intentions can be observed at comparable or slightly delayed ages as compared to children without hearing loss (Day, 1986; Mohay, 1990; Nicholas, Geers, & Kozak, 1994; Robinshaw, 1996; Schirmer, 1983; Yoshinaga-Itano, 1992). It is also generally agreed that for children who have the benefit of early identification, the earliest single- and two-word combinations, expressed in either spoken English, signed English, or ASL, follow the developmental course outlined for children with normal hearing (Bonvillian & Folven, 1993; Newport & Meier, 1986). It may be that single-word use in sign languages, such as ASL, occurs at earlier ages on average than for spoken languages; however, once language use is established, the path of development seems quite comparable, regardless of mode.

English Acquisition.   Since English is the primary instructional language in the United States for interpersonal, school, and print discourse, it will be considered first in this section. There have been few studies that have documented acquisition of English beyond the earliest stages in young children who are deaf or hard-of-hearing. Schirmer (1983) analyzed the linguistic productions of 20 children aged 3 to 5 learning manually coded English. All analyses indicated that these subjects demonstrated the same semantic categories, syntactic forms, and functional uses as children who are not hearing impaired, but at later chronological ages. J. B. Brown (1984) investigated the use of the morphological endings identified by Roger Brown (1973) as early developing forms in spoken English. Her population of children who were hard-of-hearing included some as young as 5 years of age. She found that, although the acquisition of these forms was delayed, the order of morpheme acquisition was identical for both groups. Taking into account the variations in the age of identification and intervention that would occur in such large groups of children, it is possible that individual children who are deaf or hearing impaired are not delayed at all in English morpheme performance. For example, Oshima-Takane, Cole, and Yaremko (1993) investigated first and second pronoun usage in a child who was deaf and learning spoken English. While in the 28- to 39-month age range, the child linked me/my to her mother and you to herself. This behavior is consistent with the expectation that confused pronominal use will occur in children with normal hearing at about this age (Clark, 1978).

It has long been recognized that spoken languages and, by implication, sign languages such as ASL are not monolithic. They are composed of a variety of dialects, which are of national, regional, ethnic, racial, and socioeconomic origin. Are children who are deaf or hard-of-hearing sensitive to these dialectical variations? In studies of hard-of-hearing adolescents who used nonstandard Black English Vernacular (BEV), Walton (1972) and Boutte (1975) found that the students' school language included a variety of syntactic elements that were characteristic of BEV. If older children who are deaf or hearing impaired are sensitive to dialectical differences in the use of English, then this factor needs to be considered when analyzing the language and communication efforts of younger children who come from homes where dialectical use is typical.

In addition to the semantic/syntactic aspects of the acquisition of English, studies have also examined the discourse aspects of English conversations. Nohara et al. (1995) found that the dialogues between mothers and their preteen children who were hearing impaired and had received and profited from constant amplification at young ages were no different from those between dyads of mothers and their normally hearing preteen children. The question, of course, remains as to the course of development. Beattie (1990) examined the discourse of the communication interactions of preschool-age children learning either spoken or manually coded English, as they participated in various school activities. These children exhibited turn-taking abilities consistent with English conversation; generated language productions that were socially sensitive; demonstrated strong ability to maintain conversational exchange but less skill at initiating, terminating, and tracking shifting topics during conversation; and, finally, had poor conversational repair skills. Beattie observed that his subjects who were deaf exhibited a developing sensitivity to their communication partner and to the social context. However, there was minimal use of **deictics** (relational pronouns such as *You* and *Me*), articles, and other cohesive structures, which meant that these children were probably relying on the context to carry the cohesiveness of their conversations.

With regard to communication repair strategies, Ciocci (1994) compared the responses of preschool-age children who were deaf and learning manually coded English to children with normal hearing in regard to the use of general clarification questions such as "Huh?," "What?," and "I don't understand." She found that, while all subjects were aware of the need to respond to clarification, there was a difference in the type of responses generated by the two groups of children. Children who were deaf tended to revise their utterances, whereas children who had normal hearing were just as likely to repeat as to revise. Either type of response is appropriate in English. Blaylock, Scudder, and Wynne (1995) found that with explicit training, children between ages 4 and 9 who were deaf could make use of more explicit repair questions to request clarifying information.

In a 5-month study of one hard-of-hearing child and six of his normally hearing peers during play interactions in a preschool setting, Messenheimer-Young and Kretschmer (1994) observed that the child with hearing loss displayed the same types of topicalization strategies as the normally hearing children and was just as successful in entering play sessions as long as he did not use the teacher suggestion of asking "Can I play?" He could not gain entry into play using this adult phrase, but through observation he learned to use the entry strategies of his peer group, such as simply presenting himself in the play situation and being prepared to take any role that was assigned. He was clearly able to learn valuable lessons about interpersonal communication from his peers, which is exactly what supporters of inclusion hope for in these types of day-to-day interactions.

Blennerhassett (1984) observed that an 18-month-old deaf child learning oral English was able to develop alternative discourse strategies with her mother and her father, both of whom had unique communication styles. The father usually depended on the child to indicate the topic and general direction of the conversation, whereas the mother tended to set the topic more often than the child. In both cases, the child responded with appropriate topicalization strategies, using both vocal and nonvocal means. Small (1986) reported on a child aged 3.5 who was deaf and was exposed to three different communication styles during language therapy, often during the same session. The child proved able to adapt her style to each partner by employing discourse strategies that were compatible with the expectations of the adult with whom she was interacting at that time.

All these studies confirm that children who are deaf or hearing impaired can demonstrate a variety of grammatical and discourse abilities that are very like those described for typically developing children who are learning English. These abilities can be demonstrated for both spoken and signed English modes in a variety of communication situations. Once again, the authors stress that these communication competencies can only be expressed, however, when children are continually exposed to comprehensible communication in interactive contexts that permit modes of expression suitable for each child. That is, if spoken language is chosen, the environment must support appropriately amplified conversation with a range of partners and opportunity for the child to practice speaking. If a sign language system is selected, all of those who interact with the child must be competent communicators in that system. If a system such as **Cued Speech** is selected for the reception of spoken language, then its consistent use by all those who communicate with the child is required.

Children who are deaf or hearing impaired have a much harder time learn-ing incidentally since, even if they are in a sign language environment, they cannot see communication from around a corner. In a spoken language envi-ronment, conversation is often too far away to be audible or is masked by com-peting noise. The growth of English competence is dependent on the extent and quality of each child's communication experience from the onset of lan-guage into adulthood.

ASL Acquisition.   In addition to English, many children who are deaf ac-quire ASL. Studies of children acquiring ASL confirm that although the lan-guage is received and expressed in a spatial-visual mode, its acquisition and subsequent development show similar stages and processes to those found for children acquiring spoken languages (Newport & Meier, 1986). For exam-ple, Bonvillian and Siedlecki (1996) found that the acquisition of the location aspect of ASL followed a developmental path, with highly contrastive loca-tions being acquired first. In a second study, Siedlecki and Bonvillian (1997) observed a subtle interplay between the point of contact with regard to loca-tion accuracy in the production of hand configuration, one of the four central formational features of American Sign Language. Petitto (1990) and Pizzuto (1990) both reported that the acquisition of deictic pronouns (*you* and *me*) in ASL was strikingly similar to that of young children with normal hearing. Other researchers have found that the marking system (morphological system) used to distinguish between objects and action verbs in ASL (such as *plane* and *fly*) is acquired one marker at a time, in a manner similar to the acquisition of the morphological system in languages such as Turkish (Newport, 1981; Supulla, 1982). A similar pattern was noted for the acquisition of the condi-tional construction in ASL (Snitzer Reilly, McIntire, & Bellugi, 1990a). It is still unclear, however, how young children learning ASL master the discourse requirements governing this language. Further, it is clear that ASL has as many dialectical variations as English (Maxwell & Smith-Todd, 1986). The effects, if any, of these dialectical variations have on the acquisition of ASL have yet to be resolved.

Literacy Development

In addition to interpersonal communication systems, children who are deaf or hard-of-hearing benefit from print exposure. This might not seem to be the case since limited literacy abilities continue to be observed too often in many older children and adults who are deaf (Paul & Quigley, 1990). Nor-mally hearing children who learn to read early are systematically exposed to print and allowed to experiment with it almost from the beginning of life. It has been argued by a number of researchers that children who are deaf or hard-of-hearing must have the same early access to print and be provided with opportunities to experiment with print forms in a developmentally appropriate manner if any progress is to be made in improving the literacy levels of persons who are deaf (Andrews & Gonzales, 1992; Conway, 1985; Ewoldt, 1985; Limbrick, McNaughton, & Clay, 1992; Maxwell, 1986; Rottenberg, 1992; Ruiz, 1995). Williams (1995) observed that unless a teacher believes that children who are deaf or hard-of-hearing can become literate through developmentally appropriate practice, he or she will not provide the necessary opportunities. Gaar (1989) noted that children who are deaf or hard-of-hearing, like children who are not, exhibit more emergent literacy behaviors when they are provided with interactive, literacy rich environments, both at home and in school.

The effects of early intensive exposure to literacy on children who are deaf or hard-of-hearing have been documented by a number of researchers. Conway (1985), Ewoldt (1985), and Ruiz (1995) have all demonstrated that the earliest written efforts of children who are deaf and are exposed to a literacy rich environment, are similar, both in content and form, to those produced by normally hearing children. The children who are deaf in these studies developed an understanding of ideas such as the fact that print stands for something else and that the drawings in books usually correspond to the print. Developmental writing behaviors were observed in these preschool children as well, with scribbling, drawing and strings of letters emerging just as they do in children with normal hearing.

Beyond these studies of emerging literacy, there are virtually no studies on the development of extended prose, whether in print or interpersonal discourse, involving the age group addressed by this chapter. Ewoldt (1985) did report on the early narrative stories of one student who was deaf, beginning at age 5. She noted that the child could dictate stories of more than two sentences 80 percent of the time. Using Applebee's (1978) story classification system, Ewoldt found that most of these stories could be classified as sequences, primitive narratives, unfocused chains, and finally, focused chains. At the end of the study, after a year of schooling, Ewoldt's subject could produce narratives, but few details were provided concerning the nature of these stories. Svaib (1994) traced the development of narrative structures that a 6-year-old deaf girl produced between mid-kindergarten and the end of 1st grade. Over this period of time, her stories increased in complexity through the addition of story introductions, endings, and other, more formal, aspects of story telling. Her stories also became more cohesive as events were linked together through the use of elements such as pronouns, and conjunctions, including those for causality and contrast. In addition, her syntactic complexity increased through the use of prepositional phrases, relative clauses, adverbial clauses, attributive adjectives, *that*- complementizers, and *to*-infinitives.

These findings were supported in the main by Stone's (1994) research on the personal and fictional narratives of 7- to 12-year-old children with hearing loss. Personal narratives were defined as stories about personal experiences, while fictional narratives were "pretend" or "make-believe" stories. Like Svaib, Stone found that: (a) all of his subjects, including the 7-year-olds, were able to produce sentences containing multiple propositions; (b) his subjects used primarily syntactic cohesive ties such as pronouns and conjunctions rather than semantic ones such as synonyms, complementary terms, or antonyms; and (c) his subjects used many of the conventions of storytelling, such as story introductions and orientation statements. His study adds two pieces of information to the description of narrative structure use in children with hearing loss. First, he found that stories that were generated spontaneously by the children, whether personal or fictional in nature, were structurally more complete and complex than those elicited from the child. In spontaneous stories, the children chose the topic and generated a story from their own resources. Elicited stories were patterned on materials presented to them by others such as story books. Second, he found that many of the stories, both spontaneous and elicited, lacked a clear-cut conclusion. They seemed to be a chronology of events rather than a narrative with a purpose, goal, or moral. Interestingly, age did not seem to be a factor for this element, as some of the youngest students generated the most goal-directed stories.

Clearly, exposure and interaction with print are as important for children who are deaf or hard-of-hearing as for typically developing children. Since print, unlike spoken or signed language, can be visited repeatedly to gain meaning from it, it may be an even more important communication medium for children with hearing loss. This point is emphasized because of the traditional reluctance by schools and teachers to read children's literature with young children who are deaf or to encourage them to explore drawing and writing, particularly in self-directed ways. Further, children must be engaged in extended personal and instructional conversations using a consistent mode of communication, and particularly including experiences or topics that are not teacher-directed. These points suggest direction for both parents and teachers/clinicians to be presented in the final section on intervention.

INTERVENTION

The process of intervention with children who are deaf or hard-of-hearing is not complicated, but achieving consistent success does seem to be difficult. The primary issues include: (a) insisting that the child has appropriate sensory aids, both auditory and visual, and that these aids are functioning properly and worn consistently; (b) ensuring that whatever management plans are developed are done in full collaboration with, and with input from, the child's family; (c) helping parents and other caregivers, especially those without experience with deafness, to become effective communicators with the child; (d) ensuring that the communication mode or modes chosen by the parents for the child are presented clearly, consistently, and communicatively by everyone who interacts with the child; (e) ensuring that all educational or learning environments in which the child functions also focus on the acquisition of interpersonal communication in a mode that is comprehensible to the child; and

(f) encouraging the development of literacy in as rich a way as possible, starting from the age of identification. As stated by Calderon and Greenberg (1997), there is a strong need to couple these efforts with sound action-research plans that document the efficacy and practicality of such efforts. An example of such an attempt was reported by Skarakis-Doyle and Murphy (1995), who investigated the effectiveness of a discourse-based language intervention program in establishing the modal contrast *should/must* with a 5-year-old girl who was hard of hearing. These researchers found that a focused stimulation procedure in which the clinician provided the child with intensive models of the target structures in complete grammatical utterances as part of a play activity was quite successful in establishing this modal contrast in her spontaneous language. During the course of these exchanges, the clinician also used recasts or expansions whenever the child produced a partial, but grammatically accurate, production. The researchers found that this approach was effective in improving the language abilities of this particular child. Such efforts need to be pursued with other teaching-learning techniques for children with hearing loss.

Parental issues

As we noted, most children who are deaf or hard-of-hearing are born to parents who have normal hearing. During the course of pregnancy, most of these parents have no expectation of giving birth to a child with a hearing loss. When the child is diagnosed with a hearing loss, parents generally experience normal feelings of confusion, depression, anxiety, and fear (Cole, 1992; Luterman, 1987). Such feelings, while normal, will, by their very nature, interfere with most families' ability to bond and interact with their young child. Part of any program for children who are deaf or hard-of-hearing should be directed at helping parents deal with their feelings and supporting them in establishing a relationship with their child that can foster language/communication as well as social-emotional growth. This can be accomplished by providing information about hearing impairment, providing emotional support through professional assistance, encouraging contacts with parents who have had a similar experience, and eventually exposing the family to interactions with adults who are deaf or hard-of-hearing. Unless members of the immediate family can begin to deal with their feelings and establish an emotional bond with the child, progress in language/communication development will be jeopardized. Family-centered programs for assessment and intervention are discussed in detail in a variety of excellent texts, including Adam, Fortier, Schiel, Smith, and Soland (1990), Cole (1992), and Roush and Matkin (1994).

As pointed out by Crago and Eriks-Brophy (1993), any program for parents must consider their cultural values concerning language/communication and socialization. Different cultures have very different views about how children should be reared and how language/communication is to be included in this process. Cultures vary in their views about who should interact with children, how much verbal interaction is appropriate, who initiates conversation with children and for how long, which topics are appropriate for children, and how complex the language should be when talking to children. These issues must not be overlooked when working with families. The emotional bonds established between parents, grandparents, or others involved in child rearing and the child must be embedded in the culture in which he or she spends the majority of his or her life. When we remember that within the next 10 years in the United States, as many as 65 percent of students in public schools will be from minority cultures, the issue of cultural sensitivity cannot be stressed too highly. For example, when working with a family whose cultural values reflect that children learn best when they initiate contact with adults, it could be unproductive to insist that the parents use an intervention model that requires them to actively seek out their child and engage him or her in communication.

Intervention with OME

The frequent nature of bouts of otitis media with effusion, particularly those with an associated hearing loss, suggests the need for special attention to communication development in and communication with infants, toddlers and preschool children with this problem. The following suggestions are derived from a presentation by Roberts, Roush, Medley, Swartzfarger, and Mundy (1994), with additions by the authors:

1. Secure the child's attention before speaking to make sure that he or she is listening. Gently remind the child to listen when necessary.

2. Whenever possible, get down on the child's eye level to talk. Getting close (no more than 3 feet away) and facing the child will provide clearer visual and auditory information.

3. Increase opportunities to be close by reading to the child, playing games involving conversation, or other communication activities.

4. Speak clearly and repeat important information, but use your natural way of speaking.

5. Make important information stand out by emphasizing it with intonation and stress.

6. When possible, use visual support to help the child understand what he or she is hearing. With young children you might point to objects, pictures, snapshots, or people as you talk about them. For older children, you might use print as well as talk.

7. In a preschool or school classroom, seat the child close to the teacher or main speaker, but make sure he or she can also see others who might speak (e.g., at the side of the room).

8. Be responsive to a child's attempts to talk; talk about and show an interest in the things that interest him or her. Let the child help select the books or magazines that you jointly read; encourage expression through other modes, such as writing, drawing, and movement. Use those activities for conversation topics.

9. When possible, reduce distractions by moving to a quiet area of the room or house.

10. Make the listening environment less noisy and distracting by turning off the radio or television, and moving away from noisy appliances such as air conditioners, fans, and dishwashers.

11. Discuss these suggestions with teachers, day-care workers, relatives, older siblings, or others who will be communicating with the child regularly. The more opportunity the child has to communicate and the more language he or she hears and uses, the better he or she will become at understanding and using language.

12. If the child has persistent or recurrent OME for which medical/surgical management is not indicated or if such procedures do not improve hearing, consider temporary personal amplification or sound field amplification, which can be installed in the classroom.

13. Schedule routine hearing tests to ensure that the child's hearing problem is due solely to OME and to monitor the results of medical and surgical treatment.

14. Ensure that the child has a complete speech and language evaluation from a qualified professional source so that communication problems beyond those attributed to the OME are not overlooked.

Cochlear Implants

At the opposite end of the hearing loss spectrum we find the child with profound bilateral sensorineural deafness of a congenital onset who, until recent years, could be fit only with personal hearing aids as part of auditory intervention. However, following their approval by the federal Food and Drug Administration (FDA) in 1990, cochlear implants became a permissible medical device for children as young as 2 years of age.

The multichannel cochlear implant is a device that provides, for those children with profound cochlear hearing loss and residual auditory nerve function, speech and environmental sounds recoded as electrical signals. The portion of the device that is surgically implanted (in the mastoid bone of one ear) includes a magnet, a stimulus activator, and a bundle of tightly wrapped electrodes; the electrode bundle is threaded into the cochlea. When the surgical scar is healed, an external speech processor (which may look like a body-type hearing aid or, most recently, a behind-the-ear hearing aid) with an attached pickup microphone is positioned on the external ear next to the magnet. The external speech processor, which is powered by a hearing aid battery, picks up noise and speech, recodes those sounds, and activates the internal electrodes in various electrical patterns in the cochlea. This electrical event is delivered along the auditory nerve pathways to the brain. Adults who lose hearing and receive a cochlear implant comment that the recoded speech initially sounds like that of a cartoon character. With experience, these adults soon learn to match the implant patterns to those they have heard before. The interested reader will find pictures of cochlear implants, information on function, and even audio demonstrations of recoded speech on dozens of Internet sites.

Evidence is accumulating that even the child with prelingual deafness can learn to use these electrical patterns (sensory evidence) in acquiring or improving speech and language (see Tillman, Donahue, and Shotland, 1995, for 800+ references on cochlear implants in children and adults). The cochlear implant does not, however, restore normal hearing or even leave the child with only a mild hearing loss. It does have the potential to turn a child who is profoundly deaf into a child who is severely deaf, which may be of considerable benefit to some children in the language learning years (Meyer, Svirsky, Kirk, & Miyamoto, 1998). This potential is only realized, however, with hard work and exposure to abundant speaking and listening opportunities. The FDA guidelines (and the NIH Consensus Development Conference, in 1995) advocated, as one of the criteria for implant candidacy in children, that the child should be in family and educational environments where listening and speaking are strongly encouraged. Indeed, in many auditory/oral programs and schools in the United States, children who have an implant constitute one-third to one-half of the school population. Unhappily, each implant center and/or team interprets the candidacy criteria in its own way, which results in a sizable minority of children being implanted who do not have the family or educational support systems necessary to achieve success with the device.

Progress in acquiring or improving speech intelligibility and spoken language facility is accomplished only through intense, interactive, and meaningful listening and speaking practice that is supported in all environments over a number of years. Those children who lose hearing after the onset of language and are rapidly implanted show the ability to use the recoded speech signal to continue their speech and language development in a way that is very typical of deafened adults. The majority of children who are being implanted at present, however, are prelingually deaf. The communication development processes required for children with implants are the same as those for children who are profoundly deaf and do not have an implant.

The use of cochlear implants in children is still highly controversial in North America (Balkany, Hodges, & Goodman, 1996; Lane, 1992; Rose, Vernon, & Pool, 1996). Many persons associated with Deaf Culture see the rush to obtain an implant for a deaf child as showing a lack of acceptance of that child for who he or she is on the part of parents, physicians, and speech and hearing personnel. Further, since the technology of multichannel implants is only about 15 years old, many critics argue that internal device failure rates and the reliability of the technology over a lifetime cannot be clearly understood, making the device seem experimental at best.

While the cochlear implant has made an extraordinary difference in the lives of some children who are prelingually deaf, that difference has been accomplished through the hard work of parents, teachers and the children themselves (Allum, 1996; Nevins & Chute, 1996; Tye-Murray, 1992). The cochlear implant should be understood for what it is—one piece of new technology for supporting the development of language and literacy prowess in children who are deaf.

Communication Modes

In the course of the management or intervention deliberations, the family must decide on the communication mode they wish to use with the child. Without unduly overwhelming the parents, it is important that they know the full range of options open to them. They need to explore their feelings about each mode and come to a decision that they can emotionally and practically implement. If the parents are interested, part of this discussion could involve interactions with a range of older children and adults who are deaf or hard-of-hearing and have acquired communication in various modes, whether spoken English, manually coded English, ASL, Cued Speech or any combination. A resource such as *Choices in Deafness* by Schwartz (1987) can be a valuable component to this process.

Once a decision on mode of communication has been made, it is incumbent on the early intervention professionals to help the family develop a plan that will enable them to implement their decision (Roush & Matkin, 1994). It should be recognized that any decision about communication can be modified as the child matures and demonstrates new abilities.

Spoken Language. If spoken language is the mode of choice, the parents must ensure that the child is properly amplified and that all amplification systems are constantly monitored and maintained so that he or she can hear him- or herself and others to the maximum extent possible. Simply obtaining hearing aids and placing them on the child is insufficient to the development of spoken language unless everyone communicates with the child learns to position themselves close to him or her so as to guarantee the best auditory input possible. Further, they must be able to engage the child in conversational exchanges where the communication of authentic messages occurs. It is critical that the parents not be changed into surrogate teachers; they must remain caregivers who engage in enriched conversational exchanges as they raise their child to live in their culture and in the larger society.

CASE STUDY: JOSH

Josh was a 30-month-old, shy, only child from a farming family when he was first seen for audiological evaluation. He had had an unspecified high-fever illness at 20 months of age, which resulted in a moderate to severe, bilateral, high-frequency sensorineural hearing loss. Prior to his hearing loss, Josh was producing two- to four-word utterances such as Me want some soda-pop. *The identification of his hearing loss was delayed because, although his mother was concerned about the reduction in communication following his illness, the family doctor assured the parents that he was still recovering. Since he was healthy otherwise, the family followed the doctor's lead and did not seek further evaluation. When Josh's communication failed to progress, however, his parents insisted on a referral to an ENT specialist, who quickly referred Josh for a hearing evaluation. He was fitted with binaural hearing aids and responded immediately by beginning to attempt to produce more single words and two-word combinations. His parents decided to pursue spoken English as the option of choice. He was placed in a toddler group for children who were hard of hearing. His group met twice a week for 3 hours and included individual speech and language therapy. In addition, the parents had access to a parent group for families with newly identified children. Josh made steady progress. By the time he was 3½, Josh was talking in fairly complete sentences, with some word endings, such as plurality and past tense markers, missing. Many of these efforts reflected complexity by incorporating coordination, relativization, and complementation.*

Although Josh was able to initiate topics in conversation, he sometimes had problems tracking when topics changed. After addressing this issue by having him listen and watch for subtle changes in language use, his skills improved. Once he had identified the topic, he had little difficulty sustaining conversation for at least five to seven turns. By 5 years of age he was able to engage in conversations using a variety of communication functions, including narration, persuasion, explanation, and description. Although his family did not take part in reading and writing other than for utilitarian purposes, they did agree to make a conscious effort to provide Josh with a rich print environment. Much of this involved letter writing, looking at print around the farm, and reading children's books on farm subjects or religious themes. By the time he was 5, Josh exhibited a range of preliteracy behaviors such as reading words that he knew at the store and printing versions of them in letters to his grandmother. He was referred to professionals in the local school district who were able to provide the necessary support systems to allow him to be integrated into his local school's kindergarten at age 6.

Languages Other Than Standard English. In many parts of the United States, children come from families where English is not the language of choice in daily use. For these families, interactions must be conducted in the language in which they feel most comfortable, and primary language decisions must be ones that do not exclude the family from the child's educational life (Grant, 1993). As we have noted, there are also many dialectical variations of English in the United States (Baxter & Bucci, 1994; Preston, 1986). If the acquisition of Standard American English is considered a primary goal for a child whose family uses a dialect that is distinctly different from the one used in school, consideration must be given to management of this disparity. It is possible that some families will prefer to have the child develop the dialect of the family first and that of the school later. Unless parents actively participate in this type of decision making, however, they may feel disconnected or disfranchised from the entire educational process (Jones & Kretschmer, 1986).

English Sign Languages.   Educators of the deaf and hard-of-hearing have, through the years, attempted to develop and use sign language systems that match the semantic and grammatical patterns of oral English. Three types of systems have evolved. The first employs the use of fingerspelling, which is the attempt to capture, letter by letter, the spelling of English by writing in the air, so to speak. The combined use of oral English and fingerspelling is known as the Rochester Method (Scouten, 1967). The second approach involves specially designed signed systems that attempt to match the morphological structure of oral English such as Signing Exact English (SEE). This has resulted in the construction of special signs for the word inflections found in English, both grammatical and semantic. For instance, in SEE I, when signing words such as *helped*, there is a sign for both the past tense and the core word (Gustason, Pfetzing, & Zawolkow, 1980). A variety of such systems has been developed by teachers and researchers (Anthony, 1966; Bornstein, Saulnier, & Hamilton, 1983; Wampler, 1972). The intent of these systems is for the teacher, parent, or child to speak and sign at the same time, thus providing both auditory and visual access to English. As a number of researchers, the most recent being Wilbur and Petersen (1998), have demonstrated, in actual practice it is difficult at best to maintain the simultaneous production of oral and signed English. The third tradition recognizes the problems inherent in dual presentation of English and has resulted in programs and schools utilizing Pidgin Sign English (PSE). PSE is generally produced using American Sign Language characteristics as much as possible in an English word order, without using the contrived, English-based grammatical markers, such as those in so called artificial systems such as Signing Exact English.

If a manually coded form of English is the mode of choice, then the parents and other family members must develop proficiency in that system as quickly as possible. It is critical that they use the sign system, whatever it is, consistently with their child, even when communicating between themselves whenever the child is present and observing the interaction. As with spoken language, sign language exchanges should be authentic, meaningful, and interactive. Spoken language may or may not be developed as part of the acquisition of the sign language system. The parallel development of the two systems certainly depends on the child's exposure to amplified speech as well as consistent use of a sign language system. Unfortunately, professionals who can help parents and children become truly bilingual are somewhat rare, so the family's choice regarding which system to develop will depend squarely on the resources available to learn to use a sign system in order to assist their child in language acquisition.

CASE STUDY: MARCUS

Marcus was an outgoing, 16-month-old African-American boy, the older of two children, born to a couple who were both in their late teens. He lived with both of his parents in a housing project in a large metropolitan area. His mother took care of him at home and his father held three maintenance jobs. Marcus became ill with meningitis at the age of 12 months. He was diagnosed as having a profound, bilateral sensorineural hearing loss, with responses only at the limits of the audiometer at 125 and 250 Hz in the left ear. He was fitted with amplification on a trial basis. Even though there was history of hearing loss among cousins of the mother, both parents felt that he could hear before the meningitis as he was beginning to develop oral language (which stopped after his illness).

As a result of the identification of the hearing loss, he and his family were referred to an early intervention program at the community hearing and speech center. During the initial sessions, the parents were seen by both an educational specialist familiar with hearing loss and a social worker. Discussions with the parents revealed that the mother had some familiarity with sign language and the father was willing to learn this system. It was agreed that the parents would take a course in sign language at the center and work with the amplification systems to determine how Marcus could profit from auditory input. Simultaneously, Marcus was enrolled in a twice-weekly parent-toddler program for children who are deaf. Transportation to and from home was a potential problem as the family did not have a car and did not always have the money to use public transportation. Through the social worker, the family was found to be eligible for transportation provided through their medical district.

During the course of Marcus's enrollment at the center, both parents, and especially the mother, became quite fluent in the use of signs, which followed the Black English Vernacular patterns of the family. For instance, instead of signing "is" or "are," the parent might not sign an item or might sign "be." It soon became apparent that Marcus's ability to benefit from amplification was limited at best, but he began to use single signs by 20 months. His earliest signs were similar to those found in children learning oral English. He began to put signs together by 30 months, and again these were semantically similar to those found in children learning oral English. By the time he was 38 months old, he was signing in fairly complete sentences, many of them involving complexities such as coordination and relativization. He was able to engage in conversation by topicalizing appropriately and using appropriate clarification strategies. By this age, his ability to converse had extended to approximately three to five turns on a particular topic. At the age of 40 months Marcus entered the public school in a self-contained preschool class that used total communication, namely, speech, signs, and fingerspelling.

A problem facing this family was the provision of meaningful literacy experiences. The parents could not afford the cost of children's books, nor were they close to a branch public library. In the course of discussion with the parents, it was discovered that they regularly went to the food bank. With the parents' permission, the staff of the center, in conjunction with the university program in education of the hearing impaired, convinced the food bank of the importance of providing appropriate children's literature to families (creating the "Food for Thought" program). A drive was undertaken to collect children's books from the community to donate to the food bank and Marcus's parents were able to use this resource to increase his print exposure.

American Sign Language.   When ASL becomes the mode of choice, once again, the entire family must become devoted to learning this system. Most adult ASL users employ a variety of sign systems, ranging from purely ASL with their Deaf peers to English-like sign with persons whom they do not identify as members of the Deaf Community (Hoffmeister & Moores, 1987). Thus, use of "pure" ASL in every communication situation is neither realistic nor desirable, especially if the goal of education is to help the child with deafness be able to communicate with a variety of persons, many of whom sign but do not use ASL. As with spoken and manually coded English, ASL interactions should be as authentic as possible. The importance of finding a professional who is competent in ASL and who is also able to teach and support the family as they learn cannot be overemphasized.

Literacy Development.   Regardless of interpersonal communication mode choices, parents also need to be encouraged to provide a rich literacy environment. Just having books and writing materials available is not enough. The child who is deaf or hard-of-hearing should see adults engage print routinely, whether reading (e.g., books, signs, grocery labels), writing (e.g., lists, letters), or drawing (e.g., maps). All the daily print-related activities of a family should be demonstrated. The child also needs opportunities to engage print in meaningful ways herself, through joint book-reading, having opportunities to draw, or being encouraged to write letters to grandparents and other members of the family. During these experiences, the child should have opportunities to converse about the process and its products, whether orally, manually, or through fingerspelling (Maxwell, 1988). Children need to have opportunities to relate what they have read to their own life, to ask the meaning of words, and to predict what comes next in a story or sentence. After the child writes a story or draws a picture, parents can talk with him or her about what has been expressed. Through such interactions, the child will acquire an understanding of the roles and functions of print and the ability to control print.

Once again, the use of literacy experiences must be seen in the context of cultural values. Subcultures, even within the American English community, have very different ways of viewing and using literacy (Heath, 1983). In addition, different cultures frame their literacy experiences rather differently. For example, Berman and Slobin (1994) examined the book-reading behaviors of parents who spoke English, German, Spanish, Hebrew, and Turkish, using the same wordless book, *Frog, Where Are You?* (Mayer, 1969). Although there were similarities in the language used when "reading" this book to young children, there were also significant differences, which reflect the ways in which a particular language's narrative structures are organized. When asking parents to interact around print with their children who are deaf or hard-of-hearing, we must understand the cultural values parents hold about print: How have they learned to interact around print? How does print function in the language and culture of the family?

Communication in School

It is quite common for toddlers or young children who are deaf or hard-of-hearing to be placed in preschool settings, whether regular education, self-contained settings for children with hearing loss, or noncategorical preschool programs. If the child is placed in a regular education preschool or a noncategorical setting, support services must be available. It is imperative that both the child's teachers and the other professionals with whom the child and family deal, whether audiologists, speech-language pathologists, teachers of the deaf, or interpreters, agree on the strategies for providing the richest communication experiences possible. In all cases, school placement necessitates the use of wide area amplification devices or **personal FM systems**, which must be carefully maintained and monitored. It should also include efforts to collaborate in a manner that is beneficial to the child and family and mutually satisfying to all professionals involved (Roush & Matkin, 1994).

If the child is placed in a self-contained preschool unit for children with hearing loss, the classroom teacher should be as knowledgeable about early childhood education as he or she is about managing children with hearing loss. An ability to sign and the skill to troubleshoot an amplification system are not the only requirements for teachers in preschool programs for children who are deaf or hard-of-hearing. These persons must be communication experts, of course, but they must also have a thorough understanding of how young children learn, have an appreciation for the role of literacy in the lives of young children, and demonstrate the ability to work with families to support their social, cultural and educational goals. Children in self-contained programs for the deaf or hard-of-hearing need as much opportunity to engage in authentic communication as they do at home. Not only should they learn language in school, they should begin to learn *through* language—to organize their thinking and to regulate social contact in preparation for full-time education placement. The materials made available to them should be the same materials available to any preschool child, including trade books, writing and drawing materials, computer programs, discovery math centers, and hands-on science projects. These experiences and materials should be used to foster acquisition of connected discourse. If other professionals such as SLPs or audiologists are involved in these special education programs, they should coordinate their efforts as carefully as they would with regular educators to ensure that their language or auditory "therapy" focuses on interactive communication about topics relevant to young children and not only on speech production or auditory discrimination.

SUMMARY

One of the challenges in the management of children with early language impairment is to identify physical factors that may complicate learning and to alleviate or account for those factors in the intervention process. In this chapter, we have suggested that the frequent occurrence of conductive hearing loss in young children may be one of the most overlooked, yet prominent, physical factors in this process. We urge that hearing screening be made a routine part of health and communication evaluations of infants, toddlers, and children of preschool age, particularly if they already have other identified disabilities.

We discussed in some detail the effects, or lack of effects, of childhood deafness and hearing impairment on parent-child interactions and on the acquisition of first language forms and functions. We argued that language acquisition and development in children who are deaf or hard-of-hearing should be only minimally affected if early identification and appropriate intervention occur. That is, if a child with a hearing loss is provided with comprehensible input from the earliest possible age, regardless of mode, he or she can acquire and use language in a typical way. The literature shows clearly that developmental processes are expressed whether the child is exposed to and uses spoken or signed English, ASL, or some combination of these systems. The critical issue is that the language system be tailored for the individual child's ability to receive information and that those who provide the language models do so in a consistent, interactive, and communicative way. The choice of communication mode must be one that each child's family can learn, support, and use consistently, and that educators and others around the child and family will also support. Any intervention must, of course, be provided in a culturally and linguistically sensitive way to ensure that the child who is deaf or hearing impaired not be estranged from his or her family's culture with regard to communication.

The importance of simultaneously exposing children who are deaf or hard of hearing to print and to interpersonal communication has been stressed repeatedly, particularly in view of the literacy problems known to affect this population of children in school.

APPENDIX 11-1   OTITIS MEDIA WITH EFFUSION IN YOUNG CHILDREN: SUMMARY OF CLINICAL PRACTICE GUIDELINES

Guidelines for diagnosis and hearing evaluation

1. Suspect OME in young children. Most children experience OME at least once during the preschool years. Expect this and plan to screen the hearing and middle ear function of young children once or twice a year.

2. Use pneumatic otoscopy to assess middle ear status. Pneumatic otoscopy is recommended for assessment of the middle ear because it combines visualization of the tympanic membrane (otoscopy) with a test of tympanic membrane mobility. This type of examination is routinely done by physicians specializing in ear disorders or ear, nose, and throat disorders.

3. Tympanometry may be used to confirm suspected OME. Tympanometry provides an indirect measure of tympanic membrane mobility and an estimate of middle ear air pressure. Tympanometry combined with pneumatic otoscopy improves the accuracy of OME diagnosis. Tympanometry should be used routinely as part of hearing screening along with individual pure tone screening, visual inspection of the head, neck, and external ears, and a check of history of ear pain and/or drainage.

4. A hearing evaluation should be conducted for a child with bilateral OME persisting for 3 months. After 6 weeks of OME, the hearing evaluation is an option. After 12 weeks, it is best practice. Optimally air- and bone-conduction thresholds should be established at 500, 1000, 2000, and 4000 Hz and verified by a speech reception threshold. An air-conduction pure-tone average (500, 1000, and 2000) should be calculated.

Recommendations for therapeutic interventions

1. Control environmental risk factors:
   OPTION: At all times environmental risk factors should be considered. These include unsanitary living conditions, urban environments with high pollution levels; households where one or more persons smoke, poverty, lack of regular access to health care, and poor nutrition.

2. Observation:
   OPTION: No hearing loss (i.e., 20 dB PTA or better in both ears°°) regardless of time with bilateral OME is best managed with observation rather than medical and/or surgical intervention.
   OPTION: Bilateral OME less than 3 months AND hearing loss of 20 dB or greater in one or both ears°° also suggests that observation rather than medical intervention is the best practice.

°° lower limit for normal sensitivity for young children is set at 15 dB PTA, better ear, although the Consensus Conference set the limit at 20 dB.

3. Antibiotic treatment:
   OPTION: At all times

4. Bilateral Myringotomy with tubes:
   NOT RECOMMENDED: If no hearing loss
   NOT RECOMMENDED: If Bilateral OME of less than 3 months AND hearing loss is present
   OPTION: After 3 months of OME AND hearing loss
   RECOMMENDED: After 4-6 months of bilateral OME AND hearing loss

5. NOT recommended:
   Steroids, antihistamine/decongestant, adenoidectomy (with lack of adenoid pathology), tonsillectomy with or without adenoidectomy

Adapted by permission from: Stool, S. E., Berg, A. O., Berman, S., Carney, C. J., Cooley, J. R., Culpepper, L., Eavey, R. D., Feagans, L. V., Finitzo, T., Friedman, E., et al. (1994). *Otitis media with effusion in young children. Quick reference guide for clinicians* (AHCPR Publication No. 94-0623). Rockville, Md.: Agency for Health Care Policy and Research, Public Health Service, U.S. Department of Health and Human Services.

APPENDIX 11-2   DESCRIPTION OF HEARING SCREENING PROCEDURES FOR INFANTS, TODDLERS, AND YOUNG CHILDREN TO THE AGE OF 5 YEARS.

I. Hearing Screening for neonates and infants to six months of age:

Auditory Brainstem Response (ABR) Testing

ABR screening is the most commonly used procedure, in conjunction with high risk factor registries, for screening neonates and infants up to 6 months of age. The ABR is the earliest in time of appearance of several auditory neuroelectric potentials that can be evoked by presenting brief duration clicks or other auditory signals through earphones. The response of the human auditory system to these signals is measured through electrodes placed on the scalp. The neuroelectric potentials that occur in the first 10 milliseconds after signal presentation are the ones of interest in ABR testing. Utilizing averaging computers that are capable of amplifying the extremely small voltages of the ABR and sorting or isolating them from the ongoing electrical activity of the brain, this stimulus-related response can be displayed on an oscilloscope or computer screen as a series of peaks or waves that have been named according to their order of appearance as (Jewett) waves I-VII. These waves are known to arise as a result of stimulation of the cochlea, eighth nerve, and various nuclei in the ascending and crossing pathways of the low to mid brainstem. They are referred to as "farfield" responses, which only means that the neural generators for these responses are some distance from the recording electrodes place on the surface of the head.

A variety of factors affect the appearance and measurement of ABR wave forms, including the nature of the stimuli used to evoke the waves, the age, sex, temperature and neurological condition of the subject and numerous aspects of the ABR recording instrument itself. Because ABR results correlate with behavioral audiometric thresholds, particularly for signals from 1000 to 4000 Hz, it is the test of choice to estimate sensitivity for newborns, infants, and other difficult-to-test persons such as infants and children with developmental disabilities. In this regard, however, it should be emphasized that the ABR tells us only that a certain sound intensity is capable of stimulating the auditory nerve and that the auditory brainstem pathways are capable of responding by conducting that sound to the level of the midbrain.

If an infant passes ABR screening in both ears, high-frequency sensitivity is within normal limits. If the infant does not pass, or if the response is abnormal or even absent in a neonate or infant, it may or may not mean that a hearing loss is present. It does mean that the infant should be considered at risk for hearing loss and/or other developmental problems and should receive a complete audiological assessment and associated developmental evaluation. The reader is referred to sources from the references for chapter 11 such as Gravel (1994) or Hall (1992) for detailed information on applications of ABR to infant hearing evaluation.

Behavioral Observation Screening

This procedure, which pre-dates ABR screening and still may be employed in some hospitals or well-baby clinics, involves the observation of infant responses to noisemakers or portable sound sources. Responses expected may include eye blinks, body or limb movement, changes in respiration, or other overt indicators of sound awareness. Infant responses may be recorded or rated as a way of determining pass or fail. Although this procedure may be quite useful when performed by an experienced clinician, it is both time and labor intensive and frequently overlooks infants with mild or unilateral hearing loss.

High Risk Factors

Factors in the birth history, family history, appearance of the infant, or illness history of the infant which place the child at increased risk of early onset of hearing loss are shown in Table 11-2. If one or more of these factors is present and universal hearing screening is not available, an infant will typically be referred for hearing screening using procedures such as ABR. Continued reliance on the use of a high-risk registry to identify infants and children in need of screening will identify only about half of the infants with significant hearing loss.

Immittance Measurement

Immittance measurement is an instrumental procedure for assessing the function state of the conductive or middle ear mechanism, particularly the eardrum, the ossicular chain, and the auditory tube. Referred to until recently as impedance audiometry, this procedure involves placing a small probe fitted with a rubber cuff in the external canal opening to measure directly the mechanical transfer function of sound in the external and middle ear. Successful testing does not rely on a behavioral response, nor on complete cooperation of the client. Immittance audiometry can be performed successfully on an infant or young child in approximately a minute per ear.

A small probe for measuring reflected energy must be placed to seal the external ear canal, and with most devices, this step initiates automatic measurement of tympanometry (dynamic estimate of eardrum mobility), an estimate of external and middle ear volume (air-filled or not), and finally a sample of middle ear muscle contraction. All of these measures can be interpreted to provide a description of the condition of the external ear, the tympanic membrane, and middle ear cavity, and an estimate of the function of TM, the auditory tube, and the stapedius muscle. Since immittance measures provide no information about the condition of the inner ear or auditory nerve, they cannot be used by themselves for screening, but can be a valuable adjunct to hearing screening programs for infants, pre-school, and school-age children.

Parental or Caregiver Concern

Although the documentation is not clearly available, it is probably the case that parental or caregiver concern is the primary avenue through which infants and young children are referred for hearing screening, particularly if high-risk registries and non-universal screening programs are employed. This suggests that until such time as universal hearing screening is available, parental education regarding the signs and effects of hearing loss on communication and behavior is a critical need.

Transient Evoked Otoacoustic Emissions Screening

Otoacoustic emissions are acoustic responses associated with and presumably generated by normal cochleas. In addition to coding incoming sound transmissions, it is now known that the cochlea, particularly the hair cells, simultaneously emit a sound or "echo" that is returned through the middle ear and can be recorded in the external ear canal using a small microphone. The presence of evoked OAEs indicates the presence of a healthy normally functioning cochlea. OAEs that can be evoked by very brief acoustic stimuli such as clicks and tone pips are referred to as transient evoked otoacoustic emissions (TEOAEs). The extent of research on TEOAEs in this country and abroad, particularly as a screening test of pre-neural cochlear function, confirms that this procedure is probably the rapid, cost efficient, universal hearing screening technique for which audiologists and medical personnel have been searching. If properly administered, failure of the TEOAE screening test can be caused only by an auditory disorder in the middle or inner ear. Thus, unlike ABR, this procedure will identify peripheral hearing loss of any type, degree, or configuration regardless of the infant's developmental or neurological condition.

Since 1990, the state of Rhode Island has been researching the use of TEOAEs as a universal screening tool. At present, 99 percent of hospital live births in that state are screened each month by technicians, in addition to 75,000 other infants in a nationwide research program (Mauk & White, 1995).

Otoscopic Examination

Direct visual examination of the external canal and the tympanic membrane (TM) can be used to screen for external ear anomalies and/or middle ear disease, but this method requires a very experienced clinician and is unlikely to be available for every birth. Further, although visual inspection is an important aspect of any hearing screening program, it does not yield any information about the function of the cochlea or auditory nerve.

II. Hearing Screening in infants and children from 6 months to 3 years

Any of the above-named procedures could be and are routinely utilized for hearing screening of older infants and toddlers, particularly ABR, immittance measures, high risk factors, and parental concern. In addition, pure-tone hearing screening can be used, starting at about 6 months of age if appropriate instructional techniques are employed.

Visual Reinforcement Audiometry

The procedure most commonly employed with children from 6 months to 2 years of age to determine pure-tone sensitivity is Visual Reinforcement Audiometry. In this procedure, the infant or toddler is taught to respond to frequency specific signals through head turn toward lighted, moving toys that are paired with the onset of an audible signal. That is, a connection is established for the infant between head turn at the onset of an audible signal and the reinforcement or reward of seeing an interesting toy that moves and is lit. Pure-tone stimuli of known intensity and frequency can be presented in soundfield, through a bone conduction vibrator, or via earphones. The infants or toddlers are not required to volunteer information or initiate responses themselves. Hearing sensitivity can be reliably tested using VRA in otherwise normal infants with good vision beginning at 6 months of age. VRA can also be utilized successfully with toddlers and older children with developmental delays. Its routine application, however, requires audiologists with considerable pediatric testing experience. Tangible or consumable reinforcers such as dry cereal or raisins may be used with toddlers and children to age 3.

Play Audiometry

This procedure makes hearing screening a game in which the child is taught to perform a simple motor task as a means of indicating awareness of an auditory signal. In this way, stacking rings, dropping blocks, or snapping large beads together accompanied by the social praise of the tester becomes the motivation or reinforcement for participating in hearing screening. Some children as young as 24 months of age and most by 36 months can be screened using play audiometry. A variety of interesting motor tasks should be available to maintain the child's interest. Any frequency-specific mode of testing can be utilized using play audiometry.

III. Hearing screening for children ages 3–5 years

Although there are no universally agreed-upon procedures for hearing screening in preschool age children, the following guidelines, suggested by the American Speech-Language-Hearing Association, are offered for reader information. (See American Speech-Language-Hearing Association, 1990.) ASHA's scope of practice statement requires that if the procedures are conducted by their members they must be done by members certified as audiologists, or under the direct supervision of certified audiologists.

1. Every typically developing child at age 3 through grade 3 and all children functioning at a developmental level of 3 years should have an annual hearing screening.

2. Visual inspection of head, neck, pinna, external ear canal, and TM should be carried out. Visual inspection of the external canal and TM requires an ap-

propriate light source, experience in the procedure, and properly cleaned instruments. Any unusual findings during this inspection, e.g., excessive ear wax, blood, foreign bodies, should result in immediate medical referral.

3. History from the parent, teacher or child of recent (within the last 3 months) ear pain or ear drainage should result in immediate medical referral.

4. Testing of each child in each ear with manually administered air-conduction (through earphones) pure-tone signals at the frequencies of 1000, 2000, and 4000 Hz at 20 dB hearing level should be done. This testing is typically completed using a portable audiometer, a device which allows for presentation of pure-tone signals at a variety of frequencies and intensities. A lack of response to any one of these test frequencies in either ear constitutes failure of this screening test. An immediate retest (or within 2 weeks) should be performed, however, before referral for further testing is initiated. A second failure should initiate parental notification of concern for hearing and referral for a complete audiological evaluation.

5. The second aspect of testing should be screening for external and middle ear disorders. Immittance measures and visual inspection are used for this portion of the screening. As a note, immittance measurement should only be done after careful visual inspection of the external canal and TM. Probes and probe tips utilized in screening should be cleaned appropriately after every use. Observation of any unusual conditions in the external ear or TM, including presence of a Pressure Equalization Tube, means that immittance screening should NOT be done. Specific criteria for immittance failure include a flat tympanogram and or accompanying indicators of middle ear disorder. Failure on immittance measures should result in RESCREENING in 4-6 weeks. A second failure should initiate parental notification and referral for an otologic examination.

6. Any child who fails both pure-tone and immittance screening in the same session can be referred immediately for medical evaluation.

References

Adam, A. J., Fortier, P., Schiel, G., Smith, M., & Soland, C. (1990). *Listening to learn: A handbook for parents with hearing-impaired children*. Washington, D.C.: Alexander Graham Bell Association.

Allum, D. J. (Ed.). (1996). *Cochlear implant rehabilitation in children and adults*. London: Whurr.

Anders, G. (1995, March 3–5). Beauty and the battle. *USA Weekend*, pp. 4–6.

Andrews, J. F., & Gonzales, K. (1992). Free writing of deaf children in kindergarten. *Sign Language Studies, 74*, 63–78.

Anthony, D. (1966). *Seeing essential English*. Unpublished master's thesis, Eastern Michigan University, Ypsilanti.

Applebee, A. N. (1978). *The child's concept of story*. Chicago: University of Chicago.

Baghban, M. (1984). *Our daughter learns to read and write: A case study from birth to three*. Newark, Del.: International Reading Association.

Balkany, T., Hodges, A. V., & Goodman, K. W. (1996). Ethics of cochlear implantation in young children. *Otolaryngology, Head and Neck Surgery, 114*, 748–755.

Barringer, F. (1993, May 16). Pride in a soundless world: Deaf oppose a hearing aid. *New York Times*, pp. 1, 14.

Bauer, A. M., Kretschmer, R. R., Kretschmer, L. W., & Hess, D. (1993.). *Young children in an environmentally challenged community: Communication development and related medical issues*. Cincinnati, Ohio: University of Cincinnati.

Baxter, M., & Bucci, W. (1994). Patterns of communication in Black English. In S. Friedman (Ed.), *Anxiety disorders in African Americans* (pp. 40–49). New York: Springer.

Beattie, R. G. (1990). Pragmatic language competencies of hearing impaired preschool children. *Dissertation Abstracts International, 52*(11), 3387A. (University Microfilms No. AAI90–60374).

Beattie, R. G., & Kysela, G. M. (1995). A descriptive study of communicative intentions used by hearing teachers and preschool children with hearing losses. *Journal of Childhood Communication Disorders, 17*, 32–41.

Berman, R. A., & Slobin, D. I. (Eds.). (1994). *Relating events in narrative: A crosslinguistic developmental study*. Hillsdale, N.J.: Lawrence Erlbaum.

Bess, F. H., & Paradise, J. L. (1994). Universal screening of infant hearing impairment: Not risk-free, not necessarily beneficial, and not presently justified. *Pediatrics, 86*, 330–333.

Bishop, J., & Gregory, S. (1985). Mothers and teachers looking at books with deaf children. *Child Language Teaching and Therapy, 1*, 149–161.

Blaylock, R. L., Scudder, R. R., & Wynne, M. K. (1995). Repair behaviors used by children with hearing loss. *Language, Speech, and Hearing Services in the Schools, 26*, 278–285.

Blennerhassett, L. (1984). Communicative styles of a 13-month-old hearing-impaired child and her parents. *Volta Review, 86*, 217–228.

Bonvillian, J. D., & Folven, R. J. (1993). Sign language acquisition: Developmental aspects. In M. Marschark, & M. D. Clark (Eds.), *Psychological perspectives on deafness* (pp. 229–309). Hillsdale, N.J.: Lawrence Erlbaum.

Bonvillian, J. D., & Siedlecki, T. (1996). Young children's acquisition of the location aspect of American Sign Language signs: Parental report findings. *Journal of Communication Disorders, 29*, 13–35.

Bornstein, H., Saulnier, K., & Hamilton, L. (1983). *The comprehensive Signed English dictionary*. Washington, D.C.: Gallaudet University Press.

Boutte, J. (1975). *A syntactic analysis of the oral language of ten black hearing impaired and ten black normal hearing adolescents*. Unpublished master's thesis, University of Cincinnati, Cincinnati, Ohio.

Brown, J. B. (1984). Examination of grammatical morphemes in the language of hard-of-hearing children. *Volta Review, 86*, 229–238.

Brown, R. (1973). *A first language: The early stages.* Cambridge, Mass.: Harvard University Press.

Brown, S. H., Maxwell, M. M., & Browning, L. D. (1990). Relations in public: Hearing parents and hearing impaired children. *Journal of Childhood Communication Disorders, 13*, 43–62.

Burns-Hoffman, R. (1992). A discourse analysis of variation in children's language in preschool, small group settings. *Dissertation Abstracts International, 53*(06), 1887A. (University Microfilms No. AAI92–32666).

Caissie, R., & Cole, E. B. (1993). Mothers and hearing-impaired children: Directiveness reconsidered. *Volta Review, 95*, 49–59.

Calderon, R., & Greenberg, M. (1997). The effectiveness of early intervention for deaf children and children with hearing loss (pp. 455–482). In M. J. Guralnick (Ed.), *The effectiveness of early intervention.* Baltimore: Brookes.

Cheskin, A. (1981). The verbal environment provided by hearing mothers for their young deaf children. *Journal of Communication Disorders, 14*, 485–496.

Ciocci, S. R. (1994). The use of conversational repair strategies in response to requests for clarification by deaf/hearing-impaired and hearing children. *Dissertation Abstracts International, 55*(03), 849B. (University Microfilms No. AAI94–205611).

Clark, E. V. (1978). From gesture to word: On the natural history of deixis in language acquisition. In J. S. Bruner, & A. Garton (Eds.), *Human growth and development: Wolfson College Lecturers, 1976* (pp. 85–120). Oxford, U.K.: Oxford University Press.

Cochran-Smith, M. (1984). *The making of a reader.* Norwood, N.J.: Ablex.

Cole, E. B. (1992). *Listening and talking: A guide to promoting spoken language in young hearing-impaired children.* Washington, D.C.: Alexander Graham Bell Association.

Connard, P., & Kantor, R. (1988). A partnership perspective viewing normal-hearing parent/hearing-impaired child communication. *Volta Review, 90*, 133–148.

Conway, D. (1985). Children (re)creating writing: A preliminary look at the purposes of free-choice writing of hearing-impaired kindergartners. In R. R. Kretschmer (Ed.), Learning to write and writing to learn (special issue). *Volta Review, 87*(5), 91–108.

Coplan, J. (1987). Deafness: Ever heard of it? Delayed recognition of permanent hearing loss. *Pediatrics, 79*, 206–213.

Crago, M. B., & Eriks-Brophy, A. A. (1993). Feeling right: Approaches to a family's culture. In A. L. Phillips, & E. B. Cole (Eds.), Beginning with babies: A sharing of professional experience. *Volta Review, 95*(5), 123–129.

Cross, T., Johnson-Morris, J. E., & Nienhuys, T. G. (1980). Linguistic feedback and maternal speech: Comparisons of mothers addressing hearing and hearing-impaired children. *First Language, 1*, 163–189.

da Cunha Pereira, M., & De Lemos, C. (1990). Gesture in hearing mother-deaf child interaction. In V. Volterra, & C. J. Erting (Eds.), *From gesture to language in hearing and deaf children* (pp. 178–186). Berlin: Springer-Verlag.

Day, P. S. (1986). Deaf children's expression of communicative intentions. *Journal of Communication Disorders, 19,* 367–385.

de Villiers, J., Bibeau, L., Ramos, E., & Gatty, J. (1993). Gestural communication in oral deaf mother-child pairs: Language with a helping hand? *Applied Psycholinguistics, 14,* 319–348.

Downs, M. P. (1993). Benefits of screening at birth: Economic, educational, and functional factors. In National Institutes of Health (Ed.), *Program and abstracts of the NIH Consensus Development Conference: Early identification of hearing impairment in infants and young children* (pp. 63–66). Bethesda, Md.: National Institutes of Health, National Institute on Deafness and Other Communication Disorders.

Downs, M. P. (1994). The case for detection and intervention at birth. *Seminars in Hearing, 15*(2), 76–84.

Downs, M. P., & Pike, K. (1991). The prevention of genetic deafness. *Seminars in Hearing, 12*(2), 168–174.

Dyson, A. (1989). *Multiple worlds of child writers.* New York: Columbia University, Teachers College.

Eilers, R. E., & Oller, D. K. (1994). Infant vocalization and the early diagnosis of severe hearing impairment. *Journal of Pediatrics, 124,* 199–203.

Elssman, S., Matkin, N. D., & Sabo, M. (1987). Early identification of congenital sensorineural hearing loss. *The Hearing Journal, 40,* 13–17.

Erting, C. J., Prezioso, C., & O'Grady Hynes, M. (1990). The interactional context of deaf mother-infant communication. In V. Volterra, & C. J. Erting (Eds.), *From gesture to language in hearing and deaf children* (pp. 97–106). Berlin: Springer-Verlag.

Ewoldt, C. (1985). A descriptive study of the developing literacy of young hearing-impaired children. In R. R. Kretschmer (Ed.), Learning to write and writing to learn (special issue). *Volta Review, 87*(5), 109–126.

Flexer, C. (1989). Turn on sound: An odyssey of sound field amplification. *Educational Audiology Association Newsletter, 5,* 6–7.

Flexer, C. (1994). *Facilitating hearing and listening in young children.* San Diego: Singular.

Fox, D. S. (1980). Teacher-child discourse interactions and the language of preschool hearing impaired children. *Dissertation Abstracts International, 41*(10), 4360A. (University Microfilms No. AAI81–05868.)

Fritsch, M. H., & Sommer, A. (1991). *Handbook of congenital and early onset hearing loss.* New York: Igaku-Shoin.

Gaar, S. J. (1989). Environmental factors associated with emergent literacy in deaf and hearing children. *Dissertation Abstracts International, 50*(05), 1286A. (University Microfilms No. AAI89–18007).

Grant, J. (1993). Hearing-impaired children from Mexican-American homes. In A. L. Phillips, & E. B. Cole (Eds.), Beginning with babies: A sharing of professional experience (special issue). *Volta Review, 95*(5), 131–135.

Gravel, J. S. (1994). Auditory assessment of infants. *Seminars in Hearing, 15*(2), 100–113.

Gravel, J. S., Diefendorf, A. O., & Matkin, N. D. (1994). Universal screening for infant hearing impairment [Letter to the editor]. *Pediatrics, 94,* 957–959.

Gravel, J. S., & Wallace, I. F. (1995). Early otitis media, auditory abilities, and educational risks. *American Journal of Speech-Language Pathology, 4*(3), 89–94.

Gravel, J. S., Wallace, I. F., & Abraham, S. (1991, November). *Communication sequelae of otitis media.* Presentation at the American Speech-Language and Hearing Convention, Atlanta.

Greenberg, M. T. (1980). Social interaction between deaf preschoolers and their mothers: The effects of communication method and communication competence. *Developmental Psychology, 16,* 465–474.

Greenberg, M. T., Calderon, R., & Kusche, C. (1984). Early interventions using simultaneous communication with deaf infants: The effect on communication development. *Child Development, 55,* 607–616.

Gustason, G., Pfetzing, D., & Zawolkow, E. (1980). *Signing exact English.* Los Alamitos, Calif.: Modern Signs Press.

Hall, J. W., III. (1992). *Handbook of auditory evoked responses.* Needham Heights, Mass.: Allyn & Bacon.

Harris, M., Clibbens, J., Chasin, J., & Tibbitts, R. (1989). The social context of early sign language development. *First Language, 9,* 81–97.

Hayes, D., & Northern, J. L. (Eds.). (1996). *Infants and hearing.* San Diego: Singular Press.

Heath, S. B. (1983). *Ways with words.* Cambridge, U.K.: Cambridge University Press.

Hoffmeister, R., & Moores, D. F. (1987). Code switching in deaf adults. *American Annals of the Deaf, 132,* 31–34.

Howell, R. F. (1984). Maternal reports of vocabulary development in four-year-old deaf children. *American Annals of the Deaf, 129,* 459–465.

Ince, S. (1994, January). The ear infection epidemic. *Redbook,* pp. 130, 132.

Jamieson, J. R. (1994). Instructional discourse strategies: Differences between hearing and deaf mothers of deaf children. *First Language, 14,* 153–171.

Johnson, D. (1991). Visual assessment of people who are deaf. *Asha, 33,* 32, 45–49.

Joint Committee on Infant Hearing. (1982). Position statement. *Asha, 24,* 1017–1018.

Joint Committee on Infant Hearing. (1994). 1994 position statement. *Asha, 36,* 38–41.

Jones, R. C., & Kretschmer, L. W. (1986). Attitudes of parents of black hearing impaired children.. *Language, Speech, and Hearing Services in the Schools, 19,* 41–50.

Kenworthy, O. T. (1986). Caregiver-child interaction and language acquisition of hearing-impaired children. *Topics in Language Disorders, 6,* 1–11.

Koppenhaver, D., Coleman, P., Kalman, S., & Yoder, D. (1992). The implications of emergent literacy research for children with developmental disabilities. *Journal of Speech-Language Pathology, 1*(1), 38–44.

Kurtzer-White, E., & Luterman, D. (1997, November). *Parents' perspectives on universal screening of infants for hearing loss.* Presentation at the American Speech-Language and Hearing Association National Convention, Boston.

Lane, H. (1992). *The mask of benevolence.* New York: Knopf.

Lartz, M. N., & Lestina, L. J. (1995). Strategies deaf mothers use when reading to their young deaf or hard of hearing children. *American Annals of the Deaf, 140,* 358–362.

Lartz, M. N., & McCollum, J. (1990). Maternal questions while reading to deaf and hearing twins: A case study. *American Annals of the Deaf, 135,* 235–240.

Limbrick, E. A., McNaughton, S., & Clay, M. M. (1992). Time engaged in reading: A critical factor in reading achievement. *American Annals of the Deaf, 137,* 309–314.

Luterman, D. (1987). *Deafness in the family.* Boston: Little, Brown.

Mace, A. L., Wallace, K. L., Whan, M. Q., & Stelmachowicz, P. G. (1991). Relevant factors in the identification of hearing loss. *Ear and Hearing, 12,* 287–293.

MacTurk, R. H., Meadow-Orlans, K. P., Koester, L. S., & Spencer, P. E. (1993). Social support, motivation, language, and interaction: A longitudinal study of mothers and deaf infants. *American Annals of the Deaf, 138,* 19–25.

Mahoney, G., & Neville-Smith, A. (1996). The effects of directive communications on children's interactive engagement: Implications for language intervention. *Topics in Early Childhood Special Education, 16,* 236–250.

Masataka, N. (1996). Perception of motherese in a signed language by 6-month-old deaf infants. *Developmental Psychology, 32,* 674–679.

Mauk, G. W., & White, K. R. (1995). Giving children a sound beginning: The promise of universal newborn hearing screening. *Volta Review, 97,* 5–32.

Mauk, G. W., White, K. R., Mortensen, L. B., & Behrens, T. R. (1991). The effectiveness of screening programs based on high-risk characteristics in early identification of hearing impairment. *Ear and Hearing, 12,* 312–319.

Maxwell, M. M. (1986). Beginning reading and deaf children. *American Annals of the Deaf, 131,* 14–20.

Maxwell, M. M. (1988). The alphabetic principle and fingerspelling. *Sign Language Studies, 61,* 377–404.

Maxwell, M. M., & Smith-Todd, S. (1986). Black sign language and social integration in Texas. *Language in Society, 15,* 81–93.

Mayer, M. (1969). *Frog, where are you?* New York: Dial Press.

Meadow, K. P., Greenberg, M. T., Erting, C., & Carmichael, H. (1981). Interactions of deaf mothers and deaf preschool children: Comparisons with three other groups of deaf and hearing dyads. *American Annals of the Deaf, 126*, 454–468.

Messenheimer-Young, T., & Kretschmer, R. R. (1994). "Can I play?": A hearing-impaired preschooler's requests to access maintained social interactions. *Volta Review, 96*, 5–18.

Meyer, T. A., Svirsky, M. A., Kirk, K. J., & Miyamoto, R. T. (1998). Improvements in speech perception by children with profound prelingual hearing loss: Effects of device, communication mode, and chronological age. *Journal of Speech, Language and Hearing Research, 41*, 846–858.

Mohay, H. (1990). The interaction of gesture and speech in the language development of two profoundly deaf children. In V. Volterra, & C. J. Erting (Eds.), *From gesture to language in hearing and deaf children* (pp. 187–204). Berlin: Springer-Verlag.

Musselman, C. R., & Churchill, A. (1991). A comparison of the interaction between mothers and deaf children in auditory/oral and total communication pairs. *American Annals of the Deaf, 136*, 5–16.

Musselman, C. R., & Churchill, A. (1992). The effects of maternal conversational control on the development of deaf children: A longitudinal study. *Journal of Childhood Communication Disorders, 14*, 99–118.

Musselman, C., & Churchill, A. (1993). Maternal conversational control and the development of deaf children: A test of the stage hypothesis. *First Language, 13*, 271–290.

Musselman, C. R., & Kircaali-Iftar, G. (1996). The development of spoken language in deaf children: Explaining the unexplained variance. *Journal of Deaf Studies and Deaf Education, 1*, 108–121.

Musselman, C. R., Lindsay, P. S., & Wilson, A. K. (1988). The effect of mothers' communication mode on language development in preschool deaf children. *Applied Psycholinguistics, 9*, 185–204.

National Institutes of Health. (1993). *Early identification of hearing impairment in infants and young children: Consensus development conference on early identification of hearing impairments in infants and young children.* Bethesda, Md.: National Institutes of Health, National Institute on Deafness and Other Communication Disorders.

National Institutes of Health. (1995). *NIH consensus development conference on cochlear implants in adults and children.* Bethesda, Md.: National Institute on Deafness and Other Communication Disorders.

Nevins, M. E., & Chute, P. M. (1996). *Children with cochlear implants in educational settings.* San Diego: Singular Press.

Newport, E. L. (1981). Constraints on structure: Evidence from American Sign Language and language learning. In W. A. Collins (Ed.), *Aspects of the development of competence: Minnesota symposia on child psychology: Vol. 10* (pp. 156–187). Hillsdale, N.J.: Lawrence Erlbaum.

Newport, E. L., & Meier, R. P. (1986). The acquisition of American Sign Language. In D. I. Slobin (Ed.), *The crosslinguistic study of language acquisition. Volume 1: The data* (pp. 881–938). Hillsdale, N.J.: Lawrence Erlbaum.

Nicholas, J. G., Geers, A. E., & Kozak, V. (1994). Development of communicative function in young hearing-impaired and normally hearing children. *Volta Review, 96,* 113–135.

Nienhuys, T. G., Cross, T. G., & Horsborough, K. M. (1984). Child variables influencing maternal speech style: Deaf and hearing children. *Journal of Communication Disorders, 17,* 189–207.

Nohara, M., Mackay, S., & Trehub, S. E. (1995). Analyzing conversations between mothers and their hearing and deaf adolescents. *Volta Review, 97,* 123–134.

Northern, J. L., & Downs, M. P. (1994). *Hearing in children* (5th ed.). Baltimore: Williams & Wilkins.

Northern, J. L., & Hayes, D. (1994). Universal screening for infant hearing impairment: Necessary, beneficial, and justifiable. *Audiology Today, 6*(2), 10–13.

Nozza, R. J. (1994). The effects of mild hearing loss on infant auditory function. *Infant-Toddler Intervention: The Transdisciplinary Journal, 4,* 285–298.

Nozza, R. J., Rossman, R. N., Bond, L. C., & Miller, S. L. (1990). Infant speech-sound discrimination in noise. *Journal of the Acoustical Society of America, 87,* 339–350.

Oller, D. K., Delgado, R. E., Lynch, M. P., & Steffens, M. L.(1990, November). *Transcription and categorization of child speech and infant sounds.* Short course presentation at American Speech-Language and Hearing Association Convention, Seattle.

Oller, D. K., & Eilers, R. E. (1988). The role of audition in infant babbling. *Child Development, 59,* 441–449.

Oshima-Takane, Y., Cole, E. B., & Yaremko, R. L. (1993). Pronominal semantic confusion in a hearing-impaired child. *First Language, 13,* 149–168.

Padden, C., & Humphries, T. (1988). *Deaf in America: Voices from a culture.* Cambridge, Mass.: Harvard University Press.

Padden, C., & Ramsay, C. (1993). Deaf culture and literacy. *American Annals of the Deaf, 138,* 96–99.

Paden, E. P., Novak, M. A., & Beiter, A. L. (1987). Predictors of phonological inadequacy in young children prone to otitis media. *Journal of Speech and Hearing Disorders, 52,* 232–242.

Paradise, J. L. (1981). Otitis media during early life: How hazardous to development? A critical review of the evidence (Special article). *Pediatrics, 68,* 869–873.

Paradise, J. L. (1997). Developmental outcomes in relation to early-life otitis media: Present and future directions in research. In J. E. Roberts, I. F. Wallace, & F. W. Henderson (Eds.), *Otitis media in young children* (pp. 287–306). Baltimore: Brookes.

Paterson, M. M. (1990). The first fifteen days of hearing aid wearing: Microanalysis of interactions between a 15-month-old hearing-impaired child and her French-Canadian father. *Dissertation Abstracts International, 51*(2), 503A. (University Microfilms No. AAI91–19968).

Paul, P. W., & Quigley, S. P (1990). *Education and deafness*. New York: Longman.

Paul, P. W., & Quigley, S. P. (1994). American Sign Language/English bilingual education. In P. McAnally, S. Rose, & S. Quigley (Eds.). *Language learning practices with deaf children* (2nd ed., pp. 219–253). Austin, Tex.: Pro-Ed.

Penn, T. O., & Abbott, S. E. (1997). Public health and newborn hearing screening. *American Journal of Audiology, 6*(1), 11–16.

Petitto, L. A. (1990). The transition from gesture to symbol in American Sign Language. In V. Volterra, & C. J. Erting (Eds.), *From gesture to language in hearing and deaf children* (pp. 153–161). Berlin: Springer-Verlag.

Pizzuto, E. (1990). The early development of deixis in American Sign Language: What is the point? In V. Volterra, & C. J. Erting (Eds.), *From gesture to language in hearing and deaf children* (pp. 142–152). Berlin: Springer-Verlag.

Plapinger, D. S., & Kretschmer, R. R. (1991). The effect of context on the interactions between a normally-hearing mother and her hearing-impaired child. *Volta Review, 93*, 75–87.

Power, D. J., Wood, D. J., Wood, H. A., & MacDougall, J. (1990). Maternal control over conversations with hearing and deaf infants and young children. *First Language, 10*, 19–35.

Prendergast, S. G. (1992). Capturing and maintaining deaf toddler gaze in pretend play: A comparison of dyads with deaf and hearing mothers. *Dissertation Abstracts International, 53*(10), 3496A. (University Microfilms No. AAI93–05657).

Prendergast, S. G., & McCollum, J. A. (1996). Let's talk: The effect of maternal hearing status on interactions with toddlers who are deaf. *American Annals of the Deaf, 141*, 11–18.

Preston, D. R. (1986). Five visions of America. *Language in Society, 15*, 221–240.

Ray, H., Sarff, L. S., & Glassford, F. E. (1984). Sound field amplification: An innovative educational intervention for mainstreamed learning disabled students. *The Directive Teacher, 6*, 18–20.

Reagan, T. (1990). Cultural considerations in the education of deaf children. In D. Moores, & K. Meadow-Orlans (Eds.), *Educational and development aspects of deafness* (pp. 73–84). Washington, D.C.: Gallaudet University Press.

Reichman, J., & Healey, W. C. (1983). Learning disabilities and conductive hearing loss involving otitis media. *Journal of Learning Disabilities, 16*, 272–278.

Roberts, J. E., Roush, J., Medley, L. P., Swartzfarger, J. L., & Mundy, M. R. (1994, November). *Otitis media, hearing, and language in African American children*. Mini-seminar presented at the meeting of the American Speech-Language and Hearing Association, New Orleans.

Roberts, J. E., Wallace, I. F., & Henderson, F. W. (Eds.). (1997). *Otitis media in young children*. Baltimore: Brookes.

Robinshaw, H. M. (1996). The pattern of development from non-communicative behavior to language by hearing impaired and hearing infants. *Early Child Development and Care, 120*, 67–93.

Robinshaw, H. M., & Evans, R. (1995). Caregivers' sensitivity to the communicative and linguistic needs of their deaf infants. *Early Child Development and Care, 109*, 23–41.

Rose, D. M., Vernon, M., & Pool, A. F. (1996). Cochlear implant in prelingually deaf children. *American Annals of the Deaf, 141*, 258–262.

Ross, M., Brackett, D., & Maxon, A. (1991). *Assessment and management of mainstreamed hearing-impaired children*. Austin, Tex.: Pro-Ed.

Rottenberg, C. J. (1992). Becoming literate in a preschool class: Literacy development of hearing-impaired children. *Journal of Reading Behavior, 24*, 463–479.

Roush, J., & Matkin, N. (Eds.). (1994). *Infants and toddlers with hearing loss: Family centered assessment and intervention*. Baltimore: York Press.

Ruiz, N. T. (1995). A young deaf child learns to write: Implications for literacy development. *The Reading Teacher, 49*, 206–217.

Schirmer, B. E. (1983). An analysis of the language of young hearing impaired children in terms of syntax, semantics, and use. *Dissertation Abstracts International, 44*(01), 140A. (University Microfilms No. AAI83–11521).

Schum, R. (1991). Communication and social growth: A developmental model of social behavior in deaf children. *Ear and Hearing, 12*, 320–327.

Schwartz, S. (Ed.). (1987). *Choices in deafness: A parents guide*. Washington: Woodbine House.

Scouten, E. (1967). The Rochester method: An oral multisensory approach for instructing prelingual deaf children. *American Annals of the Deaf, 112*, 50–55.

Seery, M. E., Kretschmer, R. R., & Elgas, P. M. (in press). I have something to show you: A qualitative study of the interactions of mothers and their young sons diagnosed with autism. *Infant-Toddler Intervention: A Transdisciplinary Journal*.

Shprintzen, R. J. (1997). *Genetics, syndromes, and communication disorders*. San Diego: Singular Press.

Siedlecki, T., & Bonvillian, J. D. (1997). Young children's acquisition of the handshape aspect of American Sign Language signs: Parent report findings. *Applied Psycholinguistics, 18*, 17–39.

Silberman, R. K. (1981). A comparison of visual functioning in hearing impaired and normally hearing children. *Volta Review, 83*, 95, 98–105.

Skarakis-Doyle, E., & Murphy, L. (1995). Discourse-based language intervention: An efficacy study. *Journal of Children's Communication Development, 17*, 11–22.

Small, A. R. (1986). Negotiating conversation: Interactions of a hearing impaired child with her adult communication partners in language therapy. *Dissertation Abstracts International, 49*(08), 3001A. (University Microfilms No. AAI86–27587).

Smith, R. (1998, April). *Parent perspectives on identification of hearing loss in their children*. Presentation at the National Black Speech, Language, and Hearing Association National Convention, Washington.

Smith-Gray, S., & Koester, L. S. (1995). Defining and observing social signals in deaf and hearing infants. *American Annals of the Deaf, 140,* 422–429.

Snitzer Reilly, J., McIntire, M., & Bellugi, U. (1990a). The acquisition of conditionals in American Sign Language: Grammaticalized facial expressions. *Applied Psycholinguistics, 11,* 369–393.

Snitzer Reilly, J., McIntire, M., & Bellugi, U. (1990b). Faces: The relationship between language and affect. In V. Volterra, & C. J. Erting (Eds.), *From gesture to language in hearing and deaf children* (pp. 128–141). Berlin: Springer-Verlag.

Solomon, A. (1994, August 28). Defiantly Deaf. *New York Times Magazine, 98,* 38–45, 62, 65–68.

Spencer, P. E. (1996). The association between language and symbolic play at two years: Evidence from deaf toddlers. *Child Development, 67,* 867–876.

Spencer, P. E., & Gutfreund, M. (1990). Characteristics of "dialogues" between mothers and prelinguistic hearing-impaired and normally-hearing infants. *Volta Review, 92,* 351–360.

Spencer, P. E., & Meadow-Orlans, K. P. (1996). Play, language, and maternal responsiveness: A longitudinal study of deaf and hearing infants. *Child Development, 67,* 3176–3191.

Spivak, L. (1998). *Universal newborn hearing screening.* New York: Thieme.

Stein, L. K., & Boyer, K. M. (1994). Progress in the prevention of hearing loss in infants. *Ear and Hearing, 15,* 116–125.

Stone, P. S. (1994). *A study of the development and characteristics of narrative ability in hearing-impaired children.* Unpublished doctoral dissertation, University of Cincinnati, Cincinnati, O.

Stool, S. E., Berg, A. O., Berman, S., Carney, C. J., Cooley, J. R., Culpepper, L., Eavey, R. D., Feagans, L. V., Finitzo, T., Friedman, E., et al. (1994). *Otitis media with effusion in young children. Quick reference guide for clinicians* (AHCPR Publication No. 94–0623). Rockville, Md.: U.S. Department of Health and Human Services, Agency for Health Care Policy and Research, Public Health Service.

Strome, M. (1981). Down's syndrome: A modern otorhinolaryngological perspective. *Laryngoscope, 91,* 1581–1584.

Supulla, T. R. (1982). Structure and acquisition of verbs of motion and location in American Sign Language. *Dissertation Abstracts International, 43*(05), 1647B. (University Microfilms No. AAI82–24531).

Svaib, T. A. (1994). "Once upon a time . . .": A deaf child's development of narrative skills. *Dissertation Abstracts International, 54*(12), 4427A. (University Microfilms No. AAI94–14661).

Swisher, M. V. (1984). Signed input of hearing mothers to deaf children. *Language Learning, 34,* 69–85.

Swisher, M. V. (1992). The role of parents in developing visual turn-taking in their young deaf children. *American Annals of the Deaf, 137*, 92–100.

Tanksley, C. K. (1993). Interactions between mothers and normal-hearing or hearing-impaired children. *Volta Review, 95*, 33–47.

Taylor, D. (1983). *Family literacy: Young children learning to read and write.* Exeter, N.H.: Heinemann.

Taylor, D., & Dorsey-Gaines, C. (1988). *Growing up: Learning from inner city families.* Portsmouth, N.H.: Heinemann.

Thieman-Stagge, A. (1993). *Communication interactions between a young augmentative communication device user and her parents.* Unpublished doctoral dissertation, University of Cincinnati, Cincinnati, O.

Tillman, P. S., Donahue, A., & Shotland, L. (1995). *Cochlear implants: April 1988 through March 1995.* Bethesda, Md.: National Institutes of Health, U.S. Department of Health and Human Services.

Tucker, P. (1995). *An investigation of the patterns of communication displayed by a child with severe disabilities.* Unpublished doctoral dissertation, University of Cincinnati, Cincinnati, Ohio.

Tye-Murray, N. (Ed.). (1992). *Cochlear implants and children: A handbook for parents, teachers, and speech and hearing professionals.* Washington, D.C.: Alexander Graham Bell Association for the Deaf.

Upfold, L. J. (1988). Children with hearing aids in the 1980's: Etiologies and severity of impairment. *Ear and Hearing, 9*, 75–80.

Uzuner, Y. (1993). *An investigation of a hearing mother's reading aloud efforts to her preschool age hearing and hearing impaired child before bedtime.* Unpublished doctoral dissertation, University of Cincinnati, Cincinnati, Ohio.

Van Kleeck, A. (1985). Issues in adult-child interaction: Six philosophical orientations. *Topics in Language Disorders, 5*(2), 1–15.

Vernon-Feagans, L., Menlove, E. E., & Volling, B. L. (1996). Otitis media and the social behavior of day-care-attending children. *Child Development, 67*, 1528–1539.

Volterra, V., Beronesi, S., & Massoni, P. (1990). How does gestural communication become language? In V. Volterra, & C. J. Erting (Eds.), *From gesture to language in hearing and deaf children* (pp. 205–216). Berlin: Springer-Verlag.

Walton, L. (1972). *A description of the linguistic environments and the syntactic output of ten Black hearing-impaired adolescents.* Unpublished master's thesis, University of Cincinnati, Cincinnati, Ohio.

Wampler, D. (1972). *Linguistics of visual English.* Santa Rosa, Calif.: Author. [Booklets]

Wells, G. (1986). *The meaning makers: Children learning language and using language to learn.* Portsmouth, N.H.: Heinemann.

Wernersbach, M. B. (1996). *A study of the effects of otitis media with effusion on negative ear pressure on the teacher-child interaction during bookreading.* Unpublished doctoral dissertation, University of Cincinnati, Cincinnati, Ohio.

Wernersbach, M. B. (1997). Pragmatically speaking. *Hearsay: Journal of the Ohio Speech and Hearing Association, 11*(2), 48–49.

White, K. R., Behrens, T. R., & Strickland, B. (1995). Practicality, validity, and cost efficiency of universal newborn hearing screening using transient evoked otoacoustic emissions. *Journal of Childhood Communication Disorders, 17,* 9–14.

White, S. J. (1984). The deaf imperative: Characteristics of maternal input to hearing-impaired children. *Topics in Language Disorders, 4,* 38–49.

Wilbur, R. B., & Petersen, L. (1998). Modality interactions of speech and signing in simultaneous communication. *Journal of Speech, Language, and Hearing Research, 41,* 200–212.

Williams, C. L. (1995). Preschool teachers' theoretical and pedagogical stances on the language and literacy development of deaf and hard-of-hearing children. *American Annals of the Deaf, 140,* 56–64.

Wood, D. J., & Wood, H. A. (1997). Communicating with children who are deaf: Pitfalls and possibilities. *Language, Speech, and Hearing Services in the Schools, 28,* 348–354.

Wood, D. J., Wood, H. A., Griffiths, A. J., & Howarth, C. I. (1986). *Teaching and talking with deaf children.* New York: Wiley.

Yoshinaga-Itano, C. (1992). Learning to communicate: Babies with hearing impairments make their needs known. *Volta Review, 94,* 107–129.

Yoshinaga-Itano, C. (1995a). Efficacy of early identification and early intervention. *Seminars in Hearing, 16*(2), 115–123.

Yoshinaga-Itano, C. (1995b). Universal hearing screening for infants: Simple, risk-free, beneficial, and justified [Letter to the Editor]. *Audiology Today, 7*(1), 13.

Glossary

acquired aphasia—aphasia is a multimodality language disorder characterized by reduced ability to encode and decode linguistic elements. *Acquired aphasia* indicates that the aphasia appeared after the development of language.

acquired brain injury—a general term describing injuries that includes both traumatic and non-traumatic injuries to the brain.

AIDS—Acquired Immunodeficiency Syndrome.

air conduction—when sound enters the external ear and passes through the tympanic membrane and middle ear to reach the cochlea (*see* bone conduction).

antiretroviral therapy—drug treatment to combat opportunistic infections.

Asperger's disorder—a PDD characterized by relatively high cognitive skills and good vocabulary and language structure.

associated features—characteristics that are often present in association with a particular diagnosis.

attention deficit/hyperactivity disorder (AD/HD)—a disorder characterized by a pattern of excessive impulsivity, overactivity, and inattention.

auditory agnosia—the inability to perceive the meaning of sound despite the absence of deafness.

auditory brainstem response—auditory neuroelectric potentials generated by the auditory portion of Cranial Nerve VIII, and multiple nuclei of the ascending auditory pathways.

autistic disorder—the most prototypical subtype of PDD.

behavior modification—the use of contingency management procedures to increase desirable behaviors and reduce undesirable behaviors.

behavioral disinhibition—the conceptualization of AD/HD as a deficiency in the regulation and inhibition of behaviors, with reference to operant conditioning principles.

behavioral disorder—externalizing mental disorder, causing pain or distress to others.

bone conduction—mode of sound reception achieved when a vibrating body is applied directly to the skull, bones of the face, or teeth (*see* air conduction).

***Candida* esophagitis**—yeast infection of the esophagus.

candidiasis—yeast infection of the oral cavity.

CGG repeat—a particular sequence of amino acids [cytosine (C), guanine (G), and guanine (G)] in DNA which is enlarged in the fragile X mutation.

childhood disintegrative disorder—a PDD involving the onset of symptoms after a period of normal functioning of at least two years.

closed head injury—damage caused by a blunt blow to the head or an acceleration/deceleration of the brain within the skull, producing no open wound to the head.

cognitive-behavioral strategies—metacognitive interventions incorporating verbal statements to enhance self-regulation of behaviors.

comorbidity—co-occurring with another disorder.

conductive hearing loss—hearing loss caused by a disorder or blockage of the external and/or middle ears.

cryptococcus—a yeastlike fungus that reproduces by budding.

cued speech—a system of hand cues placed at and around the speaker's mouth, designed to improve visual reception of speech by persons who have hearing loss and are attempting to speechread others.

cytomegalovirus—a group of herpes viruses.

deictics—grammatical forms in English whose meanings change depending on who is the speaker and who is the listener. Deictic forms include pronouns (you and me), verbs (come and go), adverbs (there and here), adjectives (far and near), and prepositions (to and from).

differential diagnosis—diagnostic choice among several possible diagnoses.

diplegia—paralysis corresponding to both sides of the body.

distractibility—behavioral disinhibition in the face of more interesting or stimulating activities.

dysarthria—disturbance of speech due to paralysis, incoordination, or spasticity of oral muscles.

dysphagia—difficulty in swallowing.

EEG—electroencephalogram, a record of brain potentials derived from scalp electrodes.

emotional disorder—internalizing mental disorder, causing pain or distress to oneself.

encephalopathy—any disorder of the brain.

essential features—diagnostic characteristics that must be present for a diagnosis to be made.

familial aggregation—the increased prevalence of speech, language, and learning disorders found in the families of children with SLI.

fetal alcohol effect (FAE)—A condition in which not all the physical or behavioral symptoms of FAS are displayed.

fetal alcohol syndrome (FAS)—A severe, recognizable pattern of growth disorder and central nervous system involvement, caused by prenatal exposure to alcohol.

FMR1 gene (Fragile X Mental Retardation–1 gene)—The specific gene on the X chromosome linked to the manifestations of fragile X syndrome.

full mutation—the stage of an unstable FMR1 gene in which the CGG repeat number is usually over 230 and the gene is methylated (i.e., "turned off").

genotype—The actual genetic makeup of an individual. This concept underlies the notion that more than one combination of genes may correspond to a given phenotype.

genetics clinic—A diagnostic and information clinic where genetics counselors or physicians may diagnose FAS, FAE, or fetal cocaine disorder.

head injury—damage to any part of the head. A broad term that encompasses injury from internal incidents such as stroke as well as from external forces such as a blow to the head. Head injury can imply injury to the face, scalp, skull, or brain.

HIV—Human Immunodeficiency Virus.

HIV seropositive—denoting presence of HIV.

hyperactivity—excessive motor movement and verbalization.

hyperlexia—early development of skills to decode print without commensurate ability to comprehend what is decoded.

hyperreflexia—condition where deep tendon reflexes are exaggerated.

hypogammaglobulinemia—generally decreased quantity of immunoglobulins and increased susceptibility to infections.

hypotonia—a muscle condition of diminished tone, tension, or activity.

immunocompromised—characterize an individual whose immunologic mechanism is deficient.

impulsivity—inability to delay responses to situational demands.

inattention—difficulty sustaining concentration or persisting in effort.

intentional injuries—injuries that result from others making choices that will harm another individual.

interdisciplinary—assessment in association and co-operation with other disciplines, a team process.

Landau-Kleffner syndrome—a syndrome of acquired childhood aphasia that appears in conjunction with an abnormal, paroxysmal EEG and for which there is no known cause.

late talkers—children under the age of 4 who have delayed expressive language in the presence of normal nonverbal cognitive ability, typical personality development, and adequate hearing.

lexical acquisition—the stages of knowledge, comprehension, and use of words.

linguistic deficit account—theories attributing SLI to inherited impairment of innate grammatical mechanisms.

lymphadenopathy—disease process affecting the lymph nodes.

major domains of language—the five major domains in which children with SLI are found to have deficits, namely phonology, semantic/lexical skills, morphology, syntax, and pragmatics.

mental disorder—manifestation of a behavioral, psychological, or biological dysfunction associated with distress or disability.

microencephaly—abnormal smallness of the brain.

mild traumatic brain injury—a very brief or no loss of consciousness occurs at the time of the injury.

mixed type hearing loss—a loss of hearing in which there are both conductive and sensorineural components occurring simultaneously.

moderate traumatic brain injury—a possible loss of consciousness up to 24 hours.

mosaic—a DNA finding in which an individual has more than one DNA pattern of CGG repeats and methylation. For example, the full mutation could be seen in some cell lines and the premutation in others within the same person.

multiaxial coding—a system of coding consisting of several axes on which specific psychiatric and medical conditions are coded, together with identifiable psychosocial and environmental stressors and global functioning.

myoclonus hypogammaglobulinemia—contractions of the muscles due to decreased serum globulin.

neurological soft signs—a variety of mild neurodevelopmental deficits frequently observed in children with SLI, including poor oral-motor skills, fine-motor problems, clumsiness and perceptual processing deficits.

normal distribution account—theory attributing SLI to sub-optimal functioning of some or all of the many cognitive skills subserving language, including auditory processing, phonological memory, associative ability, word retrieval, and inferencing ability.

odynophagia—painful swallowing.

open head injury—brain tissue is penetrated from the outside, as with an obvious wound to the head such as a gunshot wound or a crushing of the skull.

opportunistic infections or diseases—timely associated diseases. Infections (especially bacterial or fungal) which occur due to the opportunity afforded by an altered physiological state of the host.

oral-motor—the motor coordination, strength, and range of use for the lips, tongue, jaw, mouth, and oral cavity.

otitis media—inflamation of the middle ear.

otoacoustic emissions—acoustic responses associated with, and presumably generated by, any normal cochlea. These events are recommended for use in infant hearing screening procedures.

ototoxicity—having a toxic action of the ear.

palpebral fissures—distance from the inner to outer corners of the eyes. Too short a distance is a sign of dysmorphology or abnormal growth pattern.

paroxysmal electroencephalogram—an electroencephalogram that shows a sudden increase or recurrence of symptoms.

perceptual deficit accounts—theories attributing SLI to deficits in the auditory processing of speech, particularly grammatical morphemes.

perinatal—period occurring shortly before and after birth.

personal FM system—a type of hearing aid that utilizes a wireless microphone worn by the teacher or other person communicating with a child wearing a special receiver. The microphone/transmitter sends its signal into the classroom via an FM radio frequency, and the student's receiver, which resembles a hearing aid, is tuned to receive the transmitter signal.

pervasive developmental disorder (PDD)—a general category of disorders characterized by deficits in social interaction and communication, and a restricted range of behaviors and interests.

pervasive development disorder–not otherwise specified (PDD-NOS)—a subtype of pervasive developmental disorder characterized by symptoms of PDD which do not meet criteria for another PDD subtype.

phenotype—the observable or measurable expression of a gene or genes, i.e., how the organism appears.

philtrum—area between the nose and upper lip where two symmetrical ridges normally appear.

polymerase—term for any enzyme catalyzing a polymerization.

pragmatics—component of language involving the interpretation and use of language in varying social, physical, psychological and linguistic contexts.

premutation—the stage of an unstable FMR1 gene in which the CGG repeat number is between 50–54 and approximately 230 without methylation.

pseudobulbar palsy—a paralysis of the bulbar nerves.

psychiatric disorder—manifestation of a behavioral, psychological, or biological dysfunction associated with distress or disability; same as mental disorder.

psychosocial stressor—source of stress caused by psychosocial and/or environmental problems.

psychostimulants—medications that increase the arousal of the central nervous system.

pure tone—a type of signal produced by a tuning fork, or more commonly by an audiometer, which is a device for testing hearing. The signal must consist of a single-frequency sound, such as 256 Hertz (Hz), middle C on the piano.

pure-tone average—the simple average of the air conduction thresholds at 500, 1000, 2000 Hz computed for each ear separately. This average is commonly used to describe degree of hearing loss.

Rett's disorder—a PDD reported only in girls in which there is a regression in physical and psychosocial development.

sensorineural hearing loss—a hearing loss caused by a disorder that affects the development or function of the cochlea and the afferent auditory nerve that carries the electrical signal from the cochlea to the central auditory nervous system.

seroreverted—characterizes children born HIV-positive but who change to HIV-negative status.

severe traumatic brain injury—unconsciousness for more than 24 hours is common.

shaken baby–sudden impact—brain injury that occurs as a result of shaking an infant and impacting its head against a surface.

specific language impairment (SLI)—expressive and/or receptive language delay found when no other primary disorder is present.

speech intelligibility—clarity of speech during connected discourse.

status epilepticus—the occurrence of generalized epileptic seizures, one after the other, without recovery of consciousness between seizures.

subtypes of speech-language impairment—the two primary SLI subtypes are pure expressive subtype (prevalence 3–5%) and mixed receptive-expressive subtype (prevalence 3%).

symbolic play—play behavior of children manifested in imaginary play skills.

syntax—the order of stringing meaningful words together; the grammar of sentences.

teratogen—a substance capable of producing death, malformations, growth deficiency, or behavioral aberrations as a result of prenatal exposure.

thematic and semantic relations—meaningful relations or categories of perception, actions, and thought, often related to early linguistic features.

transcriptase—a polymerase-associated genetic transfer from DNA-dependent RNA polymerase.

transdisciplinary—when team members from various disciplines share responsibility for planning the assessment and interpreting the assessment results; typically, one individual carries out the assessment plan.

transmitting male—a male carrier of the premutation stage of the FMR1 gene who is usually unaffected but will transmit the gene to all of his daughters.

traumatic brain injury (TBI)—"an acquired injury to the brain caused by an external force, resulting in total or partial functional disability or psychosocial impairment, or both, that adversely affects a child's educational performance. The term applies to open or closed head injuries resulting in impairments in one or more areas, such as cognition; language; memory; attention; reasoning; abstract thinking; judgment; problem solving; sensory, perceptual, and motor abilities; psychosocial behavior; physical functions; information processing; and speech. The term does not apply to brain injuries that are congenital or degenerative, or brain injuries induced by birth trauma." (Federal Register, Vol. 57, no. 189).

trunkal hypertonia—extreme tension of the trunk.

unintentional injuries—injuries that result from unavoidable accidents.

virion—the complete virus particle that is structurally intact and infectious.

Index

Note: Page numbers in **bold type** reference non-text material

421